AIS 2005

ABBREVIATED INJURY SCALE 2005

Update 2008

日本語対訳版

監訳
一般社団法人 日本外傷学会

翻訳
日本外傷学会トラウマレジストリー検討委員会

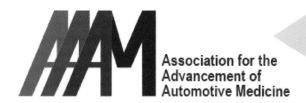

へるす出版

Copyright © 2008 the Association for the Advancement of Automotive Medicine
Japanese translation produced under license from AAAM through Japan UNI Agency, Inc.

訳者序文

　本書の前版となる AIS 90 update 98 の日本語対訳版は平成 15 年 9 月に刊行され，日本外傷診療研究機構（JTCR）が主催する AIS（Abbreviated Injury Scale）コーディングコースの教本として使用されるなど，日本外傷データバンク（JTDB）入力データの質向上に寄与してきました。このたび，外傷診療の質評価において AIS 2005 update 2008 の国際的な導入が進み，米国の National Trauma Data Bank（NTDB）も 2016 年から AIS 90 update 98 から AIS 2005 update 2008 に切り換えたことを鑑みて，我々は AIS 2005 update 2008 の翻訳を行って新版として刊行することにいたしました。多発外傷の解剖学的な重症度を示す指標は，現時点においては Injury Severity Score（ISS）が世界標準であり，ISS の算出法は AIS の重症度スコアに基づいています。したがって，AIS のコーディングは外傷の重症度評価に必要不可欠であり，米国のトラウマレジストリーである NTDB に倣って，本邦の JTDB においても近々 AIS 2005 update 2008 のコーディングを加えたいと思っております。

　AIS は Association for the Advancement of Automotive Medicine（AAAM）が中心になって 1976 年に米国で発刊され，1980 年には脳損傷，熱傷，皮膚損傷が組み入れられて AIS 80 となり，AIS 85，AIS 90，AIS 90 update 98 へと次々に改良され，AIS 2005，そして AIS 2005 update 2008 へと進化しました。AIS 2005 update 2008 は AIS 90 update 98 との対応に配慮し，臓器損傷スケールと骨折分類体系の双方に関連づけられています。また，AIS 90 update 98 と比較して損傷内容の記述の精度および洗練度が上がっている一方で，平易さにも配慮されています。さらに，一側的に発現した場合よりも両側的に発現した場合の方が，生命に対する脅威や機能障害が悪化するように改善されました。前版にない項目である Functional Capacity Index（FCI）も損傷後の機能障害評価ツールとして加わっています。その他，AIS 2005 update 2008 には新たなルールと指針が追加・収録され，本書を読んで下されば，AIS 2005 update 2008 が AIS 90 update 98 と比較して進化しているのがご理解いただけるものと拝察します。

　日本外傷データバンク（JTDB）には 2016 年 12 月現在，北海道から沖縄まで全国約 260 施設から，24 万症例以上の情報が登録されています。JTDB は AIS コーディングを中核においたデータベースです。また，2008 年より毎年，クリーニングを行った全データ（個人特定不能）を JTCR 団体施設に開示しています。その結果，JTDB 参加登録施設を中心に疫学研究が実施されており，本邦の外傷疫学研究の発展に貢献しています。JTDB のデータベースの質を維持できるか否かは，AIS のコーディング次第といって過言ではありません。正確な AIS コーディングに基づいた JTDB を用いて，本邦独自の外傷疫学研究が数多く実施され，その成果から日本の外傷診療の質が向上することを期待いたします。

2017 年 2 月

日本外傷学会トラウマレジストリー検討委員会
委員長　齋藤大蔵

AIS90 Update 98 訳者序文

　1974年Bakerらにより提唱されたInjury Severity Score（ISS）は，現在でも外傷重症度を決定するための世界的な標準となっています。ISSの計算は，Association for the Advancement of Automotive Medicine（AAAM）が刊行しているAbbreviated Injury Scale（AIS）に基づいた重症度スコアによっています。実際の損傷形態から外傷重症度としてのISSを正確に算出するには，AISの手引書（dictionary）に基づいて適切なAISスコアを決定する必要があります。AISの起源とその歴史的変遷は本書の序文を読んでいただくことにして，数回の改訂を経た最新版の『AIS90 Update98』（本書）ではコード体系は構造的に統合，洗練され，コード選択にさいしての注意書きも充実しています。また，ISS算出の基本的ルールも記載されています。

　さて，日本外傷学会では，重症外傷患者治療の標準的なプロセスとアウトカムを収集したデータバンクを構築し，外傷治療の質の向上をはかる目的で，全国的なTrauma registry（外傷患者登録）の導入を目指しています。Trauma registryを含め，外傷研究では，AISコードを適切に選択することと，ISS算出のルールを知っておくことが必要です。そこで『AIS90 Update98』の邦訳を模索していたところ，㈶日本自動車研究所によって翻訳権が獲得され，すでに邦訳が進行していることを知りました。しかし，この邦訳は，解説文を含め損傷形態の表現など医学用語の日本語への変換が不十分でした。このため，Trauma registry検討委員会は外傷の専門家の立場から，全面的にすべての訳語の見直しと訂正作業を数カ月以上にわたって行いました。

　日米の用語の対応は，基本的に日本外傷学会用語委員会編集による『外傷用語集』との整合性をもたせるように心掛けました。また，損傷形態の英語表記を残し対訳にすることで，「手引書」の使用者が正確に損傷名とそのコードを選択できるようにしました。損傷形態の一部に米国外傷外科学会のOrgan Injury Scale（OIS）が併記されていますが，詳細はインターネットURL：http://www.aast.org/injury/injury.html を参照してください。いくつかの頻出する用語の対訳については別掲の表にまとめました。手引書の内容を含め，利用者によるご意見，ご批判をいただきたいと思います。

　本書が外傷患者を診療する多くの医師と自動車事故研究者らに利用され，わが国におけるTrauma registryの成功と外傷学の発展，さらに自動車の安全設計と外傷予防に寄与することを願っています。

平成15年9月

　　　　　　　　　　　　　　　　　　　　日本外傷学会Trauma registry検討委員会
　　　　　　　　　　　　　　　　　　　　　　　　委員長　小関　一英

目　次

序
1. 今日の AIS の起源 ··· 11
2. AIS の基本理念 ··· 11
3. 現在 AIS が抱えている課題 ··· 12
4. 成果としての AIS2005 ·· 14
5. AIS，重症度，死亡率；概念上の問題 ······································· 14
6. 今後の目標と構想 ·· 16
7. AIS2005 の 2008 年改訂版 ··· 17
8. まとめ ··· 17

手引書の使い方
1. 一般的な様式 ·· 19
2. 損傷記載の変更 ··· 19
    四肢と骨盤 ·· 20
    脳 ·· 20
    顔面 ··· 21
    胸部 ··· 21
3. 両側性 ··· 21
4. AIS98 と AIS2005 の一致点 ··· 22
5. "9" 不明の意味 ··· 22
6. 臓器損傷スケール ·· 22
7. Functional Capacity Index ·· 23

AIS コード選択のルールと指針 ··· 25

AIS2005 における損傷部位の特定：ローカライザー ······················· 29

AIS2005 における受傷原因の記載 ··· 33

複数損傷の評価 ·· 37

AIS の手引書
　頭　部 ··· 39
　顔　面 ··· 62
　頸　部 ··· 73
　胸　部 ··· 79
　腹　部 ··· 92
　脊　椎 ·· 108
　　頸　椎 ··· 110
　　胸　椎 ··· 114
　　腰　椎 ··· 117
　上　肢 ·· 121
　下肢・骨盤・殿部 ··· 141
　体表（皮膚）および熱傷／その他の外傷 ··································· 170

　　索　引 ··· 175

訳者一覧

日本外傷学会トラウマレジストリー検討委員会
 齋藤 大蔵 委員長／防衛医科大学校防衛医学研究センター外傷研究部門 教授
 坂本 哲也 担当理事／帝京大学医学部救急医学講座 主任教授／帝京大学医学部附属病院 病院長
 阿部 智一 順天堂大学医学部附属浦安病院救急診療科 先任准教授
 上野 正人 うえのクリニック 院長
 内田 靖之 西大宮病院外科
 織田   順 東京医科大学救急・災害医学講座 准教授
 木村 昭夫 国立国際医療研究センター病院救命救急センター長／日本外傷学会代表理事
 阪本雄一郎 佐賀大学医学部救急医学講座 教授
 白石   淳 亀田総合病院救命救急科 部長
 田中 啓司 JA長野厚生連佐久医療センター救命救急センター 副部長
 東平日出夫 School of Primary, Aboriginal, and Rural Health Care, Faculty of Medicine, Dentistry, and Health Science, The University of Western Australia
 中原 慎二 帝京大学医学部救急医学講座 准教授
 増野 智彦 日本医科大学付属病院救命救急科 講師

同上 タスクフォース委員
 糟谷 周吾 国立成育医療研究センター病院手術・集中治療部
 加地 正人 東京医科歯科大学救急災害医学分野 講師
 西山   隆 神戸大学大学院医学研究科外科系講座災害・救急医学分野 教授
 林   宗貴 昭和大学藤が丘病院救急医学科 教授
 福田 充宏 湘南鎌倉総合病院救命救急センター 顧問
 藤田   尚 帝京大学医学部救急医学講座 准教授
 真弓 俊彦 産業医科大学救急医学講座 教授
 三宅 康史 帝京大学医学部救急医学講座 教授
 森村 尚登 東京大学大学院医学系研究科生体管理医学講座救急医学 教授
 渡部 広明 島根大学医学部 Acute Care Surgery 講座 教授
 横田順一朗 地方独立行政法人堺市立病院機構 副理事長／日本外傷学会前代表理事

ACKNOWLEDGEMENT

Dear Colleagues :

The culmination of this major revision, expansion and improvement of the Abbreviated Injury Scale 2005 is due to the commitment and contributions of many individuals and organizations around the world that have given generously of their time, resources and talents. We acknowledge and thank you for your past participation, and we encourage your future continued involvement in the various dimensions of the Abbreviated Injury Scale.

Thomas A. Gennarelli, M.D.
Elaine Wodzin
Editors, Abbreviated Injury Scale 2005

International Injury Scaling Committee (IISC)

Co-Chairs : Thomas Gennarelli*
Elaine Wodzin*

Executive Committee :

Howard R. Champion*
Ellen J. MacKenzie*
Maria Segui-Gomez (Spain)

Members-at-Large :

Jeffrey Augenstein*
Ian Civil (New Zealand)
Brad Cushing*
Thomas Esposito*
Murray Mackay (Isle of Man)

*USA

A special thanks goes to Jan Price from the Editors of AIS© 2005 for her diligence in coordinating the Update 2008. Ms. Price is AAAM's Technical Coordinator for Injury Scaling.

The AAAM especially thanks Dr. and Mrs. John D. States for their financial contribution towards the printing of AIS© 2005. Dr. States, Professor Emeritus of Orthopedics, University of Rochester, New York, was Chairman of the Committee on Injury Scaling from 1971-1981. He is also a past President of the AAAM.

Orthopedic Trauma Association (OTA)
Thanks to the OTA and its Committee on Coding and Classification for partnering with the IISC and AAAM in agreeing on a common terminology for describing joint and bone injuries, and for allowing the AAAM to use the Fracture Classification graphics. Committee members :
Larry Webb (chair), Michael Bosse, Alan Jones, James Kellam, Hans Kredor, Andrew Pollak, and Marc Swiontkowski. Special thanks to Julie Agel.

American Association of Neurological Surgeons and Congress of Neurological Surgeons Joint Section on Neurotrauma and Critical Care
Alex B. Valadka

American Association for the Surgery of Trauma
Wayne Meredith, Chairman, and Committee on Injury Assessment and Outcome

American College of Surgeons Committee on Trauma
John Weigelt and Committee on Trauma

Ophthalmological Consultant
David Steven Friedman

Maxillofacial Consultant
Paul N. Manson

National Highway Traffic Safety Administration
Stephen Luchter (retired)
William Walsh
Cathy Gotschall
Evelyn Benton
Ruth Isenberg (retired)

CIREN Teams - Field Testing
Cynthia Burch (Baltimore)
Stacy Chimento (Miami)
Carla Kohoyda-Inglis (Michigan)
Teresa Vaughan (San Diego)

AIS Course Instructors/Field Testing
USA : Jeanne Fogarty
    Donna Nayduch
    Jan Price

Canada : Maureen Brennan-Barnes
    Glenda Hicks

Australia : Christine Allsopp
    Andrea Besenyi
    Libby Carter
    Melanie Franklyn
    Lauren Jones
    David McNaughton
    Nadia Nocera
    Kerry Quinn

UK (field testing only) : Jo Barnes
    Dawn Chambers-Smith
    Laura White
    Maralyn Woodford

Editing
Special thanks for assisting with the detailed editing—
Jan Price and Yvonne Speer (USA), Christine Allsopp (Australia)

Graphics
The AAAM thanks Biodynamic Research Corporation for permission to use the following graphics, and John Martini for the development work : lung, liver, pelvis and bones of the foot.

European and Australasian Interest Groups on Injury Scaling

Christine Allsopp	Australia	Lauren Jones	Australia
Lynn Ashton	Australia	Sjaanie Koppel	Australia
Ulf Bjornstig	Sweden	Anders Kullgren	Sweden
Irene Blackberry	Australia	Klaus Langwieder	Germany
Piero Borgia	Italy	Claus Falk Larsen	Norway
Katina Bratis	Australia	Fiona Lecky	UK
Libby Braybrooks	Australia	Ari Leppaniemi	Finland
Roland Breitner	Germany	Hans Morten Lossius	Norway
Julie Brown	Australia	Murray Mackay	Isle of Man
Christian Brunet	France	Domenico Magazzu	Italy
Olle Bunketorp	Sweden	Patricia Manglick	Australia
Kim Burch	Australia	Alessandra Marinoni	Italy
Michel Burrowes	Australia	Catherine McDonald	Australia
Erica Caldwell	Australia	Trish McDougall	Australia
Raffaele Capoano	Italy	Sue Mclellan	Australia
Rhonda Carroll	Australia	David McNaughton	Australia
Libby Carter	Australia	Hugo Mellander	Sweden
Louise Carter	Australia	Mary Michaelopoulos	Australia
Claude Cavalerro	France	Jorge Mineiro	Portugal
Dominique Cesari	France	Andrew Morris	UK
Dawn Chambers-Smith	UK	S. Mulder	Netherlands
Mireille Chiron	France	Joanne Murphy	Australia
Lisa Chytra	Australia	Amina N'Diaye	France
Lisa Collins	Australia	Monique Newell	Australia
Sean Conley	Australia	Louise Niggemeyer	Australia
Mario Comelli	Italy	Nadia Nocera	Australia
Anthony Cook	Australia	Ake Nygren	Sweden
Alessandro Costanzo	Italy	Peter Oakley	UK
Andrea Costanzo	Italy	Seppo Olkkonen	Finland
Stefano DeBartolomeo	Italy	Marijke Oomens	Australia
Andrea Delprado	Australia	Per Ortenwall	Sweden
Laura DeWitt	Australia	Dietmar Otte	Germany
Soreide Eldar	Norway	Cameron Palmer	Australia
Julie Evans	Australia	Margie Peden	WHO
Fiona Fahy	Australia	Catherine Perez	Spain
Adrian Fails	UK	Antoni Plasencia	Spain
Sara Farchi	Italy	S. Prat	Spain
Sujanie Fernando	Australia	Kerry Quinn	Australia
Brian Fildes	Australia	Kellie Rees	Australia
Michael Fitzharris	Australia	Olav Roise	Norway
Melanie Franklyn	Australia	Sue Roncal	Australia
Paul Garwood	Australia	Melissa Russell	Australia
Ernestina Gomez	Portugal	Bruno Salvati	Italy
Ian Greaves	UK	Roberto Sapia	Italy
Kaylene Green	Australia	Lucien Schlosser	Germany
Herve Guillemot	France	Kari Schroder-Hansen	Norway
Linda Gutierrez	Australia	James Scully	Australia
Elizabeth Halcomb	Australia	Maria Segui-Gomez	Spain
Lasse Hantula	Finland	Joanne Sheedy	Australia
Deborah Harrison	Australia	Bernadette Shields	Australia
Melissa Hart	Australia	Andrew Short	Australia

Ali Hassan	UK	Voula Stathakis	Australia
Wolfram Hell	Germany	Bertrand Thelot	France
Morten Hestnes	Norway	Pete Thomas	UK
Celine Hill	Australia	Claes Tingvall	Sweden
Alicia Jackson	Australia	Lynn Tucker	N. Zealand
Gilles Vallet	France	Maralyn Woodford	UK
Michael Walsh	Australia	Vicki Xafis	Australia
Felix Walz	Switzerland	David Yates	UK
Rachel West	Australia	Anders Ydenius	Sweden
Laura White	UK	Fred Ziedler	Croatia
Kellie Wilson	Australia	Rachel Zordan	Australia

The AAAM acknowledges the early contributors to the development of the AIS, some of whom remain active to the present.

Members of the Committee on Injury Scaling* (between 1973 and 1998) and Advisors :

Susan P. Baker*
Bonnie L. Beaver
William F. Blaisdell
Robert W. Bryant*
Howard C. Champion*
Stephen A. Deane*
Harold A. Fenner, Jr.*
Charles F. Frey
Thomas A. Gennarelli*
Robert N. Green*
J. Alex Haller
Lee N. Hames*
Burton H. Harris
Michael Henderson*
A.C. Hering*
Donald F. Huelke*
Peter L. Lane*
Frank R. Lewis
Ellen J. MacKenzie*
Joseph C. Marsh*

Michael E. Matlack
Gerri M. McGinnis*
Eugene Moore
Kermit Morgan*
John A. Morris, Jr.*
W.D. Nelson*
J. Thomas Noga*
Leonard M. Parver
Elaine Petrucelli* (aka Wodzin)
John E. Pless*
Max L. Ramenofsky
W.J. Ruby*
G.Anthony Ryan*
Richard C. Schultz
John D. States* (chairman 1973-1981)
Joseph J. Tepas*
Donald D. Trunkey*
David C. Viano*
David E. Wesson
David W. Yates*

序

1．今日の AIS の起源

　「簡易損傷スケール」(Abbreviated Injury Scale；AIS) は，身体の損傷の重症度を示す体系として，いまから30年以上前に考案された。自動車事故による損傷の種類と重症度を分類するための標準体系が求められ，こうしたニーズに応えることがそもそもの目的であった。当初，解剖学的に定義した一連の損傷内容をいくつかのパラメータ（エネルギー散逸，生命に対する脅威，永久的機能障害，治療期間，発生率）ごとに分類することを趣旨に掲げ，1971年に AIS 初版が策定された[1]。1975年から1976年にかけて，初の損傷コード化手引書が作成・出版され，約500項目の損傷リストと，「1」（最軽症）から「6」（最重症）までの段階の重症度が収録された[2,3]。1970年代半ば頃までには，米国運輸省が資金を拠出する事故調査チームをはじめ，米国，欧州，オーストラリアのさまざまな大学や産業界の研究チームが AIS を標準指標に採用していた。

　AIS の母体である米国自動車医学振興協会（旧・米国自動車医学協会）の損傷スケーリング委員会では，常に時代の課題に対処するために AIS の改訂作業を続けてきた。こうして1980年には損傷手引書が3倍に拡充され，多くの損傷内容の記述が見直された[4]。脳損傷セクションは，当時最新の頭部損傷研究に合わせて内容が刷新された。1980年代初め，記述対象を衝撃損傷以外にも広げる取り組みが進み，1985年の AIS 改訂版には，とりわけ銃創や刺創に起因する損傷など，穿通性損傷をコード化する記述子が収録された[5]。また，この版では，AIS のコンピュータ処理を促進するため，各損傷内容に固有のコード番号を割り振る数値体系も導入された。この2本柱の改訂に加え，とくに胸部や腹部についての損傷記述子のさらなる改良や特異性向上をはかり，組織的な外傷治療の広がりや世界各地の外傷センター間の意思疎通促進のニーズに応えることになった。その後，1990年にも AIS の大改訂が実施された。この改訂では機能障害，能力障害，その他の非致死性転帰の判定にも利用でき，かつそれらを区別できるように，損傷記述子の改良と収録数の増加が行われた[6]。さらに，穿通性損傷の記述子も拡充され，小児外傷への対応もはかられた。独特の数値識別システムを改良するとともに，損傷重症度コード化の均一性と一貫性を強化するため，コード化の指針を収録した。この AIS1990は，1998年の改訂を経て，いくつかの問題点が明確になったが，この1998年の改訂は AIS1990から大きく発展するまでには至らなかった[7]。その後，現行の AIS2005年版につながるプロセスは後述する。

2．AIS の基本理念

　過去30年の間に世界で損傷疫学，車両環境，外傷治療が大きく変化しているなか，どの AIS 改訂版も可能な限り一定に保たれた原則に則っている。こうした原則には，次の考え方が浸透している。

- AIS は重症度に応じて損傷を分類する簡略な手法とする。
- 損傷を記述する用語は標準化する。
- AIS は多くの損傷原因に利用可能なものとする。

- AISはデータの詳細さの大小を問わず適合可能なものとする。
- 損傷記述子は，生理学的見地によらず，解剖学的見地から構成する。
- 1つの重症度スコアには，1つの損傷を反映する。
- 損傷ごとのAIS重症度スコアは，時間経過に影響されない単一の数値とする。
- AISは損傷を考慮するのであって，長期的な転帰は考慮しない。
- AISは単なる死亡率や生命に対する脅威の指標にとどまらない。
- AISスコアは，健康な成人における損傷重症度を反映する。
- 損傷の重症度については，全身に対する重要性との関連から記述する。

　上記の原則は，長い歴史のなかでわずかに修正が加えられている。しかし，それらの修正はいずれも損傷記述子の明瞭度を高めたり，定義を明確化したりするという場合にだけ行われた。1つ1つの原則をみればわかるように，AISの有用性と限界の両面を明示している。こうした原則に基づき，AISは次のように定義されている。

　AISは，解剖学的見地に基づき，コンセンサスから導かれたグローバルな重症度スコア化体系であり，各損傷をその重要性に応じて6段階の尺度で身体部位ごとに分類している。

3．現在AISが抱えている課題
　AISは1990年以降，実質的な改訂は実施されていない。その間，さまざまな問題が生じ，2005年の改訂状況に影響を及ぼしている。具体的には次のとおりである。

- 特殊な損傷領域における損傷スケーリングの発展について，専門医や交通事故捜査官の関心が広がっている。このため，非常に特殊な分野用に，別のスケーリング体系がいくつも出現する可能性がある。たった1つの重症度体系をありとあらゆる目的に利用できないことは十分認識されているが，特定分野用の体系がいくつも生まれることで，重症度記述言語の共通化という全体的な目標の達成が遠のいてしまうおそれがある。特定分野のコード体系は相互にも，AISとも，いかなる共通体系とも関連性が確保されない可能性が高いからである。
- さまざまなデータ収集システムで利用可能なデータ品質はますます多様化していくと思われる。これにより損傷内容の記述に極端な特異性を求めるユーザーと，データソースが比較的汎用的な損傷記述であるユーザーの二極化現象が生まれる。その結果，2つの体系を開発する必要性がはっきりする。1つは詳細度が限定的な医学情報だけをもつデータベース用の体系，もう1つは損傷について詳細な医学的記述がある体系である。
- 国によってユーザーのニーズに違いがある。
- 病院の損傷に関する記述の変更が必要である。とくにICD9-CM（国際疾病分類第9版・臨床修正版）から，まだ完成していないICD10-CMへの移行期間中においては，その必要性が明らかである。

- 非致死性損傷の長期的な転帰を重視する傾向が強まっており，損傷の全体的な負担を評価する次の重要なステップとして，何らかの合意に基づく機能障害スケールが必要になることは間違いない。
- 他の分野もさることながら，とくに自動車安全性設計の分野では，損傷した臓器内の損傷部位（左・右，近位・遠位，前方・後方など）が，損傷内容記述に含めるべき重要要素として浮上している。

こうした懸念を踏まえ，AIS改訂作業は次の総合目標に沿って進められた。

- ユーザーグループ層を明確化する。
- 国内・国外のユーザーニーズを把握する。
- ユーザーニーズに対応する損傷スケーリング体系を開発する。
- 改訂の作業中も作業後も，随時，ユーザーの懸念に対処する。
- ユーザーグループについて，差別も優遇もしないことを確約する。
- 転帰を説明する損傷手引書の作成を継続する。

こうした目標を達成するため，数年前に損傷スケーリング委員会が再編成された。任務内容をさらに練り上げたうえで，ユーザーの幅の広さに合わせて多くの専門分野から集まった多国籍構成を反映し，国際損傷スケーリング委員会（International Injury Scaling Committee；IISC）と改称した。同委員会は外傷治療と外傷の疫学・治療・予防を扱う多くの医学専門領域を対象としており，生体力学，データ収集・分析，その他の輸送・損傷の問題にかかわる学術研究機関，政府機関，産業界の代表が参加している。相互に互換性のある体系づくりをめざし，損傷や転帰のスケーリングに関心をもつ個人・団体との対応窓口が設置された。IISCは，AISによる損傷重症度を扱うだけでなく，ツールの継続的な改良を促進して非致死性損傷の転帰を的確に定義する役割も担っている。

AIS2005改訂版の計画の際，過去数年間に明らかになった多様な課題とニーズに対応するため，下記の具体的な目的を掲げた。

- 米国外傷外科学会（American Association for the Surgery of Trauma；AAST）の臓器損傷スケール[8-14]や整形外科外傷学会（Orthopaedic Trauma Association；OTA）の骨折分類体系[15]など，既存あるいは提案中の損傷スコアリング体系との互換性を高める。
- 損傷内容の記述子を引き続き精緻化し，生命に対する脅威や機能障害，身体作業能力を記述できるようにする。
- 整形外科的損傷の記述子を見直して特異性を高め，この種の損傷に対する自動車メーカーの理解を深め，自動車の設計を適切に変更するのに必要な詳細さを実現する。
- ICD10-CMとの互換性問題に対処する。
- 損傷部位表示（面，側など）を含める仕組みを導入する。

- 一側的よりも両側に受傷した場合のほうが（双方の差が全体的なレベルでないとしても）生命に対する脅威や機能障害が悪化する場合，その両側性損傷の損傷重症度コードを新たに作成する。
- 詳細な損傷データが有る場合と無い場合のいずれにおいても，できるだけ同じコードを選択できるようにする。
- コーダー間の信頼性を向上させる。
- 軍事戦闘による損傷のコード化に，どの程度まで AIS を採用できるかを決定する。

こうした目標を達成するため，IISCの会合に加え，同委員会共同議長がAASTやOTAの関係委員会のほか，ICD10-CMの担当機関である全国保健統計センター（米国）など，数多くの個人・団体と会合の機会をもった。機能障害スケーリングに関しては，ジョンズ・ホプキンス大学の研究グループと直接的な関係が築かれている。さらに，2001年10月に設立された欧州損傷スケーリング利益団体（European Interest Group in Injury Scaling；EIGIS）と2002年にオーストラリアで開始された同様のグループの関与は，改訂作業にとくに重要な役割を果たした。

4．成果としての AIS2005

AIS2005は，数年にわたる作業の産物であり，世界中の数々のグループとの会合を重ねた成果である。上記の目標は大部分が達成されている。AIS2005は，専門医が損傷の重症度と転帰を記述するのに足る精度で，医学診断と専門用語を改訂した手引書の拡張版である。また，臓器損傷スケールと骨折分類体系の双方と関連づけられている。現在，AIS2005は約2000項目の損傷記述子を収録している。必要があれば，スケールに採用された詳細な手法を用いて，身体の細かな部位の損傷を記述することが可能である。両側性損傷に対処し，爆傷などの非機械的損傷を扱う新セクションが追加された。AIS2005は，AIS98との対応がはかられている。損傷内容の記述の精度向上に関してAIS2005全体にわたって洗練度が上がっているが，平易さを求める要望を考慮し，それも担保している。AIS2005では，さまざまなデータベースやユーザーのニーズに対応するため，詳細レベルの縮約と掘り下げを強化している。コード化の詳しいルールや指示も盛り込み，コーダーの一貫性と互換性の向上をめざしている。

AIS2005の有用性検証のため，2つのコーダーグループによる実地試験を実施した。この検証作業に参加したのは，米国の衝突損傷研究エンジニアリングネットワーク（Crash Injury Research and Engineering Network；CIREN）の4チームと，4カ国から集まってAAAM（Association for the Advancement of Automotive Medicine）でトレーニングを受けたインストラクターからなる1チームだった。検証作業の結果，手引書のいくつかの分野で曖昧さを解消する必要があることが明らかになり，手引書公開に先立って適切な修正が施され，最終的に損傷スケーリング手引書の改善につながった。

5．AIS，重症度，死亡率：概念上の問題

AISでは，小数点以下のスコアで重症度を定義する。これは約30年に及ぶ AIS の歴史のなかで多くの専門家

のコンセンサスを得て作り上げられたものである。医学的な診断と治療が高度化し，AIS の用途がかつてないほど多様な原因による幅広いタイプの損傷に広がっており，重症度の決定因子が時間の経過とともに変化するため，重症度を決める正確な因子は明示的に定められていない。とはいえ，AIS の重症度については，さまざまな AIS の版で決定されているように，いくつかの重症度決定因子とは当初から関係性が保たれている。こうした因子の一部を以下にあげる。

重症度の決定項目
- 生命への脅威
- 死亡率：理論死亡率，予定死亡率，実死亡率
- エネルギー吸収／散逸量
- 組織損傷
- 入院の有無と集中治療の必要性
- 入院期間
- 治療費
- 治療の複雑度
- 治療期間
- 一時的な能力障害・永久的な能力障害
- 永久的な機能障害
- 生活の質

一部には，AIS で定義される損傷重症度は単なる死亡率の指標だとする誤った主張があり，AIS 重症度スコアの一部の変形版（各部位の AIS のなかで最もその値が高いものを示す MAIS や ISS［外傷重症度スコア］など）が死亡率に大いに関連するものの，AIS 以外の他の指標（例えば国際疾病分類第 9 版を用いた予測生存率［ICISS］など）のほうが死亡率との関連が深いと結論づけている[16]。AIS 重症度はコンセンサスに基づくものであってデータ本位ではないため，AIS から導かれるスコアは有効性が低いとの主張もある。そこで，AIS 重症度スコアと生存との相関をみるために AIS90-98 を用いて分析が実施された。全国外傷データベース（National Trauma Data Base；NTDB）を用いて，1,291,191 件の損傷を負った患者 474,025 人のデータが分析された。この NTDB は，過去数年間に米国内の外傷センターを訪れた全患者が登録されているデータベースである。ここでは，単一損傷を負った患者 181,707 人（全体の 38.3％）のデータをあげる。AIS 手引書にある損傷ごとに生存リスク比（Survival Risk Ratio；SRR）を決定した。これは，ある損傷を負った患者数に占める生存患者数の割合を，損傷ごとに求めたものである。つまり，死亡率＝1－SRR である。下記のグラフは，AIS 重症度の数値と SRR に基づいて全損傷を示したデータである。ここからいくつかの結論が明らかになる。

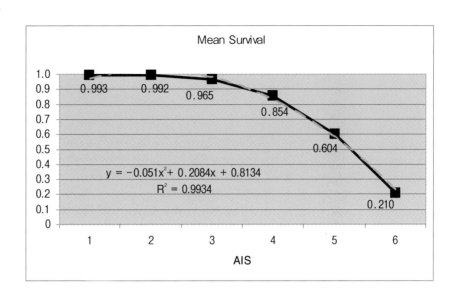

平均生存

- AIS重症度と生存（と死亡率）の間には見事な相関がみられる。
- 相関が線形でないということは，重症度が低いときは，重症度が高いときと比べて，死亡率がAIS重症度スコアの決定因子として重要ではないことを意味する。数値の低いAISスコアは，生存／死亡率以外の因子で決定される。同様に，重症度が高いときにSRRが0に等しくならない点は，死亡率が重症度スコアを決める際に考慮すべき唯一の因子ではないことを意味している。それゆえ，AISスコア6でも死と直接結びつくわけではなく，定義されているとおり，当該臓器に対する最高レベルの損傷を意味する。
- データは，R^2の相関係数＝0.9934と，ほぼ完璧に二次関数の曲線を描いている。
- この平均値からの偏差を分析すると，全AISレベルで平均値±1標準偏差からはずれる患者はわずか2.3％にとどまることがわかる。

こうしたデータから，AIS重症度スコアは死亡率の指標として有効に機能しているが，死亡率がAIS重症度の唯一の決定因子ではないと結論づけられる。

さらに，AIS重症度スコアを死亡率データだけでなくコンセンサスに基づいて決定する方式は，単一の要素（死亡率など）に全面的に依存して決定しないことから，損傷重症度という概念の価値を高めることにもなる。

6．今後の目標と構想

何をおいてもまず第一に，IISCは共同議長を通じてAIS2005の利用を直接監視し，できる限り早く広範な普及を促進する。意見・質問は **AIS@AAAM1.org** で受け付ける。

第二に，IISCは共同議長を通じてEIGISやオーストラリア損傷スケーリング利益団体（Australasian Interest Group in Injury Scaling；AIGIS）との活発な連携を維持し，世界的な規模で他のユーザーとの結びつきを深めながら，AISを損傷データ収集の唯一の国際標準として確立する。

第三に，IISC が機能障害スケーリングで積極的な役割を担う。Functional Capacity Index（FCI）は，そもそも1990年代半ばに AIS90をベースに開発されたもので，これが AIS に統合されている。FCI の詳細については，AIS 手引書と参考文献で参照できる[17-19]。

　第四に，軍事・戦闘による損傷の補遺を作成する作業が進行中である。この種の損傷のコード化には，特定損傷の重症度コードを拡充する必要があるものの，AIS を利用できると思われる。高度な外傷治療システムがある国では，特定損傷の重症度が高い理由が戦闘損傷データベースで裏づけられている。

　第五に，IISC 共同議長は AIS と ICD10－CM との互換性の問題に対処するため，全国保健統計センターが資金提供する活動に参加している。

　第六に，AAAM の AIS トレーニングプログラムは，現在，北米，オーストラリア，イタリア，日本，北欧で定着している。近いうちに，さらに数カ国への拡大が予定されている。さらに，さまざまなユーザーや多様なデータ収集システムのニーズに対応するため，別の指導法も開発予定である。
　AIS2005の普及を受けて，新たな課題が持ち上がっている。国際損傷スケーリング委員会では，こうした課題の多くについて AIS2005の2008年改訂版で対応している。

7．AIS2005の2008年改訂版
　過去３年間に AIS2005の国際的な導入が進むにつれ，いくつかの問題点が国際損傷スケーリング委員会の目にとまるようになった。そこで，利用法を明確化するとともに適切な AIS コードの付与を徹底するため，新たなルールと指針が収録された。新コードもいくつか追加され，軽微な誤りが訂正された。さらに，身体能力指数が完成し，すでに収録済みである。こうして AIS2005の2008年改訂版が誕生した。

8．まとめ
　AIS2005の2008年改訂版は，協力的な取り組みから生まれた努力の結晶である。その活動を支えたのは，さまざまな専門分野や組織，そして忘れてはならないのが，献身的にかかわった一人ひとりの力である。今回の成果は，これまでの旧版と同様，有望な研究ツールとして，今後も損傷の重症度を決定する際の究極の基準としての座は揺らがないであろう。

参考文献

1. Rating the severity of tissue damage : I. The Abbreviated Injury Scale. JAMA 215 : 277-280, 1971.
2. Joint Committee on Injury Scaling of SAE-AAAM-AMA, The Abbreviated Injury Scale (1975 revision). AAAM 1975 Proceedings, 438-466.
3. The Abbreviated Injury Scale (AIS) 1976 revision. AAAM. Morton Grove, IL, 1976.
4. The Abbreviated Injury Scale 1980 revision. AAAM. Morton Grove, IL, 1980.
5. The Abbreviated Injury Scale 1985 revision. AAAM. Arlington Heights, IL, 1985.
6. The Abbreviated Injury Scale-1990 Revision. AAAM. Des Plaines, IL, 1990.
7. The Abbreviated Injury Scale-1990 Revision, Update 1998. AAAM. Des Plaines, IL, 1998.
8. Moore EE, Shackford SR, Pachter HL, McAninch JW, Browner BD, Champion HR, Flint LM, Gennarelli TA, Malangoni MA, Ramenofsky ML and Trafton PG, Organ Injury Scaling : Spleen, Liver and Kidney, J Trauma 29(12) : 1664-1666, 1989.
9. Moore EE, Cogbill TH, Malangoni MA, Jurkovich GJ, Champion HR, Gennarelli TA, McAninch JW, Pachter HL, Shackford SR and Trafton PG, Organ Injury Scaling II : Pancreas, Duodenum, Small Bowel, Colon and Rectum, J Trauma 30(11) : 1427-1429, 1990.
10. Moore EE, Cogbill TH, Jurkovich GJ, McAninch JW, Champion HR, Gennarelli TA, Malangoni MA, Shackford SR and Trafton PG, Organ Injury Scaling III : Chest Wall, Abdominal Vascular, Ureter, Bladder and Urethra, J Trauma 33(3) : 337-339, 1992.
11. Moore EE, Malangoni MA. Cogbill TH, Shackford SR, Champion HR, Jurkovich GJ, McAninch JW and Trafton PG, Organ Injury Scaling IV : Thoracic Vascular, Lung, Cardiac and Diaphragm, J Trauma 36(3) : 299-300, 1994.
12. Moore EE, Cogbill TH, Jurkovich GJ, Shackford SR, Malangoni MA and Champion HR, Organ Injury Scaling : Spleen and Liver (1994 Revision), J Trauma 38(3) : 323-324, 1995.
13. Moore EE, Jurkovich GJ, Knudson MM, Cogbill TH, Malangoni MA, Champion HR, and Shackford SR, Organ Injury Scaling VI : Extrahepatic Biliary, Esophagus, Stomach, Vulva, Vagina, Uterus (Nonpregnant), Uterus (Pregnant), Fallopian Tube and Ovary, J Trauma 39(6) : 1069-1070, 1995.
14. Moore EE, Malangoni MA, Cogbill TH, Peterson NE, Champion HR, Jurkovich GJ, and Shackford SR, J Trauma 41(3) : 523-524, 1996.
15. Fracture and Dislocation Compendium, Orthopaedic Trauma Association Committee on Coding and Classification, J Orthopaedic Trauma 10 (suppl. 1) : 1-155, 1996.
16. Meredith JW, Evans G, Kilgo PD, MacKenzie EJ, Osler T, McGwin G, Col S, Esposito T, Gennarelli TA, Hawkins M, Lucas C, Mock C, Rontondo MRL and Champion HR, A Comparison of the Abilities of the Nine Scoring Algorithms in Predicting Mortality, J Trauma 53(4) : 621-629, 2002.
17. MacKenzie EJ, Damiano A, Miller T and Luchter S, The Development of the Functional Capacity Index, J Trauma 41(5) : 799-807, 1996.
18. MacKenzie EJ, McCarthy ML, Luchter S, Ditunno JF, Forrester-Staz C, Gruen GS, Mario DW, Schwab CW and the Pennsylvania Trauma Study Group. (2002(b) ; Validating the Functional Capacity Index, Quality of Life Research 11(8) : 797-808.
19. Segui-Gomez M, Application of the Functional Capacity Index to NASS CDS Data. Final Report to NHTSA. DOT HS 808 492.

手引書の使い方

1．一般的な様式

　AIS2005の本手引書は旧版と同様のフォーマットを継続している。そしてその9つの章は以下のように分かれている。「頭部（頭蓋と脳）」「顔面（目と耳を含む）」「頸部」「胸部」「腹部」「脊椎（頸椎・胸椎・腰椎）」「上肢」「下肢・骨盤・殿部」「体表（皮膚）および熱傷／その他の外傷」。これらの章は，37ページに記載されているInjury Severity Score（ISS）の6身体部位とは異なっている。

　AISを新たに使用する者は，AIS身体区分と，ISSを計算する際の身体部位の相違点に注意してほしい。

　AIS98にあるように，各々の損傷は，6桁の固有数値（UNI）として小数点の左側（小数点前コードとして知られている）に記述されてきた。AIS2005はそれを継承し，AIS98で記載された6桁のUNIをそのまま使用できるようにしてある。その結果，とくに損傷カテゴリーが再構成もしくは拡張されたところでは，いくつかのUNIは数値順に記載されていない。

　少数点の右の1桁の数値（小数点後コードとして知られている）はAIS重症度コードであり，以下の長年用いられているランクに一致している。

AISコード	内容
1	軽症（Minor）
2	中等症（Moderate）
3	重症（Serious）
4	重篤（Severe）
5	瀕死（Critical）
6	救命不能（Maximal）（現在の医療レベルでは）

2．損傷記載の変更

　「上肢」と「下肢」の章は，構造と個々の損傷のレベルが大いに見直された。比較的小幅ではあるが，銘記すべき程度に現行の臨床・診断のプロトコールや命名法が反映されるように，「頭部」「顔面」「胸部」の章も見直された。「頸部」「腹部」「脊椎」「体表（皮膚）および熱傷／その他の外傷」の章には，ほとんど変更がない。

　例外は，「その他の外傷」の区分にいままでのAISに含まれていない新たな外傷のカテゴリーが加わったことである。

　いくつかの損傷AIS重症度コードも変更され，手引書をとおして脚注として説明されている。**重症度コードの変更は独断的に行われたものではない。**

つまり，それらは，生命を脅かすという観点からのみならず，序文でも述べたように，組織傷害全体を同定するという AIS の長年の主張に基づく観点からも，現行の臨床的な実証により明らかにされた損傷の相対的重症度に基づいている。**AIS，重症度そして死亡率；概念上の問題である**。ごく少数例ではあるが，損傷の記載が示しているより高い AIS 重症度を，間違って過去にコードしたことに対処するため，損傷記述では，損傷部の大きさや範囲をより細かく区別されている。

これらの変更は以下のパラグラフで重点的に述べられている。

<u>四肢と骨盤</u> - IISC と OTA のコーディングと分類の委員会は，骨格および関節損傷の現行の臨床的記述を反映した共通用語の開発に，この数年間共同作業してきた。これらの手間のかかる整形外科損傷の記述は，四肢や骨盤損傷においてより詳細な情報の集積を促進した。その情報は，自動車開発技師の損傷がどのようにして起こり，どのようにすれば予防が可能かということに対する理解や，バイオメカニクス研究者の現時点での要求を満たし，利用しやすく，要望に応えるものであった。さらに，それらにより，多くの四肢や骨盤損傷が，相対的に生命を脅かすものか，長期もしくは生涯の機能障害をもたらすものかが区別された。それゆえ，この改良された整形外科損傷分類は，将来の AIS に基づく障害スケールの基盤となりうる。

1．したがって，長幹骨骨折は，骨折部位（近位部，骨幹部，遠位部）で分類される。近位部と遠位部の骨折は，関節に及んでいるか否かでさらに分類され，骨幹部骨折は，開放性の度合いで分類される。この重要な分類の改訂は，損傷の詳細記述が必要か，可能かにかかわらず，正確にコード化するための能力を保ちつつ，上下肢に個々の損傷のいくつもの記述追加をもたらした。

2．骨盤は，骨盤輪と寛骨臼に分類された。骨盤輪は，個々の骨に及ぶ骨折がいくつあろうと，AIS コード選択では一つの解剖学的構造物である。旧版 AIS98 の AIS のパラメータと違って，全般的に骨盤輪の重症度は，積み重なった複数の骨折の影響のみならず，構造破綻の結果による骨盤輪の安定性と不安定性に依存している。

3．AIS2005 では，"転位"という骨折記載は削除されている。というのは，これらの損傷は，軟部組織で覆われていない（開放骨折など）か，重度粉砕でなければ，臨床上問題とならないからである。同様に単純な"閉鎖"骨折は，臨床的に重要ではなく，しばしば患者の診療録には個別に記載されていない。したがって"閉鎖"という骨折の記載もまた削除されている。AIS コード選択で，"閉鎖"や"転位"とだけ記載されている骨折は，詳細不明（NFS）という記述にあてはめるべきである。

<u>脳</u> - 「頭部」の章の損傷記述の変更には，脳挫傷，血腫，脳裂傷・裂創，穿通性損傷の大きさの，より詳細な分類が含まれている。

1．震盪損傷セクション全体が削除され，現代的な神経損傷の用語を反映した損傷記述の合理化されたセクションに置き換えられた。

　この新しい一連の損傷記述は，この種の脳損傷のコード選択の制度を改善するであろう。過去において，意識消失によって特徴づけられていた脳損傷のコード選択は，しばしば問題となっていた。というのも，利用できる情報から知ることが限られていたり，強調されすぎて不適切なコード選択につながる事故現場や来院時の患者の神経学的状況に依存していたからである。

2．この種の損傷に対する AIS 利用者のよりよい理解と DAI と診断記載があるときの適切なコード選択を助けるために，びまん性軸索損傷の詳細な解説を，「頭部」の章に提示してある。

3．脳腫脹と浮腫の微妙な相違について記載した。

顔面－眼（臓器と骨による眼窩の両方），ある種の顔面骨（とくに頬骨）の損傷記載が拡張された。LeFort 骨折の 3 形態が，損傷定義とともに図示されている。

胸部－肺挫傷と肺裂傷の記述の変更がなされ，爆風傷という新しいカテゴリーが加わった。左肺の図には，改訂された挫傷と裂傷・裂創の記述を助けるために，コード選択者により肺葉の描画が加わった。

1．肋骨骨折の AIS コード選択は，動揺があるかないかという重症度における最も重要な区別をもって単純化した。

2．食道と気管の損傷は，「頸部」と「胸部」の両方の章に含まれることになった。特定できる部位の情報がない場合には，どちらかの身体部位にこれらの損傷があるとみなすように指導する。

3．重要な AIS2005 の変更は，血胸や気胸といった外傷のコード選択が，関連する解剖学的に記載された損傷に加えて，別々に行われるルールになったことである。

3．両側性

　AIS の旧版では，コード選択の原則としての両側性は，ごくわずかな損傷記述（例えば，複数の脳挫傷，両側性声門損傷，両側性肺挫傷・裂傷）や上顎骨，下顎骨，胸郭，骨盤といった単一の解剖学的構造における骨折のコード選択に限られていた。AIS2005 では，両側性の原則をいくつかの個々の損傷記述にまでひろげ，両側性損傷に対し，致命傷や組織傷害，後遺症の点からそれがあると，片側の場合より重症な外傷状況を表すように，単一の重症度コードを割りつけた。全例ではないが一部の例において，両側性の場合，AIS 重症度コードが一つ高いレベル（つまり，より重症）となり，複数損傷を負った患者の全体的評価にかかわってくる。

4．AIS98 と AIS2005 の一致点

1. 2つのオプションが，AIS98 と AIS2005 間の重要度コードを一致させるために利用できる。損傷記述右側の第一カラム（⇒ AIS98 と示してある）は，もし損傷記述の変更がなければ，AIS98 と AIS2005 の記述は，そのまま一致するか，変更が重要でなければ，最もよく一致する AIS98 が示してある。損傷記述右側の第二カラム（⇐ AIS98 と示してある）は，AIS98 損傷記述にマッチする AIS2005 が示してある。もしこの第二カラムに"該当なし"と表示してあれば，AIS2005 上のこの損傷コードは，AIS98 にないことを意味している。

2. ほとんどすべての AIS2005 は，AIS98 とマッチしうる。例外は AIS2005 における全く新たないくつかの記載（例えば，顔面損傷，体幹部離断）や他の外傷の新たな記載（例えば，溺水，低体温症）や，9 というコードで記載される詳細不明損傷である。

5．"9"不明の意味

AIS2005 では身体部位での外傷分類を容認するが，重症度コードがない少数の詳細不明損傷の記述を導入している。例えば，顔面詳細不明における血管損傷は，6 桁の UNI はあるが 9 コードとして示されている（つまり AIS コード 220099.9）。このことは，詳細不明損傷は，疫学的目的では勘定に入れるが，AIS 重症度レベルの頻度情報としては認めないということである。

6．臓器損傷スケール

1. AIS98 では，損傷記載と米国外傷外科学会の臓器損傷スケール（OIS）のグレードを一体化して，OIS 記載と AIS 書式は適切に統合された。この過程は AIS2005 でも発展され，AIS と OIS 間の統一された用語を育成している。OIS グレードは［イタリック体のカギカッコ］で記載されている。しかしながら，OIS の一部の記述は，そう診断することが患者の臨床を行うために重要であるかもしれないが，現段階での AIS にとっては詳細すぎているため，両システムの完全なる統合は不可能である。

2. 一方，OIS と AIS の関連は，可能な限り発展するであろうが，2つの点において両システムが違うことを知っておく価値がある。第一に，概念的に OIS は，1（最も軽症）から 6（最も重症）までの重症度の尺度スケールでの，個々の臓器の解剖学的破綻に基づいた分類の枠組みである。OIS における損傷重症度は，単に救命率に基づいているのに対し，AIS は，前述したように多くの他の損傷重症度の観点を取り込んでいる。したがって，OIS における 1－6 のグレードは，AIS における 1－6 の重症度と乖離している。

3. 第二に，OIS グレードは，同じ臓器に複数の損傷があると，1 グレードずつ重症度が上がる。例えば OIS グレード 2 の脾臓裂傷は裂傷・裂創が複数あるとグレード 3 に上昇する。AIS では，胸部および腹部の記載された各々の損傷は，極めてまれな例外を除き，別々にコードが選択される。

4．IISC と AAST は継続的に連携している。

7．Functional Capacity Index

1．Functional Capacity Index（FCI）は，身体状況の好ましさに基づく尺度である。これは，個人や集団のレベルにおける致死的ではない損傷後の機能障害を表現するために開発された（Mackenzie ら 1996）。全体的な損傷の機能障害評価ツールとして概念づけられており，ほとんどの損傷形態に利用できる。FCI は，食事，排尿排便，性行為，歩行，手，屈曲と起き上がり，視力，聴力，会話，認知の 10 の項目で機能を表す。とくに注目すべきは，文献に用いられている他の長期予後評価スケールには通常欠けている認知機能を含んでいることである。

2．各項目内で，各々の負傷者は，機能レベルの変数（何の障害もないレベルから全く実行できないまで）を用いて格付けされる。これらのレベルは，完全な機能がある a から b／c／d／e／f（項目による）―最も悪い機能もしくは不能までの順で表わされる。10 のアルファベットの組み合わせ（一項目一文字）が機能障害のプロフィールを形成する。例えば，"aaaaaaaaaa" は，10 項目すべてにおいて完璧な機能をしめす。一方，"abadaaaaaa" は排便排尿障害（b は，服薬や器具を用いれば問題ないか，薬の使用にかかわらず 1 週間に 1 回以下のアクシデントと定義されている）と歩行障害（d は介助や器具があってもなくても短距離に限られる；150 ヤードは歩けないが，より短い距離（つまり＜ 150 ヤード）あれば，介助や器具の有無によらず歩行できる）以外は，問題のないことを示す。ある人の機能障害を評価したい場合には，提供されている医療評価を用いるかジョンスホプキンス大学の Mackenzie 医師によって開発された質問用紙による自己評価を用いる。他のほとんどの長期予後評価スケールと同様，質問用紙を利用し，異なった時点での患者のプロフィールを作成することができるため，良くなっていようが悪くなっていようが，その期間での推移を評価できる。

3．プロフィールの情報は，若干解析が困難である。致死的な損傷とそうでない損傷の連携した評価を可能にする必要性から解析がさらに複雑になるのだが，多属性効用理論活用を導入した。これは項目固有のスコアを，米国国民の利便性標本から得られた，個々の機能障害を抱えて生きるとどんなに大変かという意見を用い，選好性に基づいたアルゴリズムへと統合したものである。他の選好性健康評価尺度と同様，この統合スコアの範囲は，0（最も好ましくない；死）から 100（全く障害のない，最も好ましい状態）までである。

4．損傷研究においてありがちのことだが，われわれは損傷記述のデータはもっているが，患者の機能障害を評価する仕組みをもちあわせてはいない。このため FCI の異なった利用法が開発され，これは AIS に基づく予測 Functional Capacity Index（pFCI－AIS）とよばれている。この利用法について，専門家の委員が招集され，コンセンサスを得るために反復プロセス法が使われた。反復プロセス前段では，専門家は AIS98 手引書にある AIS コードを各々調べ，一つの損傷だけで適切な治療とリハビリテーショ

ンが行われ，その年まで生存した18～65歳の症例において，受傷1年後に最もなりやすい機能状態のコンセンサスに達した。このコンセンサスをとる作業は，その後AIS2005手引書においても繰り返された。

　選好性に基づくスコアとプロフィールを一致（一つが各々のAIS2005小数点前コードに）させるようにコンピューター解析するためにこのアルゴリズムが使われた。これらのスコアは5（完全な状態）から1（考えうる最悪の状態）の，5つのカテゴリーにまとめられた。このカテゴリーは，本手引書（AIS 2005 update 2008）に発表されている。**FCIスコアの1－5は，AISの1－5のスコア（AIS 1は軽症であり，6は現時点では治療不能）とは逆の順になっていることを銘記すべきである。すべてのAIS 6の損傷はFCIスコア1であり，すべてのAISコード9（損傷の重症度不明を表す）にはFICスコアは与えられていない。**AIS98とAIS2005のコードをFCIに変換ができて利用可能なソフトウエアが公開されている。www.unav.es/ecip（ECIP 2008a, ECIP 2008b）

参考文献

1. Mackenzie EJ, Damiano A, Miller T, Luchter S. 1996. The development of the Functional Capacity Index J Trauma 41（5）：799-807.
2. European Center for Injury Prevention, University of Navarra. 2008a. Algorithm to calculate the Functional Capacity Index（version 2.0）using AIS-98. STATA version.
3. European Center for Injury Prevention, University of Navarra. 2008b. Algorithm to calculate the Functional Capacity Index（version 2.0）using AIS-05. STATA version.

注：Functional Capacity Indexスコアは，機能障害を測定し，このツールを現場で試用することを奨励するために，AIS手引書に含まれている。しかしながら，FCIは，AAAMで開発されたものではない。

AIS コード選択のルールと指針

　コード選択のルールと指針は，臓器・構造・身体部位の各文頭，および各章の最初に集約されている。また，ほとんどすべての損傷診断には同義語や詳細な記載情報が加えられていて，利用者が損傷診断と AIS 記載を一致させやすくなっている。

　臓器に特異的なコード選択ルールに加えて，いくつかの一般的なコード選択の取り決めが普及している。コード選択の整合性と互換性を確立するためには例外なく適応されるべきである。それらは以下のものである。

- **控えめにコード選択する**。すべての利用できる記載に基づく損傷の重症度に対して疑問が生じた場合は，その損傷カテゴリーにおいて最も重症でないものとする。

- **AIS 6** は，AIS において重症度レベル 6 に決められた特定の損傷についてのみ適用すること。AIS 6 は，患者が死亡したからといって，単純に選択してはならない。

- **損傷の実証** − AIS コードを選択するにあたって，損傷は診断的もしくは放射線学的手技，外科手術，剖検などのかたちで実証しなければならない（**穿通性損傷**における例外参照）。"ルールアウト" や "疑い" "可能性" といった語句のついた場合は無視してよい。同様に，治療だけの記載では，損傷の重症度を決定することはできない。

- **出血量**は損傷の重症度になり，全血液量の 20％喪失は，AIS において重症度レベルを区別するのに用いられてきた。もし複数の損傷が 20％以上の出血量を有する場合，最も重症な臓器損傷によると判断する。すべての損傷が同等の重症度の場合は，血液喪失は，そのうちの一つによるものとする。

　経験則として 1000ml の血液喪失は平均的な成人で 20％に相当する。20％の血液喪失の想定するうえで，以下の表は，とくに小児において一助となるであろう。

体重／kg	20％の出血量／ml
100	1500
75	1125
50	750
25	375
10	150
5	75

- **血管の分枝**は，命名されていなければ，もしくは個々の欠陥記載のリストになければ，コード化されていない。

・穿通創 – AIS コードでは，穿通損傷は，その下にある臓器や構造のダメージの有無にかかわらず，銃創や刺創，杙創のような突かれることによる外傷によって生じる損傷と定義されている。

1．放射線学的もしくは手術，剖検による検証を必要とする深部構造を巻き込まない穿通創の重症度は，視診でも実証しうる。

2．銃創や刺創では，その下にある損傷した構造や臓器について AIS コードが設定してある。その上にある皮膚の創については，コードを選択しない。

3．銃創が骨折を引き起こしていれば，開放骨折のコードを選択する。

4．銃創の射入孔と射出孔は，両者で一つの損傷としてコードを選択する。同じ一身体部位に複数の損傷がある場合には，もしそれが連続していない別々の創と判断されたなら，各々についてコードを選択する。

・鈍的損傷 – AIS コードでは，その定義からして被覆している軟部組織の損傷を織り込み済みの開放骨折を除き，すべての軟部組織損傷は別々にコードを選択する。

・詳細不明（NFS）は，詳細な情報が不明なときの損傷をコード選択するのに用いられる。AIS2005 では，詳細不明（NFS）は"開放"と記載されていない四肢損傷にも用いられる。例えば"閉鎖"大腿骨骨折は，大腿骨骨折詳細不明（NFS）のコードに設定されている。
　　損傷不明は，特定の臓器や構造に損傷はあるが，詳細な損傷形態がわからないことを意味する。
　　重症度不明は，特定の損傷（例えば裂傷・裂創）を負ったが，重症度に特定されていないか不明なことを意味する。例えば，腎裂傷・裂創のほか何も情報がない場合は，腎裂傷・裂創詳細不明（NFS）のコードが選択される。

・**軟部組織皮膚損傷（鈍的または穿通）** – 皮膚損傷の分類では，データベースは，必要とされる詳細情報の量によって変化する。しかしながら，ISS 算出における整合性と両立性を維持するためには，以下のルールを用いるべきである。

－皮膚損傷単独（つまり内損傷がない）の場合，該当する AIS 章に基づいてコード選択されるべきである。
－皮膚損傷が内損傷を合併していたなら，各々該当する AIS 章（例外：開放骨折）に従って両者ともコードを選択する。内損傷には該当する ISS 身体部位が定まり，皮膚損傷には，ISS 身体部位として体表が当てはまる［情報が利用可能で臨まれたものであるならば，すべての記載のある皮膚損傷は，別々にコード選択されるべきである］。

- **様式に関する手引き** – AIS には，手引書で用いられるプロトコールでは，コード選択する側の理解を助けるために，特別な様式がある。
  - **外枠と太字文書**は AIS コード選択ルールと慣習を表している。
  - **[ ]** は，包含するもしくは除外する情報を示す。
  - **( )** は，同義語もしくは時に非臨床用語が書かれている。
  - **セミコロン**は，重症度が類似する損傷記述の間に用いる。
  - **太字体**は，解剖学的構造を確定する。
  - **イタリック字体**は，固有名詞が付いている解剖学的構造や損傷，OIS グレードに用いる。

コード選択のルールと慣習は明確化されるであろうし，定期的に更新される。AIS を用いる者には AAAM のウェブサイト（AAAM.org）を時々チェックするよう指導する。

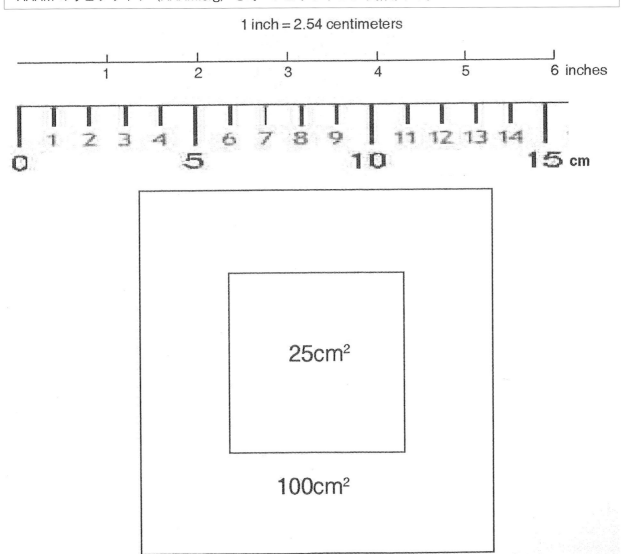

AIS2005における損傷部位の特定：ローカライザー

人体の内外の損傷部位を特定しようとする取り組みのなかで，AIS2005では，コーダーがより詳しく損傷部位を特定する必要が生じた場合に，コーダーが識別選択可能な損傷部位を特定できるローカライザーシステムを導入した。コーダー全員やすべてのデータシステムにおいて，このような正確さが必要とされるわけではない。ある身体区分においては，損傷位置をコード選択するのには適さない場合に，ローカライザーは損傷部位の特定のために使われる。このシステムは柔軟性をもってつくられていて，それぞれの研究者が工夫して，特定のデータに適したローカライザーを追加できる余地をもたせてある。

このシステムはローカライザー1（L1）とローカライザー2（L2）から構成される。

これらはそれぞれ2桁の数字で，損傷を表すAISの小数点以下第1位の重症度の後にくる。したがって，これらのローカライザーを用いた場合，小数点以下は最大で5桁である。つまり，小数点以下第1位はAIS重症度，残りの4桁はL1とL2となる。

もしL1とL2が損傷部位の特定に用いられなかった場合，L1とL2はそれぞれ「00」となる。

1．ローカライザー1（L1）

<u>ローカライザー1の2桁の数値は損傷の位置がどの側（どの面）にあるかを示す。</u>

- <u>01-07はより一般的に用いられる数値である。</u>片側，複数の個所，漠然とした場所（上部，下部）が特定されている場合，あるいはコード選択するのが望ましい場合に用いられる。右側，左側は多くの部位に用いられる。同じ損傷が体の両側にあり，AISの項目に「両側」がない場合には「04」の記号が付けられる。あるいは，データ収集の要求に則って，それぞれの損傷に対し，別々に「01」と「02」の記号を付けることもできる。体の正中線上に損傷が生じた場合，もしくは左右両方に損

ローカライザーの記載		ローカライザー1：L1
右		01
左		02
正中		03
両側		04
複数（多発）		05
上部		06
下部		07
		08
		09
右	前（前頭部）	10
右	中央（頭頂部）	11
右	後（後頭部）	12
右	下部（側頭部・下位）	13
右	上部（上位）	14
右	複数（多発）	15
右		16
右		17
右		18
右		19
左	前（前頭部）	20
左	中央（頭頂部）	21
左	後（後頭部）	22
左	下部（側頭部・下位）	23
左	上部（上位）	24
左	複数（多発）	25
左		26
左		27
左		28
左		29
両側	前（前頭部）	30
両側	中央（頭頂部）	31
両側	後（後頭部）	32
両側	下部（側頭部・下位）	33
両側	上部（上位）	34
両側	複数（多発）	35
両側		36
両側		37

傷があって,「正中線上に損傷がある」と記述することが適切な場合に「03」を付ける。「06」と「07」は基本的には歯や顎の損傷限定の記号だが,必要があれば他の部位に使用することもできる。

- 「10-29」はより限定的な記号である。

    体の右側か左側かを含む損傷部位をより詳細に特定する必要がある場合に使われる。損傷部位は,損傷面に応じて腹側（前面），正中部,背側（後面），下部,上部,複数側に分類される。ただし,特定が望ましい場合に限る。

    大脳に関しては,10-13, 20-23, 30-33は前頭葉,頭頂葉,後頭葉,側頭葉に対応する記号である。適当なら他の部位にも適応することもできる。13-14, 23-24, 33-34は下部上部に対応する記号としても使用する。

- 30-37の記号は,体の左右両方に損傷がある場合に10-29と同様に使用される。あるいは10-29の記号を必要に応じて2つの別々の記号として付けることもできる。もちろんこれらの記号はAIS手引書で両側損傷が規定されたものには使用できない。

- 38-99の記号は,ユーザーが研究の際に必要があれば加えることができる。

ローカライザーの記載		L2
頸椎	C1	01
	C2	02
	C3	03
	C4	04
	C5	05
	C6	06
	C7	07
胸椎	T1	08
	T2	09
	T3	10
	T4	11
	T5	12
	T6	13
	T7	14
	T8	15
	T9	16
	T10	17
	T11	18
	T12	19
腰椎	L1	20
	L2	21
	L3	22
	L4	23
	L5	24

2．ローカライザー2（L2）

2つ目の記号L2は,より詳細に損傷部位を特定するために,L1とともに使用される。L1と同様にL2も2桁の数値でコード選択する者の裁量で,必要に応じて使用できる。

- 00-24は損傷を受けた脊椎および脊柱の部位を表すために用いられる。
    - 1カ所の損傷ならばその部位を適切にL2のコードを選択する。
    - より詳細な限定がない場合にはL2の前のL1のコードは「00」となる。例えば,詳細不明なT6の胸椎骨折の場合は,L1とL2を合わせて,

「0013」とコードする。

○より詳細な損傷部位が特定されるときにはL2の前に適切なL1を付けなければならない。したがって，T6の損傷が右側だとわかっている場合，L1とL2を合わせて，「0113」となる。また，左の前面が損傷している場合には，「2013」となる。

○椎体間に損傷がある場合（椎間板の損傷や脱臼など）には上位の椎体の記号を付けなければならない。したがって，例えば，C5-6の脱臼の場合にはC5レベルの記号「05」を付ける。同様にC3-4の脊髄損傷（脊椎骨の損傷ではない）には「03」を付ける。繰り返すが，適切なL1をこのL2の前に付ける。

● L2のコード25-28は手指足指の損傷部位に対して用いられる。示指は25，中指は26，環指は27，小指は28となる。母指（足）について番号がないのはAIS手引書で独立した損傷として定義されているからである。適切なL1のコードとともに使用されるべきで，詳細不明の場合には「00」とコード選択される。

● 29-30は空き番号になっており，コーダーの必要に応じて使用できる。

● 31-42のL2はそれぞれの肋骨に対応する番号である。

○損傷している肋骨は1本のとき，これらのL2は適切なL1によって損傷の位置（側）を記述した後に用いられる（したがって，L1は00-03，10-14，20-24のいずれかになる）。

○損傷している肋骨が複数ある場合，

1）L2＝00としてL1を複数部位として選択する（訳者注：1500，2500，3500）。

2）L1の損傷部位を右01，左02，両側04として選択し，さらにL2の31－42を選択する。

3）AISの重症度を反映しなくなるが，それぞれ

ローカライザーの記載		L2
手指／足指	2	25
	3	26
	4	27
	5	28
		29
		30
肋骨	1	31
	2	32
	3	33
	4	34
	5	35
	6	36
	7	37
	8	38
	9	39
	10	40
	11	41
	12	42
歯	中央門歯	43
	側方門歯	44
	犬歯	45
	第一小臼歯	46
	第二小臼歯	47
	第一大臼歯	48
	第二大臼歯	49
	第三大臼歯	50

の肋骨損傷についてL1とL2を記載する。

○ 複数の肋骨が損傷していて，その数がはっきりしないときは，L2に関して最も損傷が大きい肋骨に対する番号を付け，その前のL1は適切なもの（00，05-07，15，25）を付ける。

- <u>43-50は歯の損傷に対する番号である。</u>

同じ名前をもつ歯（例えば，犬歯や第一大臼歯）は4カ所にある。損傷した歯が右上部，左上部，右下部，左下部のどれにあたるかに応じ，L1には13，14，23，24のいずれかを付ける。

複数の歯の損傷に対しては「複数」に対応するL1と「L2＝00」を合わせて用いる。

- <u>51-81は体表の損傷に対して用いられる番号である。</u>

これらのローカライザーは外面的な損傷や皮膚や皮下組織の損傷に最も有用である。したがってこれらは挫傷，擦過傷，裂傷・裂創，熱傷などに対してもL1とセットで使用できる。これらの部位とは，ある特定の体組織（例えば耳，鼻など）や，具体的ではない，日常的によく使用される名前の部位（例えば腹部，体幹部，背部など）などである。これらの部位とは詳細に定義されるようなものではないが，使用者が特定の要求に応じて定義できる。

- <u>L2の番号の82-99は空き番号で</u>，個人の使用者の必要に応じて使用できる。

以下に小数点前のAISコードと小数点以下の重症度とL1とL2のローカライザーの使用例をあげる。

ローカライザーの記載	L2
頭皮	51
額	52
顔面	53
眼	54
眼瞼	55
耳	56
鼻	57
口唇	58
首	59
肩	60
腕	61
肘	62
前腕	63
手首	64
手	65
手指	66
体幹	67
背部	68
側腹部	69
胸部	70
腹部	71
殿部	72
生殖器	73
会陰	74
腰殿部	75
大腿	76
膝	77
脚	78
足首	79
足	80
足指	81

損傷の記述	完全なAISのコード
軽傷な右前額部の表層の裂傷・裂創	110602.11051
小さい右の側頭部の硬膜外血腫	140632.41300
15分の意識消失を伴う脳震盪	161004.20000
左耳の擦り傷	210202.10256
右の第3肋骨の複数カ所の骨折	450201.11533
肝右葉の後面の2cmの裂傷	541822.21200
C4の右椎弓と関節面の骨折	650217.20104
左足指の銃創	816030.10281
両側の大腿骨骨幹部骨折（単純）	853251.30400

AIS2005における受傷原因の記載

　AIS2005ではCOI（受傷原因）を4桁の数値で表せるようになっている。

　このCOIコード記載は任意で，それぞれのAISコードに関係するCOI情報を要求されているコーダーによって使用されるべきものである。それぞれのAISにCOI情報を入れて記載するには，小数点以下5桁の重症度とL1とL2のローカライザーの後に，4桁の数値で表される。

　4桁のCOIは以下の方法で使用される。

- 4桁のCOIの最初の1桁は，損傷の性質を記す。
  - 0＝意図的でない損傷
  - 1＝意図的な損傷
- 2桁目と3桁目の数値は損傷の原因についてのものである。これらの原因については使用者の必要に応じて，より一般的により具体的に記述される可能性があるため，別表に記載した（p34, 35の表）。
- 4桁目の数値はほとんどの場合"0"となるが，必要に応じて特殊な場合に用いられる。以下に乳児用・幼児用チャイルドシート使用時の記載例をあげた。乗用車の事故でチャイルドシートがかかわっていた場合に用いられる。

1桁目のCOI	
非意図的	0
意図的	1

4桁目のCOI	
乳児用チャイルドシート	2
乳児用チャイルドシート前部座席	3
乳児用チャイルドシート後部座席	4
幼児用チャイルドシート前部座席	5
幼児用チャイルドシート後部座席	6
ブースターシート（補助席）	7

	2桁目3桁目のCOI
鈍的外傷	01
輸送手段	02
道路交通	03
乗客	04
大型トラック	05
運転手	06
助手席同乗者	07
その他	08
小型トラック	09
運転者	10
助手席同乗者	11
その他	12
バン，SUV	13
運転者	14
前部の左右の同乗者	15
前部のその他	16
中央右	17
中央の中央	18
中央左	19
後部右	20
後部中央	21
後部左	22
乗用車	23
運転者	24
助手席の同乗者	25
前部のその他	26
後部右	27
後部中央	28
後部左	29
その他	30
自動2輪	31
運転者	32
同乗者	33
原付自動2輪	34
運転者	35
同乗者	36
自転車	37
運転者	38
同乗者	39
その他の人動力車両	40
運転者	41
同乗者	42
歩行者	43
その他	44

項目				番号
		道路交通以外の乗り物		45
			列車鉄道	46
			乗員乗客	47
			歩行者	48
			飛行機	49
			旅客機	50
			小型機, 個人所有機	51
			軍用機	52
			船舶	53
			乗員乗客	54
			衝突された側	55
			動物	56
			乗員	57
			乗客	58
		乗り物以外		59
			暴行	60
			人的（殴る蹴る）	61
			武器	62
			落下物との衝突	63
			墜落, 転落	64
			身長より低位より	65
			身長より高位より	66
			20m以上の高所から	67
			スポーツ	68
			ボクシング	69
			ダイビング	70
			個人競技	71
			モータースポーツ	72
			スキー, スノーボード	73
			水泳, 潜水	74
			チームスポーツ	75
			その他	76
		その他		77
穿通損傷				78
	銃創	拳銃		79
		一般ライフル		80
		軍用ライフル		81
				82
	刺創			83
	咬創	人間		84
		動物		85
				86
	その他の刺創機械による損傷			87
	その他			88
爆発				89
	鉱山			90
	爆破装置			91
	超加圧力のみ			92
その他				93
	建物の倒壊			94
	地震地滑り土砂崩れ			95
	洪水			96
	ハリケーン（訳者注：台風も）竜巻			97
（空欄・未定）				98
（空欄・未定）				99

複数損傷の評価

1. 伝統を踏襲して，AIS 自身は複数部位損傷の合併効果を評価するものではない。
   最大 AIS（Maximum AIS or MAIS）と損傷重症度スコア（Injury Severity Score or ISS）の 2 通りの評価方法が広く使われ続けている。

2. MAIS とは，複数の損傷がある患者の重症度の最も高い（最も重症な）AIS コードのことである。MAIS はとくに自動車衝突事故を研究している人たちの間で最も広く使われ，特定の身体部位あるいは全身の損傷の記載に最も幅広く使用されている。MAIS は特定の損傷の頻度や相対的な重症度の比較にとくに有用である。自動車のデザインの変更（例えばエアバッグなど）により，損傷の頻度を減らしたり，公共政策の変更（シートベルト着用の義務化など）にも有用である。

3. ISS は臨床分野で広く使われている。外傷疾病登録の重症度評価の道具として最も重要なものである。ISS は 3 つの身体部位の最も重症な AIS スコアの 2 乗の和である。New ISS（NISS）はここ数年 ISS に代わる新しいシステムとして提案されている。NISS はすべての身体部位において最も重症な AIS スコア 3 つの 2 乗の和である。NISS の提唱者は ISS より優れていると主張したが，現在までのところそれほど広く用いられていない。

4. <u>ISS の計算のためには</u>，最も重症度の高い身体部位 3 つから AIS 重症度スコアを採り，それぞれを 2 乗し，2 乗した 3 つの数値を足し合わせる。ISS は以下の 6 つの身体部位を用いて求める。

---

1. 頭部および頸部
2. 顔面
3. 胸部
4. 腹部および骨盤内臓器
5. 四肢および骨盤
6. 体表

頭部または頸部の損傷には，脳や頸髄の損傷，頭蓋骨や頸椎の骨折が含まれる。狭圧外傷は頭部に割り振られる。

顔面損傷には口目耳鼻および顔面骨損傷が含まれる。

胸部損傷と腹部および骨盤内臓器損傷には，それぞれを取り囲む「腔」に含まれるすべての内臓が含まれる。胸腔には横隔膜，肋骨胸郭そして胸椎が含まれる。腰椎の損傷は腹部骨盤内臓器に含まれる。溺水は胸部の損傷に含むものとする。

四肢および骨盤，肩甲帯は，捻挫，骨折，脱臼，切断を含む。

体表の損傷にはその場所にかかわらず裂傷・裂創，挫傷，剥離，熱傷を含む。穿通性損傷は AIS 辞書に特別な記載がある場合を除き，全域の体表の損傷に入れられる。低体温症，電撃傷，全身損傷も（173, 174 ページにあるように）体表に含まれる。

5．繰り返しになるが AIS の身体区分と ISS の身体部位は一致していない。AIS では頸部は頭部と別の身体区分だが，ISS では同じ身体部位である。ISS では頸椎は「頸部」に，胸椎は「胸部」に，腰椎は「腹部および骨盤内臓器」に分類される。しかし AIS では脊椎はすべて「脊椎」に分類される。

6．ISS スコアは 1 から 75 の範囲にある。75 は，AIS 5 が 3 つもしくは AIS 6 から導かれる。他の損傷がみつかろうが，どんな AIS 6 も自動的に ISS 75 となる。しかしながら，たとえ他の損傷が加わることにより ISS が変わらないとしても，すべての損傷のコード選択をするべきである。AIS では，いくつかの損傷記載は，9 に設定される。このような記載は，損傷の存在を示すが，損傷を特定することはない。したがって ISS を計算するときに用いることはできない。

頭 部
（頭蓋と脳）

HEAD (cranium and brain)

AIS 2005	Injury Description	⇒ AIS98	⇐ AIS98	FCI

WHOLE AREA

> Use one of the following two descriptors when such vague information, including traumatic brain injury or closed head injury, is the only information available. While these descriptors identify the occurrence of a head injury, they do not specify its severity.

100099.9	**Injuries to the Head** NFS	115099.9	115099.9	
100999.9	Died of head injury without further substantiation of injuries or no autopsy confirmation of specific injuries.	115999.9	115999.9	
110009.1	**Head Injury NFS involving only headache**	160402.1	160402.1	5
113000.6	**Crush Injury**	113000.6	113000.6	1

> Must involve massive destruction of skull, brain and intracranial contents.

> Code a penetrating injury to a specific anatomical site (e.g., brain stem, cerebellum or cerebrum) if site is known. If site is unknown or if more than one site is injured, code to one of the following three descriptors. If the skull is not penetrated, code as scalp laceration. Code a single gunshot wound with both entry and exit wounds as one injury. Assign the following three descriptors to Head/Neck body region for calculating an ISS.

116000.3	**Penetrating Injury to Skull** NFS[a]	116002.3	116002.3	5
116002.3	superficial ; ≤ 2cm beneath entrance	116002.3	116002.3	5
116004.5	major ; >2cm penetration	116004.5	116004.5	2

---

[a] New descriptor in AIS 2005

頭部（頭蓋と脳）

AIS 2005	損傷内容	⇒ AIS98	⇐ AIS98	FCI

全 域

> 外傷性脳損傷，閉鎖性頭部損傷など不確実な情報しか得られない場合には，以下の2つのコードのうちいずれかを選択する。これらのコードは頭部損傷の存在を示すものであり，その重症度を明示したものではない。

100099.9	頭部損傷　詳細不明	115099.9	115099.9	
100999.9	頭部以外に原因が特定できない，もしくは剖検によっても頭部以外に原因が特定できないもの	115999.9	115999.9	
110009.1	頭部損傷（頭痛のみを訴える）詳細不明	160402.1	160402.1	5
113000.6	挫滅損傷	113000.6	113000.6	1

> 頭蓋骨ならびに頭蓋内臓器の広範囲損傷を含むもの。

> 穿通性損傷は解剖学的に部位が特定可能であれば（例：脳幹，小脳，大脳），それらについても個別にコードを選択する。部位が不明な場合，もしくは複数カ所である場合には，以下の3つのコードから選択する。また，穿通創が頭蓋骨まで達していない場合には頭皮裂傷・裂創として扱う。一発の銃創で，射入口と射出口のあるものは，一つの損傷として扱う。ISSを算出する場合には，以下の3つのコードを頭部・頸部の身体部位として割り当てる。

116000.3	穿通性損傷（頭蓋骨に達する）詳細不明[a]	116002.3	116002.3	5
116002.3	表在性；創の深さが2cm以下	116002.3	116002.3	5
116004.5	深い；創の深さが2cmを超える	116004.5	116004.5	2

---

[a] AIS2005に加えられた新しいコード。

HEAD (cranium and brain)

AIS 2005	Injury Description	⇒ AIS98	⇐ AIS98	FCI
	Use the following section for blunt soft tissue injury to the scalp (head). Assign to External Body Region for calculating an ISS.			
110099.1	**Scalp** NFS	110099.1	110099.1	5
110202.1	abrasion	110202.1	110202.1	5
110402.1	contusion ; subgaleal hematoma if >6 months old	110402.1	110402.1	5
110403.2	subgaleal hematoma in infants ≤ 6 months old[a]	110402.1[b]	None	5
110404.3	blood loss > 20% by volume in infants ≤ 6 months old[a]	110402.1[b]	None	5
110600.1	laceration NFS	110600.1	110600.1	5
110602.1	minor ; superficial	110602.1	110602.1	5
110604.2	major ; >10cm long and into subcutaneous tissue	110604.2	110604.2	5
110606.3	blood loss >20% by volume	110606.3	110606.3	5
110800.1	avulsion NFS	110800.1	110800.1	5
110802.1	superficial ; minor ; tissue loss ≤ 100cm^2	110802.1	110802.1	5
110804.2	major ; tissue loss >100cm^2	110804.2	110804.2	5
110806.3	blood loss >20% by volume	110806.3	110806.3	5
110808.3	total scalp loss	110808.3	110808.3	5

VESSELS, INTRACRANIAL

Vessel injuries are coded separately from other injuries to the brain, except for crush-type injury, major penetrating injury to the skull or penetrating injury to the brain stem, cerebrum or cerebellum which include all accompanying brain injuries. If a vessel is not named specifically, code as Vascular Injury in Head NFS. Thrombosis includes any injury to a vessel resulting in its occlusion (e.g., intimal tear, dissection).

120099.9	**Vascular Injury in Head** NFS[f]		None	None

---

[a] New descriptor in AIS 2005
[b] Change in severity code in AIS 2005
[f] New descriptor in AIS 2005 that allows classification of trauma by body region, but does not allow assigning a severity code.

頭部（頭蓋と脳）

AIS 2005	損傷内容	⇒ AIS98	⇐ AIS98	FCI
	以下は，頭皮（頭部）での鈍的軟部損傷である。ISSを算出する場合には体表部として割り当てる。			
110099.1	**頭皮**　詳細不明	110099.1	110099.1	5
110202.1	擦過傷	110202.1	110202.1	5
110402.1	挫傷：6カ月を超える乳児では帽状腱膜下血腫	110402.1	110402.1	5
110403.2	6カ月以下の乳児では帽状腱膜下血腫[a]	110402.1[b]	なし	5
110404.3	出血量が全血液量の20％を超える[a]	110402.1[b]	なし	5
110600.1	裂傷・裂創　詳細不明	110600.1	110600.1	5
110602.1	小；表在性	110602.1	110602.1	5
110604.2	大；長さが10cmを超え，かつ皮下組織まで達する	110604.2	110604.2	5
110606.3	出血量が全血液量の20％を超える	110606.3	110606.3	5
110800.1	剥離　詳細不明	110800.1	110800.1	5
110802.1	表在性：小；100cm²以下の組織欠損	110802.1	110802.1	5
110804.2	大；100cm²を超える組織欠損	110804.2	110804.2	5
110806.3	出血量が全血液量の20％を超える	110806.3	110806.3	5
110808.3	全頭皮剥離	110808.3	110808.3	5

血管，頭蓋内

血管損傷は，他の脳損傷とは別に選択する。ただし，挫滅損傷や頭蓋骨まで達する広範な穿通性脳損傷，脳幹・小脳・大脳に至る穿通性脳損傷は個々の脳損傷に含める。もし，どの主要血管か特定できない場合には，頭部内血管損傷詳細不明のコードを選択する。血栓症は血管の閉塞をまねく血管損傷をすべて含む（例：内膜損傷，解離など）。

120099.9	**頭部内血管損傷**　詳細不明[f]		なし	なし

---

[a] AIS2005に加えられた新しいコード。
[b] AIS2005で重症度に変更あり。
[f] AIS2005に加えられた新しいコード。外傷の存在部位を示すことができる。ただし重症度はない。

HEAD (cranium and brain)

AIS 2005	Injury Description	⇒ AIS98	⇐ AIS98	FCI
120199.3	**Artery** NFS[a]	121299.3	None	5
120299.3	**Anterior cerebral artery** NFS	120299.3	120299.3	2
120202.5	laceration	120202.5	120202.5	5
120204.3	thrombosis ; occlusion	120204.3	120204.3	2
120205.4	bilateral[c]	120204.3[b]	None	1
120206.3	traumatic aneurysm	120206.3	120206.3	2
120499.4	**Basilar artery** NFS	120499.5[b]	120499.5[b]	1
120402.5	laceration	120402.5	120402.5	5
120404.5	thrombosis ; occlusion	120404.5	120404.5	1
120406.5	traumatic aneurysm	120406.5	120406.5	1
121099.3	**Internal carotid artery** NFS	121099.3	121099.3	1
121002.5	laceration	121002.5	121002.5	5
121003.6	bilateral[c]	121002.5[b]	None	1
121004.4	thrombosis ; occlusion	121004.4	121004.4	1
121005.5	bilateral[c]	121004.4[b]	None	1
121006.3	traumatic aneurysm	121006.3	121006.3	5
121499.3	**Middle cerebral artery** NFS	121499.3	121499.3	1
121402.5	laceration	121402.5	121402.5	5
121404.4	thrombosis ; occlusion	121404.4	121404.4	1
121405.5	bilateral[c]	121404.4[b]	None	1
121406.3	traumatic aneurysm	121406.3	121406.3	5

[a] New descriptor in AIS 2005
[b] Change in severity code in AIS 2005
[c] In previous editions of AIS, with few exceptions, each injury was coded separately. AIS 2005 introduces "bilateral" for certain injury descriptions. Some bilateral injuries may affect severity levels and, therefore, the ISS for patients with those injuries.

頭部（頭蓋と脳）

AIS 2005	損傷内容	⇒ AIS98	⇐ AIS98	FCI
120199.3	**動脈** 詳細不明[a]	121299.3	なし	5
120299.3	**前大脳動脈** 詳細不明	120299.3	120299.3	2
120202.5	裂傷・裂創	120202.5	120202.5	5
120204.3	血栓症；閉塞	120204.3	120204.3	2
120205.4	両側性[c]	120204.3[b]	なし	1
120206.3	外傷性動脈瘤	120206.3	120206.3	2
120499.4	**脳底動脈** 詳細不明	120499.5[b]	120499.5[b]	1
120402.5	裂傷・裂創	120402.5	120402.5	5
120404.5	血栓症；閉塞	120404.5	120404.5	1
120406.5	外傷性動脈瘤	120406.5	120406.5	1
121099.3	**内頸動脈** 詳細不明	121099.3	121099.3	1
121002.5	裂傷・裂創	121002.5	121002.5	5
121003.6	両側性[c]	121002.5[b]	なし	1
121004.4	血栓症；閉塞	121004.4	121004.4	1
121005.5	両側性[c]	121004.4[b]	なし	1
121006.3	外傷性動脈瘤	121006.3	121006.3	5
121499.3	**中大脳動脈** 詳細不明	121499.3	121499.3	1
121402.5	裂傷・裂創	121402.5	121402.5	5
121404.4	血栓症；閉塞	121404.4	121404.4	1
121405.5	両側性[c]	121404.4[b]	なし	1
121406.3	外傷性動脈瘤	121406.3	121406.3	5

[a] AIS2005に加えられた新しいコード。
[b] AIS2005で重症度に変更あり。
[c] 旧版の AIS では一部の例外を除き両側損傷はそれぞれ別にコード選択をしていた。AIS2005では，"両側"を導入した。いくつかの両側損傷は重症度が変化し，その結果 ISS が変わることがある。

HEAD (cranium and brain)

AIS 2005	Injury Description	⇒ AIS98	⇐ AIS98	FCI
121699.3	**Other artery NFS** [branch of anterior, posterior or middle cerebral artery or branch of basilar or vertebral artery]	121699.3	121699.3	
121602.4	laceration	121602.4	121602.4	
121604.3	thrombosis ; occlusion	121604.3	121604.3	
121606.3	traumatic aneurysm	121606.3	121606.3	
121899.3	**Posterior cerebral artery** NFS	121899.3	121899.3	2
121802.5	laceration	121802.5	121802.5	3
121804.3	thrombosis ; occlusion	121804.3	121804.3	2
121805.4	bilateral[c]	121804.3[b]	None	1
121806.3	traumatic aneurysm	121806.3	121806.3	5
122899.3	**Vertebral artery** NFS	122899.3	122899.3	5
122802.5	laceration	122802.5	122802.5	5
122803.6	bilateral[c]	122802.5[b]	None	1
122804.3	thrombosis ; occlusion	122804.3	122804.3	5
122805.4	bilateral[c]	122804.3[b]	None	1
122806.3	traumatic aneurysm	122806.3	122806.3	5

---

[b] Change in severity code in AIS 2005

[c] In previous editions of AIS, with few exceptions, each injury was coded separately. AIS 2005 introduces "bilateral" for certain injury descriptions. Some bilateral injuries may affect severity levels and, therefore, the ISS for patients with these injuries.

AIS 2005	損傷内容	⇒ AIS98	⇐ AIS98	FCI
121699.3	**その他の動脈**　詳細不明［前，中，後　大脳動脈，脳底動脈，椎骨動脈の各分枝］	121699.3	121699.3	
121602.4	裂傷・裂創	121602.4	121602.4	
121604.3	血栓症；閉塞	121604.3	121604.3	
121606.3	外傷性動脈瘤	121606.3	121606.3	
121899.3	**後大脳動脈**　詳細不明	121899.3	121899.3	2
121802.5	裂傷・裂創	121802.5	121802.5	3
121804.3	血栓症；閉塞	121804.3	121804.3	2
121805.4	両側性[c]	121804.3[b]	なし	1
121806.3	外傷性動脈瘤	121806.3	121806.3	5
122899.3	**椎骨動脈**　詳細不明	122899.3	122899.3	5
122802.5	裂傷・裂創	122802.5	122802.5	5
122803.6	両側性[c]	122802.5[b]	なし	1
122804.3	血栓症；閉塞	122804.3	122804.3	5
122805.4	両側性[c]	122804.3[b]	なし	1
122806.3	外傷性動脈瘤	122806.3	122806.3	5

[b] AIS2005で重症度に変更あり。
[c] 旧版の AIS では一部の例外を除き両側損傷はそれぞれ別にコード選択をしていた。AIS2005では，"両側"を導入した。いくつかの両側損傷は重症度が変化し，その結果 ISS が変わることがある。

HEAD (cranium and brain)

AIS 2005	Injury Description	⇒ AIS98	⇐ AIS98	FCI
122299.3	**Sinus** NFS[d]	122299.3	122299.3	5
122202.4	laceration	122202.4	122202.4	5
122204.3	thrombosis ; occlusion	122204.3	122204.3	5
120602.4	**Carotid-cavernous fistula**	120602.4	120602.4	3
120603.4	bilateral[c]	120602.4	None	2
	Do not code internal carotid artery injury separately.			
120899.3	**Cavernous sinus** NFS	120899.3	120899.3	3
120802.4	laceration	120802.4	120802.4	3
120804.5	open laceration (bleeding externally) or segmental loss	120804.5	120804.5	3
120806.3	thrombosis ; occlusion	120806.3	120806.3	3
122099.4	**Sigmoid sinus** NFS	122099.4	122099.4	1
122002.4	laceration	122002.4	122002.4	1
122003.5	bilateral[c]	122002.4[b]	None	1
122004.5	open laceration (bleeding externally) or segmental loss	122004.5	122004.5	2
122005.6	bilateral[c]	122004.5[b]	None	2
122006.4	thrombosis ; occlusion	122006.4	122006.4	2
122007.5	bilateral[c]	122006.4[b]	None	1
123099.4	**Straight sinus** NFS[a]	122299.3[b]	None	
123002.4	laceration[a]	122202.4	None	
123003.5	open laceration (bleeding externally) or segmental loss[a]	122202.4[b]	None	
123004.5	thrombosis ; occlusion[a]	122204.3[b]	None	

[a] New descriptor in AIS 2005
[b] Change in severity code in AIS 2005
[c] In previous editions of AIS, with few exceptions, each injury was coded separately. AIS 2005 introduces "bilateral" for certain injury descriptions. Some bilateral injuries may affect severity levels and, therefore, the ISS for patients with these injuries.
[d] Major vein and sinus were combined as one descriptor in AIS 98. In AIS 2005, they are separate descriptors ; hence, the duplication of AIS 98 matching codes.

頭部（頭蓋と脳）

AIS 2005	損傷内容	⇒ AIS98	⇐ AIS98	FCI
122299.3	**静脈洞**　詳細不明[d]	122299.3	122299.3	5
122202.4	裂傷・裂創	122202.4	122202.4	5
122204.3	血栓症；閉塞	122204.3	122204.3	5
120602.4	**内頸動脈−海綿静脈洞瘻**	120602.4	120602.4	3
120603.4	両側性[c]	120602.4	なし	2
	別個に内頸動脈損傷のコードを選択してはならない。			
120899.3	**海綿静脈洞**　詳細不明	120899.3	120899.3	3
120802.4	裂傷・裂創	120802.4	120802.4	3
120804.5	開放性裂傷・裂創（体外に出血）または部分欠損	120804.5	120804.5	3
120806.3	血栓症；閉塞	120806.3	120806.3	3
122099.4	**S状静脈洞**　詳細不明	122099.4	122099.4	1
122002.4	裂傷・裂創	122002.4	122002.4	1
122003.5	両側性[c]	122002.4[b]	なし	1
122004.5	開放性裂傷・裂創（体外に出血）または部分欠損	122004.5	122004.5	2
122005.6	両側性[c]	122004.5[b]	なし	2
122006.4	血栓症；閉塞	122006.4	122006.4	2
122007.5	両側性[c]	122006.4[b]	なし	1
123099.4	**直静脈洞**　詳細不明[a]	122299.3[b]	なし	
123002.4	裂傷・裂創[a]	122202.4	なし	
123003.5	開放性裂傷（体外に出血）または部分欠損[a]	122202.4[b]	なし	
123004.5	血栓症；閉塞[a]	122204.3[b]	なし	

---

[a] AIS2005に加えられた新しいコード。
[b] AIS2005で重症度に変更あり。
[c] 旧版のAISでは一部の例外を除き両側損傷はそれぞれ別にコード選択をしていた。AIS2005では、"両側"を導入した。いくつかの両側損傷は重症度が変化し、その結果ISSが変わることがある。
[d] AIS98では主要な静脈と静脈洞は1つのコードにまとめられていたが、AIS2005では別々のものとする。したがって、AIS98の該当コードを反復入力する。

HEAD (cranium and brain)

AIS 2005	Injury Description	⇒ AIS98	⇐ AIS98	FCI
122499.3	**Superior longitudinal (saggital) sinus** NFS	122499.4[b]	122499.4[b]	5
122402.4	laceration	122402.4	122402.4	5
122404.5	open laceration (bleeding externally) or segmental loss	122404.5	122404.5	5
122406.4	thrombosis ; occlusion[e]	122406.4	122406.4	2
122407.4	anterior half of sinus[a]	122406.4	None	2
122408.5	posterior half of sinus[a]	122406.4[b]	None	1
122699.3	**Transverse sinus** NFS	122699.4[b]	122699.4[b]	2
122602.4	laceration	122602.4	122602.4	5
122603.5	bilateral[c]	122602.4[b]	None	5
122604.5	open laceration (bleeding externally) or segmental loss[e]	122604.5	122604.5	5
122605.6	bilateral[c]	122604.5[b]	None	1
122607.6	torcular[a]	122604.5[b]	None	
122606.4	thrombosis ; occlusion	122606.4	122606.4	2
122608.5	bilateral[c]	122606.4[b]	None	1
122399.3	**Vein** NFS[a]	121299.3	None	5
122599.3	**Vein, major** NFS [includes *Galen, Labbe, Trolard, Rosenthal* or *internal cerebral*][d]	122299.3	122299.3	5
122502.4	laceration	122202.4	122202.4	5
122504.3	thrombosis ; occlusion	122204.3	122204.3	2
122799.3	**Vein, non-major** NFS[a] [any named vein that is not major]	121299.3	None	
122702.4	laceration[a]	121202.4	None	
122704.3	thrombosis ; occlusion[a]	121204.3	None	

[a] New descriptor in AIS 2005
[b] Change in severity code in AIS 2005
[c] In previous editions of AIS, with few exceptions, each injury was coded separately. AIS 2005 introduces "bilateral" for certain injury descriptions. Some bilateral injuries may affect severity levels and, therefore, the ISS for patients with these injuries.
[d] Major Vein and Sinus were combined as one descriptor in AIS 98. In AIS 2005, they are separate descriptors ; hence, the duplication of AIS 98 matching codes.
[e] In AIS 98, this injury description had only one severity level. In AIS 2005, it has several.

頭部（頭蓋と脳）

AIS 2005	損傷内容	⇒ AIS98	⇐ AIS98	FCI
122499.3	上矢状洞　詳細不明	122499.4[b]	122499.4[b]	5
122402.4	裂傷・裂創	122402.4	122402.4	5
122404.5	開放性裂傷・裂創（体外に出血）または部分欠損	122404.5	122404.5	5
122406.4	血栓症；閉塞[e]	122406.4	122406.4	2
122407.4	前半部[a]	122406.4	なし	2
122408.5	後半部[a]	122406.4[b]	なし	1
122699.3	横静脈洞　詳細不明	122699.4[b]	122699.4[b]	2
122602.4	裂傷・裂創	122602.4	122602.4	5
122603.5	両側性[c]	122602.4[b]	なし	5
122604.5	開放性裂傷・裂創（体外に出血）または部分欠損[e]	122604.5	122604.5	5
122605.6	両側性[c]	122604.5[b]	なし	1
122607.6	静脈洞交会[a]	122604.5[b]	なし	
122606.4	血栓症；閉塞	122606.4	122606.4	2
122608.5	両側性[c]	122606.4[b]	なし	1
122399.3	静脈　詳細不明[a]	121299.3	なし	5
122599.3	主要な静脈　詳細不明［ガレン，ラーベ，トロラード，ローゼンタル，内大脳静脈を含む］[d]	122299.3	122299.3	5
122502.4	裂傷・裂創	122202.4	122202.4	5
122504.3	血栓症；閉塞	122204.3	122204.3	2
122799.3	その他の静脈　詳細不明[a]［名称があっても主要でない］	121299.3	なし	
122702.4	裂傷・裂創[a]	121202.4	なし	
122704.3	血栓症；閉塞[a]	121204.3	なし	

[a] AIS2005に加えられた新しいコード。
[b] AIS2005で重症度に変更あり。
[c] 旧版のAISでは一部の例外を除き両側損傷はそれぞれ別にコード選択をしていた。AIS2005では，"両側"を導入した。いくつかの両側損傷は重症度が変化し，その結果ISSが変わることがある。
[d] AIS98では主要な静脈と静脈洞は1つのコードにまとめられていたが，AIS2005では別々のものとする。したがって，AIS98の該当コードを反復入力する。
[e] AIS98ではこの損傷コードは1つだけであったが，AIS2005においては複数個ある。

HEAD (cranium and brain)

AIS 2005	Injury Description	⇒ AIS98	⇐ AIS98	FCI
	NERVES, CRANIAL			
	Because of limitations in diagnostic capabilities, cranial nerve injuries may be described only by the type of dysfunction that exists in normal nerve activity. Unless contusion or laceration is specified, code total loss of nerve function (paralysis) as a laceration and partial loss of function (paresis) as a contusion. Do not increase the severity for multiple injuries to the same nerve. Certain nerve injuries have a higher AIS code when they occur bilaterally ; these are specifically indicated. Nerve injuries are coded separately from other injuries to the brain, except for crush-type or massive penetrating brain injuries which are inclusive of all injuries to the brain. If a nerve is not named specifically, code as cranial nerve NFS.			
	Use one of the following three descriptors if specific nerve is not named.			
130299.2	**Cranial nerve** NFS	130299.2	130299.2	5
130202.2	contusion	130202.2	130202.2	5
130204.2	laceration	130204.2	130204.2	5
130499.2	I (Olfactory nerve, tract) NFS	130499.2	130499.2	5
130402.2	contusion	130402.2	130402.2	5
130404.2	laceration	130404.2	130404.2	5
130699.2	II (Optic nerve-intracranial and intracanalicular segments) NFS [includes chiasm and tracts]	130699.2	130699.2	3
	Code intraorbital segment under Face. If segment is unknown, code under Head.			
130602.2	contusion	130602.2	130602.2	3
130604.2	bilateral	130604.2	130604.2	3
130606.2	laceration	130606.2	130606.2	3
130608.2	bilateral	130608.2	130608.2	2

AIS 2005	損傷内容	⇒ AIS98	⇐ AIS98	FCI

脳神経

診断上の限界により確定が困難な場合があるので，脳神経損傷はその脳神経の本来の機能が障害され，異常所見があるときのみ記載する。脳神経の挫傷あるいは裂傷・裂創が確認されない限り，神経機能の完全消失（麻痺）を裂傷・裂創，不完全消失（麻痺）を挫傷としてコードを選択する。同一神経への複数の損傷により重症度を上げてはならない。両側の損傷の場合，別途高い AIS コードを選択する。脳神経損傷は脳に加わる他の外傷とは別にコードを選択する。ただし，脳の挫滅や重度の穿通性脳損傷の場合はすべてのタイプの脳損傷を含むため，この限りではない。どの脳神経の損傷か特定できない場合は詳細不明のコードを選択する。

損傷した脳神経が特定できない場合に，以下の3つから1つを選択する。

130299.2	**脳神経** 詳細不明	130299.2	130299.2	5
130202.2	挫傷	130202.2	130202.2	5
130204.2	裂傷・裂創	130204.2	130204.2	5
130499.2	Ⅰ（嗅神経，嗅覚路）　詳細不明	130499.2	130499.2	5
130402.2	挫傷	130402.2	130402.2	5
130404.2	裂傷・裂創	130404.2	130404.2	5
130699.2	Ⅱ（視神経－頭蓋内と視神経管内）詳細不明 [視交叉と視索を含む]	130699.2	130699.2	3

眼窩内の視神経損傷は顔面損傷としてコードを選択する。損傷部位が特定されない場合には頭部損傷としてコードを選択する。

130602.2	挫傷	130602.2	130602.2	3
130604.2	両側	130604.2	130604.2	3
130606.2	裂傷・裂創	130606.2	130606.2	3
130608.2	両側	130608.2	130608.2	2

HEAD (cranium and brain)

AIS 2005	Injury Description	⇒ AIS98	⇐ AIS98	FCI
130899.2	**III (Oculomotor nerve)** NFS	130899.2	130899.2	3
130802.2	contusion or compression [includes injury due to transtentorial herniation]	130802.2	130802.2	5
130804.2	laceration	130804.2	130804.2	3
131099.2	**IV (Trochlear nerve)** NFS	131099.2	131099.2	3
131002.2	contusion	131002.2	131002.2	5
131004.2	laceration	131004.2	131004.2	3
131299.2	**V (Trigeminal nerve)** NFS	131299.2	131299.2	3
131202.2	contusion	131202.2	131202.2	5
131204.2	laceration	131204.2	131204.2	3
131499.2	**VI (Abducens nerve)** NFS	131499.2	131499.2	3
131402.2	contusion	131402.2	131402.2	5
131404.2	laceration	131404.2	131404.2	3
131699.2	**VII (Facial nerve)** NFS	131699.2	131699.2	3
131602.2	contusion	131602.2	131602.2	5
131604.2	laceration	131604.2	131604.2	3
131605.3	bilateral[c]	131604.2[b]	None	2
131899.2	**VIII (Vestibulocochlear nerve)** NFS [includes **auditory, acoustic and vestibular nerves**]	131899.2	131899.2	4
131802.2	contusion	131802.2	131802.2	5
131804.2	laceration	131804.2	131804.2	4
131806.3	bilateral	131806.2[b]	131806.2[b]	2

---

[b] Change in severity code in AIS 2005
[c] In previous editions of AIS, with few exceptions, each injury was coded separately. AIS 2005 introduces "bilateral" for certain injury descriptions. Some bilateral injuries may affect severity levels and, therefore, the ISS for patients with these injuries.

AIS 2005	損傷内容	⇒ AIS98	⇐ AIS98	FCI
130899.2	Ⅲ （動眼神経） 詳細不明	130899.2	130899.2	3
130802.2	挫傷または圧迫［テント切痕ヘルニアによる損傷を含む］	130802.2	130802.2	5
130804.2	裂傷・裂創	130804.2	130804.2	3
131099.2	Ⅳ （滑車神経） 詳細不明	131099.2	131099.2	3
131002.2	挫傷	131002.2	131002.2	5
131004.2	裂傷・裂創	131004.2	131004.2	3
131299.2	Ⅴ （三叉神経） 詳細不明	131299.2	131299.2	3
131202.2	挫傷	131202.2	131202.2	5
131204.2	裂傷・裂創	131204.2	131204.2	3
131499.2	Ⅵ （外転神経） 詳細不明	131499.2	131499.2	3
131402.2	挫傷	131402.2	131402.2	5
131404.2	裂傷・裂創	131404.2	131404.2	3
131699.2	Ⅶ （顔面神経） 詳細不明	131699.2	131699.2	3
131602.2	挫傷	131602.2	131602.2	5
131604.2	裂傷・裂創	131604.2	131604.2	3
131605.3	両側[c]	131604.2[b]	なし	2
131899.2	Ⅷ （前庭・蝸牛神経） 詳細不明 ［聴神経，前庭神経を含む］	131899.2	131899.2	4
131802.2	挫傷	131802.2	131802.2	5
131804.2	裂傷・裂創	131804.2	131804.2	4
131806.3	両側	131806.2[b]	131806.2[b]	2

[b] AIS2005で重症度に変更あり。
[c] 旧版の AIS では一部の例外を除き両側損傷はそれぞれ別にコード選択をしていた。AIS2005では，"両側"を導入した。いくつかの両側損傷は重症度が変化し，その結果 ISS が変わることがある。

HEAD (cranium and brain)

AIS 2005	Injury Description	⇒ AIS98	⇐ AIS98	FCI
132099.2	IX (Glossopharyngeal nerve) NFS	132099.2	132099.2	2
132002.2	contusion	132002.2	132002.2	5
132004.2	laceration	132004.2	132004.2	2
132299.2	X (Vagus nerve) NFS [excludes injury in neck, thorax or abdomen]	132299.2	132299.2	3
132202.2	contusion	132202.2	132202.2	5
132204.2	laceration	132204.2	132204.2	3
132499.2	XI (Spinal accessory nerve) NFS	132499.2	132499.2	5
132402.2	contusion	132402.2	132402.2	5
132404.2	laceration	132404.2	132404.2	5
132699.2	XII (Hypoglossal nerve) NFS	132699.2	132699.2	2
132602.2	contusion	132602.2	132602.2	5
132604.2	laceration	132604.2	132604.2	2

頭部（頭蓋と脳）

AIS 2005	損傷内容	⇒ AIS98	⇐ AIS98	FCI
132099.2	Ⅸ（舌咽神経）詳細不明	132099.2	132099.2	2
132002.2	挫傷	132002.2	132002.2	5
132004.2	裂傷・裂創	132004.2	132004.2	2
132299.2	Ⅹ（迷走神経）詳細不明 　　［頸部，胸郭，腹部における損傷を除く］	132299.2	132299.2	3
132202.2	挫傷	132202.2	132202.2	5
132204.2	裂傷・裂創	132204.2	132204.2	3
132499.2	Ⅺ（副神経）詳細不明	132499.2	132499.2	5
132402.2	挫傷	132402.2	132402.2	5
132404.2	裂傷・裂創	132404.2	132404.2	5
132699.2	Ⅻ（舌下神経）詳細不明	132699.2	132699.2	2
132602.2	挫傷	132602.2	132602.2	5
132604.2	裂傷・裂創	132604.2	132604.2	2

HEAD (cranium and brain)

CODING RULES : Brain

Time to Code

Given current imaging and other radiological techniques in trauma care, virtually all brain injuries can be diagnosed within the first 24 hours. Surgical and other interventions, such as administering anticoagulants, can increase the size of a contusion or hemorrhage which would artificially inflate its severity. Therefore, coding of brain injuries should be done at 24 hours or at initial confirmed diagnosis if later than 24 hours.

Coma

Under Cerebrum, several descriptors of imaging findings include coma as a modifier (i.e., intraventricular hemorrhage, ischemic brain damage directly related to head trauma, subarachnoid hemorrhage and subpial hemorrhage). If a patient sustains more than one of these documented findings involving coma, assign the coma only once to the finding that will result in the highest AIS code. If there is no difference in the AIS code, add the coma to only one of the findings and code the other finding(s) as not further specified (NFS).

Example :
Coma > 6 hours, but no substantiated DAI
Trauma-related ischemic brain damage   140683.5
Subarachnoid hemorrhage   140693.2

Diffuse Axonal Injury

Patients with a substantiated clinical or pathological diagnosis of DAI may also have other imaging findings noted (e.g., intraventricular hemorrhage, petechial hemorrhage). In such cases, only the substantiated DAI is assigned an AIS severity code.

Example :
Mild DAI (LOC 6-24 hours)   161008.4
Intraventricular hemorrhage   do not code

Note that a diagnosis of DAI must meet specific coding rules described in the text "Diffuse Axonal Injury" (page 60). Substantiated DAI by definition includes prolonged coma.

コード選択のルール：脳

コードを選択するタイミング
外傷初療における最近の画像や放射線学的技術により，すべての脳外傷は最初の24時間以内に視覚的に診断できる。外科手術や他の治療，例えば抗凝固薬を投与されている場合，脳挫傷や血腫のサイズが増大する可能性があり，それにより本来の結果より重症化しうる。そのため，脳外傷のコードを選択する場合には，24時間の時点，24時間以降の場合には最初に診断した時点で行うべきである。

昏睡
大脳の項で，画像所見による分類のなかに，選択肢として昏睡が含まれるものがある（すなわち，脳室内出血，頭部外傷に直接由来する虚血性脳障害，くも膜下出血，軟膜下出血）。昏睡で，さらに上述した所見を複数もつ場合には，もっとも高いAISコードのみに昏睡コードを割り当てる。もしAISコードの重症度に差がない場合には，そのうちの1つのみに昏睡のコードを割り当て，他の所見は詳細不明のコードを選択する。

例：
昏睡が6時間を超えたが，確定したびまん性軸索損傷はない
外傷に関連した虚血性脳障害　　　　140683.5
くも膜下出血　　　　　　　　　　　140693.2

びまん性軸索損傷

臨床的にあるいは病理学的にびまん性軸索損傷を示す患者では，たいてい他の画像所見も併せ持つ（例：脳室内出血や実質内出血）。そのような場合には，確定したびまん性軸索損傷のみにAISの重症度コードを割り当てられる。

例：
軽症DAI（意識消失時間が6〜24時間）　　161008.4
脳室内出血　　　　　　　　　　　　　　　コードしない

DAIの診断は"びまん性軸索損傷"（本手引書60ページ）の特別な振り分けコードのルールに合致しなければならない。定義に則ったDAIには遷延性昏睡が含まれる。

HEAD (cranium and brain)

AIS 2005	Injury Description	⇒ AIS98	⇐ AIS98	FCI
	INTERNAL ORGANS			
	Injuries to Internal Organs (i.e., brain stem, cerebellum or cerebrum) must be verified by CT, MRI, surgery, x-ray, angiography or autopsy. Clinical diagnosis alone is not adequate for substantiating the existence of an anatomic lesion for coding purposes.			
140299.5	**Brain stem [hypothalamus, medulla, midbrain, pons]** NFS	140299.5	140299.5	1
140202.5	compression [includes transtentorial (uncal) or cerebellar tonsillar herniation]	140202.5	140202.5	1
140204.5	contusion	140204.5	140204.5	1
140208.5	infarction	140208.5	140208.5	1
140210.5	injury involving hemorrhage	140210.5	140210.5	1
140212.6	laceration	140212.6	140212.6	1
140214.6	massive destruction (crush-type injury)	140214.6	140214.6	1
140216.6	penetrating injury	140216.6	140216.6	1
140218.6	transection	140218.6	140218.6	1
	Use Cerebellum section only if cerebellum, infratentorial or posterior fossa are named. Otherwise, code under Cerebrum.			
140499.3	**Cerebellum** NFS	140499.3	140499.3	5
140402.3	contusion, single or multiple, NFS [include perilesional edema for size]	140402.3	140402.3	5
140407.2	tiny ; < 1 cm diameter[a]	140403.3[b]	None	5
140403.3	small ; superficial ; ≤15cc ; 1-3cm diameter	140403.3	140403.3	5
140404.4	large ; 15-30cc ; >3cm diameter	140404.4	140404.4	3
140405.5	extensive ; massive ; total volume >30cc	140405.5	140405.5	2

---

[a] New descriptor in AIS 2005
[b] Change in severity in AIS 2005

頭部（頭蓋と脳）

AIS 2005	損傷内容	⇒ AIS98	⇐ AIS98	FCI

脳

> 脳の損傷（すなわち脳幹，小脳，大脳）はCT，MRI，手術，X線検査，血管撮影または病理解剖により特定しなければならない。臨床診断のみでは十分とはいえないので，具体的な解剖学的な所見を用いて，正確なコードを選択する必要がある。

AIS 2005	損傷内容	⇒ AIS98	⇐ AIS98	FCI
140299.5	**脳幹[視床下部，延髄，中脳，橋]** 詳細不明	140299.5	140299.5	1
140202.5	圧迫[テント切痕（拘回）ヘルニア，小脳扁桃ヘルニアを含む]	140202.5	140202.5	1
140204.5	挫傷	140204.5	140204.5	1
140208.5	脳梗塞	140208.5	140208.5	1
140210.5	出血を含む損傷	140210.5	140210.5	1
140212.6	裂傷・裂創	140212.6	140212.6	1
140214.6	高度損傷（脳挫滅型損傷）	140214.6	140214.6	1
140216.6	穿通損傷	140216.6	140216.6	1
140218.6	離断	140218.6	140218.6	1

> 小脳，テント下，後頭蓋窩などの記載があったときのみ小脳の項を割り振る。それ以外では，大脳の項でコードを選択する。

AIS 2005	損傷内容	⇒ AIS98	⇐ AIS98	FCI
140499.3	**小脳** 詳細不明	140499.3	140499.3	5
140402.3	挫傷，1カ所でもそれ以上でも，詳細不明[損傷周囲の浮腫を含む]	140402.3	140402.3	5
140407.2	微小；直径1cm未満[a]	140403.3[b]	なし	5
140403.3	小；表在性；15ml以下；直径1～3cm	140403.3	140403.3	5
140404.4	大；15～30ml；直径3cmを超える	140404.4	140404.4	3
140405.5	広範囲；大量；合計30mlを超える	140405.5	140405.5	2

---

[a] AIS2005に加えられた新しいコード。
[b] AIS2005で重症度に変更あり。

HEAD (cranium and brain)

AIS 2005	Injury Description ⇒ AIS98	⇐ AIS98	FCI	
	Cerebellum (continued)			
140410.3	hematoma (hemorrhage) NFS	140410.4[b]	140410.4[b]	5
	Use above descriptor for "extra axial" unless further described as epidural or subdural.			
140414.3	epidural or extradural NFS [include perilesional edema for size]	140414.4[b]	140414.4[b]	5
140416.2	tiny ; <0.6cm thick[a]	140418.4[b]	None	5
140418.4	small ; moderate ; ≤30cc or ≤15cc if ≤age 10 ; 0.6-1cm thick	140418.4	140418.4	5
140422.5	large ; massive ; extensive ; >30cc or >15cc if ≤age 10 ; >1cm thick	140422.5	140422.5	1
140426.3	intracerebellar including petechial and subcortical NFS [include perilesional edema for size]	140426.4[b]	140426.4[b]	5
140428.2	tiny ; <0.6cm diameter [includes radiographic "shearing" lesions][a]	140430.4[b]	None	5
140430.4	small ; ≤15cc ; 0.6-3cm diameter	140430.4	140430.4	5
140434.5	large ; >15cc ; >3cm diameter	140434.5	140434.5	2
140438.3	subdural NFS	140438.4[b]	140438.4[b]	5
140440.2	tiny ; <0.6cm thick[a]	140442.4[b]	None	5
140442.4	small ; moderate ; ≤30cc or ≤15cc if ≤age 10 ; 0.6-1cm thick	140442.4	140442.4	5
140446.5	large ; massive ; extensive ; >30cc or >15cc if ≤age 10 ; >1cm thick	140446.5	140446.5	2
140474.3	laceration [not from penetrating injury] NFS[e]	140474.4[b]	140474.4[b]	5
140473.3	≤2cm length or depth	140474.4[b]	None	5
140472.4	>2cm length or depth	140474.4	None	3

[a] New descriptor in AIS 2005
[b] Change in severity code in AIS 2005
[e] In AIS 98, this injury description had only one severity level. In AIS 2005, it has several.

AIS 2005	損傷内容	⇒ AIS98	⇐ AIS98	FCI
	小脳（続き）			
140410.3	血腫（出血）詳細不明	140410.4[b]	140410.4[b]	5
	"硬膜外""硬膜下"などの追加記載がない限り，実質外のものとしてこのコードを選択する。			
140414.3	硬膜外　詳細不明［損傷周囲の浮腫を含む］	140414.4[b]	140414.4[b]	5
140416.2	微小；厚さが0.6cm未満[a]	140418.4[b]	なし	5
140418.4	小；中程度；皮質下30ml以下（10歳以下では15ml以下）；厚さが0.6～1cm	140418.4	140418.4	5
140422.5	大；広範囲；大量；30ml以上（10歳以下では15mlを超える）；厚さが1cmを超える	140422.5	140422.5	1
140426.3	実質内と皮質下を含む小脳内　詳細不明［損傷周囲の浮腫を含む］	140426.4[b]	140426.4[b]	5
140428.2	微小；厚さが0.6cm未満［画像診断による剪断損傷を含む］[a]	140430.4[b]	なし	5
140430.4	小；15ml以下；直径0.6～3cm	140430.4	140430.4	5
140434.5	大；15mlを超える；直径3cmを超える	140434.5	140434.5	2
140438.3	硬膜下　詳細不明	140438.4[b]	140438.4[b]	5
140440.2	微小；厚さが0.6cm未満[a]	140442.4[b]	なし	5
140442.4	小；中等症；30ml以下（10歳以下では15ml以下）；厚さが0.6～1cm	140442.4	140442.4	5
140446.5	大；広範囲；大量；30mlを超える（10歳以下では15mlを超える）；厚さが1cmを超える	140446.5	140446.5	2
140474.3	裂傷・裂創［穿通外傷によるものは除く］詳細不明[e]	140474.4[b]	140474.4[b]	5
140473.3	長さまたは深さが2cm以下	140474.4[b]	なし	5
140472.4	長さまたは深さが2cmを超える	140474.4	なし	3

[a] AIS2005に加えられた新しいコード。
[b] AIS2005で重症度に変更あり。
[e] AIS98ではこの損傷コードは1つだけであったが，AIS2005においては複数個ある。

HEAD (cranium and brain)

AIS 2005	Injury Description	⇒ AIS98	⇐ AIS98	FCI
	Cerebellum (continued)			
140478.3	penetrating injury NFS[e]	140478.5[b]	140478.5[b]	5
140477.3	≤2cm deep	140478.5[b]	None	5
140476.5	>2cm deep	140478.5	None	2
140489.9	trauma-associated findings not related either to intervention or to anatomically-described head injury NFS[f]	None	None	
140450.3	brain swelling/edema NFS	140450.3	140450.3	5
	Must be directly related to head injury, not anoxia or perilesional. Read "Brain Edema and Brain Swelling" below for coding guidance.			
140458.3	infarction (acute due to traumatic vascular occlusion)	140458.3	140458.3	2
140462.3	ischemic brain damage directly related to head trauma	140462.3	140462.3	5
140466.2	subarachnoid hemorrhage	140466.3[b]	140466.3[b]	5
140470.2	subpial hemorrhage	140470.3[b]	140470.3[b]	5

Brain Edema and Brain Swelling

The terms brain edema (BE) and brain swelling (BS) are often confused because in many regions of the world, they are intentionally used interchangeably. However, in other regions BE and BS are considered to be separate entities. Thus, the following definitions are offered.

Brain Swelling is a generic description of a swollen brain whereas brain edema represents a specific type of brain swelling, that due to increased brain water content. In BE, the increased water may either be inside of cells or between cells. Both BE and BS may be documented by any of the following depending on the data source: increased brain weight (pathological observations), swelling of the brain beyond the usual dural margin (at surgery), imaging studies that demonstrate any of the following: obscuration of the grey-white matter junctions; compression or obliteration of the ventricles; narrowing or obliteration of the basal cisterns.

Brain Edema is best distinguished from brain swelling by the presence of: hypodensity (more black than normal brain) on CT imaging, or hypointensity on T1 or hyperintensity on T2 or flair MRI imaging. Thus, brain edema should only be diagnosed if these conditions exist. Otherwise, the diagnosis of brain swelling should be made (isodense or slightly hyperdense on CT or isodense on MRI).

---

[b] Change in severity code in AIS 2005
[e] In AIS 98, this injury description had only one severity level. In AIS 2005, it has several.
[f] New descriptor in AIS 2005 that allows classification of trauma by body region, but does not allow assigning a severity code.

頭部（頭蓋と脳）

AIS 2005	損傷内容	⇒ AIS98	⇐ AIS98	FCI
	小脳（続き）			
140478.3	穿通性損傷　詳細不明[e]	140478.5[b]	140478.5[b]	5
140477.3	深さが2cm以下	140478.5[b]	なし	5
140476.5	深さが2cmを超える	140478.5	なし	2
140489.9	診断・治療や解剖によって得られたものではない頭部外傷に関連する所見　詳細不明[f]	なし	なし	
140450.3	脳腫脹／脳浮腫　詳細不明	140450.3	140450.3	5
	これは低酸素や損傷周囲の脳浮腫ではなく，頭部外傷に直接関係するものでなくてはならない。正しいコードのために，下記の"脳浮腫と脳腫脹"の項を参照。			
140458.3	脳梗塞（急性のもので外傷による血管閉塞を原因とする）	140458.3	140458.3	2
140462.3	頭部外傷と直接関連する虚血性脳障害	140462.3	140462.3	5
140466.2	くも膜下出血	140466.3[b]	140466.3[b]	5
140470.2	軟膜下出血	140470.3[b]	140470.3[b]	5

脳浮腫と脳腫脹

　脳浮腫と脳腫脹という言葉は，しばしば世界各国で時に意識的に分け隔てなく使用されて混乱を生じてきた。しかし，この2つの単語は別の病態と認識され使用されている地域もある。この混乱を避けるために，以下の分類が提案されている。

　脳腫脹は，腫脹した脳の総称として記載されるのに対し，脳浮腫は脳の水分量の増大という脳腫脹の特殊な型として表現される。脳浮腫の原因は，細胞内や間質での水分貯留による。データにもよるが，脳腫脹も脳浮腫も，脳重量の増大（病理学的所見），硬膜の折り返しを超える脳の腫脹（術中），そして白質-灰白質境界の不鮮明化，脳室の圧迫や消失，脳底槽の圧迫や消失などの画像検査所見によって表現される。

　脳浮腫は，CTでは低吸収域として正常脳よりも暗く映ることで，またMRIではT1で低信号，T2とFLAIRで高信号を示すことによって，脳腫脹は脳腫瘍と明確に区別可能となる。したがって，脳浮腫はこのような病態が明らかに存在するときのみ診断が可能である。それ以外では，脳腫脹としてコードを選択する（CTでは等吸収域からやや高吸収域，MRIでは等信号）。

---

[b] AIS2005で重症度に変更あり。
[e] AIS98ではこの損傷コードは1つだけであったが，AIS2005においては複数個ある。
[f] AIS2005に加えられた新しいコード。外傷の存在部位を示すことができる。ただし重症度はない。

HEAD (cranium and brain)

AIS 2005	Injury Description	⇒ AIS98	⇐ AIS98	FCI
140699.3	**Cerebrum** NFS [includes **basal ganglia, thalamus, putamen, globus pallidius**]	140699.3	140699.3	5
	Use Cerebrum section for supratentorial, anterior or middle cranial fossa ; also use if trauma is vaguely described as "brain injury".			
140602.3	contusion NFS [include perilesional edema for size]	140602.3	140602.3	5
140604.3	single NFS	140604.3	140604.3	5
140605.2	tiny ; <1cm diameter[a]	140604.3[b]	None	5
140606.3	small ; superficial ; ≤30cc or ≤15cc if ≤age 10 ; 1-4cm diameter or 1-2cm diameter if ≤age 10 ; midline shift ≤5mm	140606.3	140606.3	5
140608.4	large ; deep ; 30-50cc or 15-30cc if ≤age 10 ; >4cm diameter or 2-4cm diameter if ≤age 10 ; midline shift >5mm	140608.4	140608.4	2
140610.5	extensive ; massive ; total volume >50cc or >30cc if ≤age 10	140610.5	140610.5	1
140611.3	multiple NFS	140611.3	140611.3	3
140612.3	multiple, on same side but NFS	140612.3	140612.3	5
140613.2	tiny ; each <1cm diameter[a]	140612.3[b]	None	5
140614.3	small ; superficial ; total volume ≤30cc or ≤15cc if ≤age 10 ; midline shift ≤5mm	140614.3	140614.3	5
140616.4	large ; total volume 30-50cc or 15-30cc if ≤age 10 ; midline shift >5mm	140616.4	140616.4	1
140618.5	extensive ; massive ; total volume >50cc or >30cc if ≤age 10	140618.5	140618.5	1
140620.3	multiple, at least one on each side but NFS	140620.3	140620.3	3
140621.2	tiny ; each <1cm diameter[a]	140622.3[b]	None	5
140622.3	small ; superficial ; total volume ≤30cc or ≤15cc if ≤age 10	140622.3	140622.3	3
140624.4	large ; total volume 30-50cc or 15-30cc if ≤age 10	140624.4	140624.4	1
140626.5	extensive ; massive ; total volume >50cc or >30cc if ≤age 10	140626.5	140626.5	1

[a] New descriptor in AIS 2005
[b] Change in severity code in AIS 2005

頭部（頭蓋と脳）

AIS 2005	損傷内容	⇒ AIS98	⇐ AIS98	FCI
140699.3	大脳　詳細不明［基底核，視床，被殻，淡蒼球を含む］	140699.3	140699.3	5

大脳の項目は，テント上か，前または中頭蓋窩の損傷に対して選択する。また，単に"脳損傷"と記載された損傷に対しても選択する。

AIS 2005	損傷内容	⇒ AIS98	⇐ AIS98	FCI
140602.3	挫傷　詳細不明［損傷周囲の浮腫を含む］	140602.3	140602.3	5
140604.3	単発性　詳細不明	140604.3	140604.3	5
140605.2	微小；直径1cm未満[a]	140604.3[b]	なし	5
140606.3	小；表在性；30ml以下（10歳以下では15ml以下）；直径1～4cm（10歳以下では1～2cm）；正中偏位5mm以下	140606.3	140606.3	5
140608.4	大；深在性；30～50ml（10歳以下では15～30ml）；直径4cmを超える（10歳以下では2～4cm）；正中偏位が5mmを超える	140608.4	140608.4	2
140610.5	広範囲；大量；合計50mlを超える（10歳以下では30mlを超える）	140610.5	140610.5	1
140611.3	多発性　詳細不明	140611.3	140611.3	3
140612.3	多発性，片側　詳細不明	140612.3	140612.3	5
140613.2	微小；いずれも直径1cm未満[a]	140612.3[b]	なし	5
140614.3	小；表在性；合計30ml以下（10歳以下では15ml以下）；正中偏位が5mm以下	140614.3	140614.3	5
140616.4	大；合計30～50ml（10歳以下では15～30ml）；正中偏位が5mmを超える	140616.4	140616.4	1
140618.5	広範囲；大量；合計50mlを超える（10歳以下では30mlを超える）	140618.5	140618.5	1
140620.3	多発性，両側　詳細不明	140620.3	140620.3	3
140621.2	微小；いずれも直径1cm未満[a]	140622.3[b]	なし	5
140622.3	小；表在性；合計30ml以下（10歳以下では15ml以下）	140622.3	140622.3	3
140624.4	大；合計30～50ml（10歳以下では15～30ml）	140624.4	140624.4	1
140626.5	広範囲；大量；合計50mlを超える（10歳以下では30mlを超える）	140626.5	140626.5	1

---

[a] AIS2005に加えられた新しいコード。
[b] AIS2005で重症度に変更あり。

HEAD (cranium and brain)

AIS 2005	Injury Description	⇒ AIS98	⇐ AIS98	FCI
	Cerebrum (continued)			
140628.4	diffuse axonal injury (DAI) NFS [24 hours > requires coma > 6 hours or, if fatal within 6 hours, diagnosis is made by pathological examination][e]	140628.5[b]	140628.5[b]	1
140625.4	DAI confined to white matter or basal ganglia	140628.5[b]	None	1
140627.5	DAI involving corpus callosum	140628.5	None	1
	If white matter/basal ganglia <u>and</u> corpus callosum are involved, code only the more severe ; do not code both. If coma exceeds 24 hours and diagnosis meets coding rules for DAI, use 161011.5, 161012.5 or 161013.5 no matter what anatomic description is recorded. Read "Diffuse Axonal Injury" (page 60) for coding guidance.			
140629.3	hematoma (hemorrhage) NFS	140629.4[b]	140629.4[b]	5
	Use above descriptor for "extra axial" unless described as epidural or subdural.			
140630.3	epidural or extradural NFS [include perilesional edema for size]	140630.4[b]	140630.4[b]	5
140631.2	tiny ; <0.6cm thick[a]	140632.4[b]	None	5
140632.4	small ; moderate ; ≤50cc or ≤25cc if ≤age 10 ; 0.6-1cm thick	140632.4	140632.4	5
140634.5	bilateral	140634.5	140634.5	5
140636.5	large ; massive ; extensive ; >50cc or >25cc if ≤age 10 ; >1cm thick	140636.5	140636.5	1

---

[a] New descriptor in AIS 2005
[b] Change in severity code in AIS 2005
[e] In AIS 98, this injury description had only one severity level. In AIS 2005, it has several.

頭部（頭蓋と脳）

AIS 2005	損傷内容	⇒ AIS98	⇐ AIS98	FCI
	大脳（続き）			
140628.4	びまん性軸索損傷　詳細不明［6時間を超え24時間以下の昏睡か，もしくは6時間以内の死亡の場合は病理学的診断が必要］[e]	140628.5[b]	140628.5[b]	1
140625.4	びまん性軸索損傷　大脳白質か基底核に限局したもの	140628.5[b]	なし	1
140627.5	びまん性軸索損傷　脳梁に及ぶもの	140628.5	なし	1

> 大脳白質か基底核かつ脳梁にも及ぶものであれば，重症度の高いほうだけをコード選択し，両方は選択しない。たとえどんな解剖学的記述が記録されていても，昏睡が24時間を超えDAIのコード選択のルールに合致するときは，161011.5，161012.5または161013.5を選択する。"DAI"の項目（60ページ）を参照。

140629.3	血腫（出血）詳細不明	140629.4[b]	140629.4[b]	5

> 上のコードは脳実質外の血腫であるが，硬膜外血腫あるいは硬膜下血腫と特定できる根拠がない場合に使用する。

140630.3	硬膜外　詳細不明［損傷周囲の浮腫を含む］	140630.4[b]	140630.4[b]	5
140631.2	微小；厚さ0.6cm未満[a]	140632.4[b]	なし	5
140632.4	小；中程度；50ml以下（10歳以下では25ml以下）；厚さ0.6〜1cm	140632.4	140632.4	5
140634.5	両側	140634.5	140634.5	5
140636.5	大；大量；広範囲；50mlを超える（10歳以下では25mlを超える）；厚さ1cmを超える	140636.5	140636.5	1

---

[a] AIS2005に加えられた新しいコード。
[b] AIS2005で重症度に変更あり。
[e] AIS98ではこの損傷コードは1つだけであったが，AIS2005においては複数個ある。

HEAD (cranium and brain)

AIS 2005	Injury Description	⇒ AIS98	⇐ AIS98	FCI
	Cerebrum (continued)			
	hematoma			
140638.3	intracerebral NFS [include perilesional edema for size]	140638.4[b]	140638.4[b]	5
140639.2	tiny ; single or multiple <1cm diameter[a]	140640.4[b]	None	5
140642.2	petechial hemorrhage (s) [includes radiographic "shearing" lesions][e]	140642.4[b]	140642.4[b]	5
140643.2	not associated with coma >6 hours	140642.4[b]	None	5
140645.4	associated with coma >6 hours	140642.4	None	1
	If DAI diagnosis is made, code as diffuse axonal injury to cerebrum, AIS codes 140628.4, 140625.4 or 140627.5, as appropriate, based on substantiation of injury. Do not code here. Read "Diffuse Axonal Injury" (page 60) for coding guidance.			
140640.4	small ; ≤30cc or ≤15cc if ≤age 10 ; 1-4cm diameter or ≤1cm if ≤age 10 ; subcortical hemorrhage[e,g]	140640.4	140640.4	5
140647.3	not associated with coma >6 hours	140640.4[b]	None	5
140649.4	associated with coma >6 hours	140640.4	None	1
	If DAI diagnosis is made, code as diffuse axonal injury to cerebrum, AIS codes 140628.4, 140625.4 or 140627.5, as appropriate, based on substantiation of injury. Do not code here. Read "Diffuse Axonal Injury" (page 60) for coding guidance.			
140646.5	bilateral	140646.5	140646.5	1
140648.5	large ; >30cc or >15cc if ≤age 10 ; >4cm or >1cm diameter if ≤age 10	140648.5	140648.5	1
140641.5	bilateral [each >4cm][c]	140648.5	None	1
140650.3	subdural NFS	140650.4[b]	140650.4[b]	5
140651.3	tiny ; <0.6cm thick [includes tentorial (subdural) blood one or both sides][a]	140652.4[b]	None	5
140652.4	small ; moderate ; ≤50cc or ≤25cc if ≤age 10 ; 0.6-1cm thick	140652.4	140652.4	5
140654.4	bilateral [both sides 0.6-1cm thick]	140654.5[b]	140654.5[b]	3
140656.5	large ; massive ; extensive ; >50cc or >25cc if ≤age 10 ; >1cm thick	140656.5	140656.5	1
140655.5	bilateral [at least one side >1cm thick][c]	140656.5	None	1

AIS 2005	損傷内容	⇒ AIS98	⇐ AIS98	FCI
	大脳（続き）			
	血腫（出血）			
140638.3	脳内血腫　詳細不明［損傷周囲の浮腫を含む］	140638.4[b]	140638.4[b]	5
140639.2	微小；単発性または直径1cm未満の多発性のもの[a]	140640.4[b]	なし	5
140642.2	点状出血［放射線学的"剪断"損傷を含む］[e]	140642.4[b]	140642.4[b]	5
140643.2	6時間を超える昏睡と関連がないもの	140642.4[b]	なし	5
140645.4	6時間を超える昏睡と関連があるもの	140642.4	なし	1
	DAIの診断がなされているときは，上記をコード選択せず，損傷の実際に応じて大脳のびまん性軸索損傷として140628.4か140625.4もしくは140627.5をコード選択する。"DAI"の項目（60ページ）を参照。			
140640.4	小；30ml以下（10歳以下では15ml以下）；直径1～4cm（10歳以下では1cm以下）；皮質下出血[e, g]	140640.4	140640.4	5
140647.3	6時間を超える昏睡と関連がないもの	140640.4[b]	なし	5
140649.4	6時間を超える昏睡と関連があるもの	140640.4	なし	1
	DAIの診断がなされているときは，上記をコード選択せず，損傷の実際に応じて大脳のびまん性軸索損傷として140628.4か140625.4もしくは140627.5をコード選択する。"DAI"の項目（60ページ）を参照。			
140646.5	両側	140646.5	140646.5	1
140648.5	大；30mlを超える（10歳以下では15mlを超える）；直径4cmを超える（10歳以下では1cmを超える）	140648.5	140648.5	1
140641.5	両側［それぞれ4cmを超える］[c]	140648.5	なし	1
140650.3	硬膜下　詳細不明	140650.4[b]	140650.4[b]	5
140651.3	微小；厚さ0.6cm未満［一側または両側のテントの（硬膜下）出血を含む］[a]	140652.4[b]	なし	5
140652.4	小；中程度；50ml以下（10歳以下では25ml以下）；厚さ0.6～1cm	140652.4	140652.4	5
140654.4	両側［両側とも厚さ0.6～1cm］	140654.5[b]	140654.5[b]	3
140656.5	大；大量；広範囲；50mlを超える（10歳以下では25mlを超える）；厚さ1cmを超える	140656.5	140656.5	1
140655.5	両側［少なくとも一側は厚さ1cmを超える］[c]	140656.5	なし	1

HEAD (cranium and brain)

AIS 2005	Injury Description	⇒ AIS98	⇐ AIS98	FCI

> In cases of bilateral subdural hematoma where one side is tiny (i.e., < 0.6cm thick) and the other side is ≥0.6cm thick, code only the larger one.

---

[a] New descriptor in AIS 2005
[b] Change in severity code in AIS 2005
[c] In previous editions of AIS, with few exceptions, each injury was coded separately. AIS 2005 introduces "bilateral" for certain injury descriptions. Some bilateral injuries may affect severity levels and, therefore, the ISS for patients with those injuries.
[e] In AIS 98, this injury description had only one severity level. In AIS 2005, it has several.
[g] Subcortical hemorrhage was a separate descriptor (140644.4) in AIS 98.

AIS 2005	損傷内容	⇒ AIS98	⇐ AIS98	FCI

> 両側の硬膜下血腫で，一側は微小（すなわち，厚さ0.6cm未満）で対側は厚さ0.6cm以上のような場合，大きいほうのみをコード選択する。

---

[a] AIS2005に加えられた新しいコード。
[b] AIS2005で重症度に変更あり。
[c] 旧版のAISでは一部の例外を除き両側損傷はそれぞれ別にコード選択をしていた。AIS2005では，"両側"を導入した。いくつかの両側損傷は重症度が変化し，その結果ISSが変わることがある。
[e] AIS98ではこの損傷コードは1つだけであったが，AIS2005においては複数個ある。
[g] 皮質下出血はAIS98では別個のコード（140644.4）であった。

HEAD (cranium and brain)

AIS 2005	Injury Description	⇒ AIS98	⇐ AIS98	FCI
	Cerebrum (continued)			
140688.3	laceration NFS [not from penetrating injury][e]	140688.4[b]	140688.4[b]	5
140687.3	≤2cm length or depth	140688.4[b]	None	5
140686.4	>2cm length or depth	140688.4	None	2
140690.3	penetrating injury NFS[e]	140690.5[b]	140690.5[b]	1
140691.3	≤2cm deep	140690.5[b]	None	5
140692.5	>2cm deep	140690.5	None	1
140689.9	trauma-associated findings not related either to intervention or to anatomically-described head injury NFS[f]	None	None	

Use the following descriptors for brain swelling or brain edema directly related to head trauma, not anoxia or perilesional. Read "Brain Edema and Brain Swelling" (page 51) for coding guidance.

AIS 2005	Injury Description	⇒ AIS98	⇐ AIS98	FCI
140660.3	brain swelling NFS[h]	140660.3	140660.3	5
140662.3	mild ; compressed ventricles without compressed brain stem cisterns	140662.3	140662.3	5
140664.4	moderate ; compressed ventricles and brain stem cisterns	140664.4	140664.4	1
140666.5	severe ; absent ventricles or brain stem cisterns	140666.5	140666.5	1
140668.3	brain edema NFS[h]	140660.3	140660.3	5
140670.3	mild ; compressed ventricles without compressed brain stem cisterns	140662.3	140662.3	5
140672.4	moderate ; compressed ventricles and brain stem cisterns	140664.4	140664.4	2
140674.5	severe ; absent ventricles or brain stem cisterns	140666.5	140666.5	1
140701.9	hypoxic or ischemic brain damage secondary to systemic hypoxemia, hypotension or shock not directly related to head trauma[f]	None	None	
140702.9	not associated with coma >24 hours[f]	None	None	
140703.9	associated with coma >24 hours not secondary to primary brain injury ; bilateral ; multifocal[f]	None	None	

---

[b] Change in severity code in AIS 2005
[e] In AIS 98, this injury description had only one severity level. In AIS 2005, it has several.
[f] New descriptor in AIS 2005 that allows classification of trauma by body region, but does not allow assigning a severity code.
[h] Brain swelling and brain edema were combined as one descriptor in AIS 98. In AIS 2005, they are separate descriptors ; hence the duplication of AIS 98 matching codes.

AIS 2005	損傷内容	⇒ AIS98	⇐ AIS98	FCI
	大脳（続き）			
140688.3	裂傷・裂創　詳細不明［穿通性損傷ではないもの］[e]	140688.4[b]	140688.4[b]	5
140687.3	創が2cm以下の長さまたは深さのもの	140688.4[b]	なし	5
140686.4	創が2cmを超える長さまたは深さのもの	140688.4	なし	2
140690.3	穿通性損傷　詳細不明[e]	140690.5[b]	140690.5[b]	1
140691.3	2cm以下の深さのもの	140690.5[b]	なし	5
140692.5	2cmを超える深さのもの	140690.5	なし	1
140689.9	医療行為や解剖学的記載のある頭部損傷に関係のない外傷に関連した所見　詳細不明[f]	なし	なし	

> 次の脳腫脹と脳浮腫については，頭部外傷に直接関係のある場合に限り使用する．低酸素によるものや，損傷周囲の腫脹／浮腫に対しては使用しない．"脳浮腫と脳腫脹"の項目（51ページ）を参照．

AIS 2005	損傷内容	⇒ AIS98	⇐ AIS98	FCI
140660.3	脳腫脹　詳細不明[h]	140660.3	140660.3	5
140662.3	軽症；脳室の圧迫はあるが脳幹周囲槽の圧迫はない	140662.3	140662.3	5
140664.4	中等症；脳室と脳幹周囲槽の圧迫がある	140664.4	140664.4	1
140666.5	重症；脳室または脳幹周囲槽の消失がある	140666.5	140666.5	1
140668.3	脳浮腫　詳細不明[h]	140660.3	140660.3	5
140670.3	軽症；脳室の圧迫はあるが脳幹周囲槽の圧迫はない	140662.3	140662.3	5
140672.4	中等症；脳室と脳幹周囲槽の圧迫がある	140664.4	140664.4	2
140674.5	重症；脳室または脳幹周囲槽の消失がある	140666.5	140666.5	1
140701.9	頭部外傷には直接関係がなく，全身性の低酸素血症や低血圧症，ショックによる二次性の低酸素性あるいは虚血性の脳損傷[f]	なし	なし	
140702.9	24時間を超える昏睡と関連がないもの[f]	なし	なし	
140703.9	24時間を超える昏睡と関連があり，初期の脳損傷に続発するものではないもの；両側性；多発性[f]	なし	なし	

---

[b] AIS2005で重症度に変更あり．
[e] AIS98ではこの損傷コードは1つだけであったが，AIS2005においては複数個ある．
[f] AIS2005に加えられた新しいコード．外傷の存在部位を示すことができる．ただし重症度はない．
[h] 脳腫脹と脳浮腫はAIS98では1つのものとしていた．AIS2005では別々のものとする．したがってAIS98のコードでは重複する．

HEAD (cranium and brain)

AIS 2005	Injury Description	⇒ AIS98	⇐ AIS98	FCI
	Cerebrum (continued)			
140676.3	infarction [acute due to traumatic vascular occlusion]	140676.3	140676.3	1
140678.2	intraventricular hemorrhage[e]	140678.4[b]	140678.4[b]	5
140675.2	not associated with coma >6 hours	140678.4[b]	None	5
140677.4	associated with coma >6 hours	140678.4	None	1
	If DAI diagnosis is made, code as diffuse axonal injury, AIS codes 161007.4, 161008.4, 161011.5, 161012.5 or 161013.5 as appropriate based on substantiation of the injury. Do not code this finding. Read coding rules for coma (page 48) and "Diffuse Axonal Injury" (page 60) for coding guidance.			
140680.3	ischemic brain damage directly related to head trauma[e]	140680.3	140680.3	1
140681.3	not associated with coma >6 hours	140680.3	None	
140683.5	associated with coma >6 hours	140680.3[b]	None	
	If DAI diagnosis is made, code as diffuse axonal injury, AIS codes 161007.4, 161008.4, 161011.5, 161012.5 or 161013.5 as appropriate based on substantiation of the injury. Do not code this finding. Read coding rules for coma (page 48) and "Diffuse Axonal Injury" (page 60) for coding guidance.			
140682.3	pneumocephalus directly related to head trauma	140682.3	140682.3	1
140693.2	subarachnoid hemorrhage NFS[e]	140684.3[b]	140684.3[b]	5
140694.2	not associated with coma >6 hours	140684.3[b]	None	5
140695.3	associated with coma >6 hours	140684.3	None	1
	If DAI diagnosis is made, code as diffuse axonal injury, AIS codes 161007.4, 161008.4, 161011.5, 161012.5 or 161013.5 as appropriate based on substantiation of the injury. Do not code this finding. Read coding rules for coma (page 48) and "Diffuse Axonal Injury" (page 60) for coding guidance.			
140696.2	subpial hemorrhage NFS[e]	140686.3[b]	140686.3[b]	5
140697.2	not associated with coma >6 hours	140686.3[b]	None	5
140698.3	associated with coma >6 hours	140686.3	None	1
	If DAI diagnosis is made, code as diffuse axonal injury, AIS codes 161007.4, 161008.4, 161011.5, 161012.5 or 161013.5 as appropriate based on substantiation of the injury. Do not code this finding. Read coding rules for coma (page 48) and "Diffuse Axonal Injury" (page 60) for coding guidance.			

頭部（頭蓋と脳）

AIS 2005	損傷内容	⇒ AIS98	⇐ AIS98	FCI
	大脳（続き）			
140676.3	梗塞［外傷性血管閉塞による急性のもの］	140676.3	140676.3	1
140678.2	脳室内出血[e]	140678.4[b]	140678.4[b]	5
140675.2	6時間を超える昏睡と関連がないもの	140678.4[b]	なし	5
140677.4	6時間を超える昏睡と関連があるもの	140678.4	なし	1

> DAIの診断がなされているときは，上記をコード選択せず，損傷の実際に応じてびまん性軸索損傷として161007.4か161008.4, 161011.5, 161012.5もしくは161013.5をコード選択する。昏睡の項目（48ページ）と"DAI"の項目（60ページ）を参照。

140680.3	頭部外傷に直接起因する虚血性脳損傷[e]	140680.3	140680.3	1
140681.3	6時間を超える昏睡と関連がないもの	140680.3	なし	
140683.5	6時間を超える昏睡と関連があるもの	140680.3[b]	なし	

> DAIの診断がなされているときは，上記をコード選択せず，損傷の実際に応じてびまん性軸索損傷として161007.4か161008.4, 161011.5, 161012.5もしくは161013.5をコード選択する。昏睡の項目（48ページ）と"DAI"の項目（60ページ）を参照。

140682.3	頭部外傷に直接起因する気脳症	140682.3	140682.3	1
140693.2	くも膜下出血　詳細不明[e]	140684.3[b]	140684.3[b]	5
140694.2	6時間を超える昏睡と関連がないもの	140684.3[b]	なし	5
140695.3	6時間を超える昏睡と関連があるもの	140684.3	なし	1

> DAIの診断がなされているときは，上記をコード選択せず，損傷の実際に応じてびまん性軸索損傷として161007.4か161008.4, 161011.5, 161012.5もしくは161013.5をコード選択する。昏睡の項目（48ページ）と"DAI"の項目（60ページ）を参照。

140696.2	軟膜下出血　詳細不明[e]	140686.3[b]	140686.3[b]	5
140697.2	6時間を超える昏睡と関連がないもの	140686.3[b]	なし	5
140698.3	6時間を超える昏睡と関連があるもの	140686.3	なし	1

> DAIの診断がなされているときは，上記をコード選択せず，損傷の実際に応じてびまん性軸索損傷として161007.4か161008.4, 161011.5, 161012.5もしくは161013.5をコード選択する。昏睡の項目（48ページ）と"DAI"の項目（60ページ）を参照。

HEAD (cranium and brain)

AIS 2005	Injury Description	⇒ AIS98	⇐ AIS98	FCI
140799.3	**Pituitary** injury	140799.3	140799.3	5

---

[b] Change in severity code in AIS 2005
[e] In AIS 98, this injury description had only one severity level. In AIS 2005, it has several.
[f] New descriptor in AIS 2005 that allows classification of trauma by body region, but does not allow assigning a severity code.

AIS 2005	損傷内容	⇒ AIS98	⇐ AIS98	FCI
140799.3	下垂体損傷	140799.3	140799.3	5

[b] AIS2005で重症度に変更あり。
[e] AIS98ではこの損傷コードは1つだけであったが，AIS2005においては複数個ある。
[f] AIS20005に加えられた新しいコード。外傷の存在部位を示すことができる。ただし重症度はない。

HEAD (cranium and brain)

AIS 2005	Injury Description	⇒ AIS98	⇐ AIS98	FCI
	SKELETAL			
	Skull fractures are divided into base and vault. Code all skull fractures under vault unless specified as base. If a single skull fracture involves both base and vault, code the more severe. If both are of equal severity, code the fracture to point of origin. Code associated brain, vascular and nerve injuries separately.			
150000.2	**Skull** fracture NFS[a]	150400.2	None	5
	The skull base includes the following bones : orbital roof ; ethmoid ; sphenoid ; basilar process of occipital bone ; petrous, squamous and mastoid portions of temporal bone. The following clinical signs may be used to corroborate a diagnosis of a basilar skull fracture : hemotympanum ; perforated tympanic membrane with blood in canal ; mastoid hematoma ("*Battle's* sign") ; CSF otorrhea ; rhinorrhea ; periorbital ecchymosis ("racoon eyes").			
150200.3	**Base (basilar)** fracture NFS	150200.3	150200.3	5
150202.3	without CSF leak	150202.3	150202.3	5
150204.3	with CSF leak	150204.3	150204.3	5
150206.4	complex ; open with torn, exposed or loss of brain tissue ; comminuted ; ring ; hinge	150206.4	150206.4	5
	The skull vault includes the following bones : frontal, occipital, parietal and temporal.			
150400.2	**Vault** fracture NFS	150400.2	150400.2	5
150402.2	closed ; simple ; undisplaced ; diastatic ; linear	150402.2	150402.2	5
150404.3	comminuted ; compound but dura intact ; depressed ≤2cm ; displaced	150404.3	150404.3	5
150406.4	complex ; open with torn, exposed or loss of brain tissue	150406.4	150406.4	5
150408.4	massive ; large areas of skull depressed >2cm	150408.4	150408.4	5

---

[a] New descriptor in AIS 2005

頭部（頭蓋と脳）

AIS 2005	損傷内容	⇒ AIS98	⇐ AIS98	FCI

骨格

頭蓋骨骨折は，頭蓋底骨折と頭蓋冠骨折に分けられる。頭蓋底骨折と記載されていない限り，頭蓋冠骨折としてコードを選択する。単一の頭蓋骨骨折が頭蓋底と頭蓋冠の両方に及ぶときは，より重症であるほうをコード選択する。両者が同じ重症度であれば，骨折の始点であるほうを選択する。また，合併する脳損傷や血管損傷，神経損傷は別個にコード選択する。

150000.2	**頭蓋骨**骨折　詳細不明[a]	150400.2	なし	5

頭蓋底には，眼窩上壁，篩骨，蝶形骨，後頭骨の基底突起，錐体骨，側頭骨と乳様部を含む。鼓室内出血，外耳道への出血を伴う鼓膜穿孔，乳様突起の血腫（"Battle's sign"），髄液耳漏，髄液鼻漏，眼窩周囲の斑状出血（"raccoon eyes"）といった臨床症状は，頭蓋底骨折の診断を裏づけるのに用いてよい。

150200.3	**頭蓋底**骨折　詳細不明	150200.3	150200.3	5
150202.3	髄液漏を伴わない	150202.3	150202.3	5
150204.3	髄液漏を伴う	150204.3	150204.3	5
150206.4	複雑；硬膜の裂傷，脳組織の露出あるいは脱出を伴う開放骨折；粉砕骨折；環状骨折；蝶番骨折	150206.4	150206.4	5

頭蓋冠には，前頭骨，後頭骨，頭頂骨，側頭骨の鱗部を含む。

150400.2	**頭蓋冠**骨折　詳細不明	150400.2	150400.2	5
150402.2	閉鎖性；単純；偏位なし；縫合離開；線状	150402.2	150402.2	5
150404.3	粉砕；硬膜損傷は伴わないが骨折部が露出しているもの；2cm以下の陥没；偏位あり	150404.3	150404.3	5
150406.4	複雑；脳組織の裂傷，露出あるいは脱出を伴う開放骨折	150406.4	150406.4	5
150408.4	広範囲；大きな面積にわたって2cmを超える陥没	150408.4	150408.4	5

---

[a] AIS2005に加えられた新しいコード。

Diffuse Axonal Injury

Diffuse axonal injury (DAI) is a clinicopathological complex defined as immediate and prolonged coma due to widespread damage to axons and other neuronal processes in the brain. For practical purposes, "prolonged" represents more than six hours. Coma is defined as the absence of eye opening to painful stimuli AND no following of commands AND no word utterances. For intubated patients, coma can be diagnosed based on the absence of eye opening to painful stimuli AND no following of commands. For intubated patients where local injury or hemorrhage prevents eye opening, coma can be diagnosed solely on the basis of no following of commands. If chemical paralysis or sedation preclude evaluation of these three responses, the diagnosis of coma cannot be made.

Other entities can be confused with DAI, but are not incorporated by the name DAI, including:
- imaging findings often found with DAI (see below) that are not associated with the clinical criteria of DAI or have unknown clinical findings,
- traumatic axonal damage associated with ischemia, hemorrhage or contusion irrespective of the clinical findings,
- any condition with coma less than six hours in duration.

Acceptable means of diagnosing DAI include:
- a neuropathological examination of the brain that demonstrates widespread damage to axons in the white matter of the cerebral hemispheres or cerebellum that is not associated with contusion, infarct, ischemia or mass lesions (intracerebral hematoma/hemorrhage),
- a clinical diagnosis of DAI made by a combination of clinical observations and a brain imaging study with CT or MRI. DAI can be diagnosed by a physician when a patient sustains coma from the time of the traumatic event AND remains in post-traumatic coma for more than six hours AND there is no ischemic damage (prolonged hypotension or infarction on imaging) or mass lesion (epidural, subdural or intracerebral hematoma) to explain the coma on imaging studies. Similar coma lasting less than six hours is called concussion (of various levels of severity).

DAI cannot be diagnosed on the basis of clinical observations only. There must be imaging validation. The presence of small contusions or small intracerebral hemorrhages does not preclude the diagnosis of DAI, if, in the judgment of the physician, these are insufficient in size or in location to be responsible for the observed coma. Similarly, imaging studies alone are insufficient to make the diagnosis of DAI unless clinical observations confirm that coma longer than six hours is present and there are no mass lesions to explain the coma.

Several imaging findings are commonly associated with DAI, but in themselves cannot make the diagnosis of DAI in the absence of clinical findings of immediate and prolonged coma. These include:
- small or petechial hemorrhages in the cerebral white matter, basal ganglia, thalamus, corpus callosum, fornix, septum pellucidum, periventricular regions or dorsal brainstem. These may be called "tissue tear hemorrhages", "shear lesions", "Strich lesions" or simply petechial hemorrhages.
- Small hemorrhages in the parasaggital frontal or parietal lobes. These may be called "gliding contusions".
- Intraventricular hemorrhage.
- Evidence of small (petechial-sized) areas of non-hemorrhagic damage on sophisticated imaging studies such as magnetic transfer imaging or diffusion tensor imaging or other MRI methods that may be developed that show regions of axonal damage.

For patients who die within 24 hours, the diagnosis of DAI can be made only if:
- Coma has been present since the traumatic event AND,
- Imaging shows one or more small hemorrhages (sometimes called "tissue tear hemorrhages", "shearing lesions" or petechiae) in the central (deepest) third of the brain (i.e., not cortical or subcortical).

びまん性軸索損傷

びまん性軸索損傷（DAI）は，脳における軸索と他の神経突起の広範囲損傷による受傷直後から遷延する昏睡の臨床病理学的な総称である。実際には，"長時間に及ぶ"は6時間以上を意味する。昏睡は，痛み刺激に対して開眼しない，かつ命令に従わない，かつ発語がない状態と定義される。挿管されている患者に関しては，痛み刺激に対して開眼しない，かつ命令に従わない状態をもって昏睡と診断してよい。局所損傷や出血で開眼の評価ができない挿管患者に関しては，命令に対して従わない状態だけをもって昏睡と診断してよい。麻薬や鎮静により，これら3つの反応に対する評価に値しないときは，昏睡の診断はできない。

次にあげるようなものは，DAI と紛らわしいことがあるが，DAI と名づけてはならない。
- 臨床的に DAI に合致しないものや臨床所見が不明な場合，画像所見から DAI（以下参照）と診断してはならない。
- 臨床所見によらず虚血や出血，挫傷による外傷性の軸索への損傷。
- 6時間に満たないすべての昏睡。

次にあげるようなものは，DAI を診断する根拠としてよい。
- 神経病理学的検査では，挫傷や梗塞，虚血，占拠性病変（脳実質内の血腫や出血）に関係のない大脳半球または小脳の白質における軸索の広範囲損傷である。
- DAI の臨床診断は，臨床経過と CT や MRI による画像所見の両者から診断される。DAI は，昏睡が受傷時から持続し，かつ6時間以上の昏睡継続，かつ虚血による損傷（遷延した低血圧や画像で捉えられるような梗塞）や画像上昏睡を説明しうるような占拠性病変（硬膜外血腫や硬膜下血腫，脳内血腫）がないという条件を満たせば，医師によって診断してよい。

DAI は臨床所見のみでは診断できない。画像による検証が必須である。小さな挫傷や小さな脳内出血を認めたとしても，それらの大きさや場所が実際の昏睡の原因として不十分と医師が判断する場合は，DAI の診断を妨げるものではない〈訳者注：DAI が併存している可能性がある〉。同様に，臨床所見で昏睡が6時間以上継続していることと，昏睡を説明しうるような占拠性病変がないことを確認しない限り，画像検査のみでは DAI の診断をするには不十分である。

一般的には DAI を連想させる次のような画像所見があるが，受傷直後から遷延する昏睡なしに，これらの画像所見のみでは DAI の診断はできない。
- 大脳白質や基底核，視床，脳梁，脳弓，透明中隔，脳室周囲部，脳幹背側の小さな出血または点状出血。これらは，"組織裂傷による出血"や"剪断損傷"，"Strich（シュトリヒ）病変"単純な点状出血とよばれることがある。
- 前頭葉または頭頂葉の矢状縫合近傍の小さな出血。これらは"滑走挫傷"とよばれることがある。
- 脳室内出血。
- 磁気転写画像や拡散テンソル画像，軸索損傷の部位が明らかになるよう開発された他の MRI の撮像方法のような高度な画像検査で捉えられる小さな（点状の大きさ）範囲の非出血性損傷であることの証明。

24時間以内に死亡した場合の DAI の診断は，次の条件に合致する場合にのみ可能である。
- 受傷時から続く昏睡であること。
- かつ，1つ以上の小さな出血（"組織裂傷による出血"や"剪断損傷"，点状出血とよばれることがある）が，脳の中央部（最深部）（すなわち，皮質や皮質下ではない部位）に画像で確認できること。

HEAD (cranium and brain)

AIS 2005	Injury Description	⇒ AIS98	⇐ AIS98	FCI
	CONCUSSIVE INJURY[i]			
161000.1	**Cerebral Concussion**, NFS	161000.2[b]	161000.2[b]	5
161001.1	mild concussion ; no loss of consciousness	161000.2[b]	161000.2[b]	5

> Use 161000.1 and 161001.1 where there is convincing evidence of head injury **and** where the medical diagnosis is given as "concussion" with no other description or clarification.

> Code loss of consciousness (LOC) only where there is convincing evidence of head trauma **and** the diagnosis of loss of consciousness is made by a physician or recorded by a physician based on EMS corroboration. The Glasgow Coma Score (GCS) is only one indicator of brain injury and should never be used as the sole indicator. Self-reported LOC or reports of bystanders are insufficient for coding and should be disregarded.

161002.2	brief loss of consciousness NFS	160406.2	None	5
161003.2	loss of consciousness < 1 hour NFS	160202.2	160202.2	5
161004.2	loss of consciousness ≤30 mins	160202.2	160202.2	5
161005.2	loss of consciousness 31-59 mins	160202.2	160202.2	5
161006.3	loss of consciousness 1-6 hours (severe concussion)	160206.3	160206.3	5

> Use this category to code a substantiated diagnosis of DAI if no anatomical description is recorded or if coma exceeds 24 hours and meets the coding rules for DAI. Read "Diffuse Axonal Injury" (page 60) for coding guidance.

161007.4	**Diffuse Axonal Injury** (prolonged traumatic coma LOC >6 hours not due to mass lesion) NFS	160210.4	None	5
161008.4	LOC 6-24 hours (mild DAI)	160814.4	160814.4	5
161011.5	LOC >24 hours NFS	160818.5	160818.5	5
161012.5	without brainstem signs (moderate DAI)	160818.5	160818.5	1
161013.5	with brainstem signs (severe DAI)	160824.5	160824.5	1

> Brainstem signs : decerebrate ; decorticate

---

[b] Change in severity code in AIS 2005
[i] This section "Concussive Injury" reflects contemporary neurotrauma terminology in describing these types of brain injury. It replaces the sections "Length of Unconsciousness" and "Level of Consciousness" in AIS 98. Because this revision uses a significantly different framework for describing concussive injuries and diffuse axonal injury, the matching codes between AIS 2005 and AIS 98 are "best" choices.

頭部（頭蓋と脳）

AIS 2005	損傷内容	⇒ AIS98	⇐ AIS98	FCI
	震盪損傷[i]			
161000.1	**脳震盪** 詳細不明	161000.2[b]	161000.2[b]	5
161001.1	軽症脳震盪；意識消失なし	161000.2[b]	161000.2[b]	5

> 161000.1と161001.1については，頭部外傷であることの説得力のある証拠があり，かつ医学的診断が単純に"脳震盪"だけで他に記載や説明がない場合に選択する。

> 意識消失（LOC）は，頭部外傷であることの説得力のある証拠があり，かつ意識消失の診断が医師または救急隊員による証言に基づく医療従事者による記録である場合に限りコードを選択する。Glasgow Coma Score（GCS）は，脳損傷の1つの指標にすぎず，唯一の指標として使用してはならない。自己申告による意識消失や目撃者の意見はコード選択するには不十分であり無視すべきである。

AIS 2005	損傷内容	⇒ AIS98	⇐ AIS98	FCI
161002.2	短時間の意識消失　詳細不明	160406.2	なし	5
161003.2	1時間未満の意識消失　詳細不明	160202.2	160202.2	5
161004.2	30分以下の意識消失	160202.2	160202.2	5
161005.2	31〜59分の意識消失	160202.2	160202.2	5
161006.3	1〜6時間の意識消失（重症脳震盪）	160206.3	160206.3	5

> DAIと確定診断されたもののうち，解剖学的記載がなかったり，昏睡が24時間を超えDAIのコード選択のルールに合致する場合は，以下DAIと確定診断されたもののうち，解剖学的記載がなかったり，昏睡が24時間を超えDAIのコード選択のルールに合致する場合は，以下のなかからコードを選択する。"DAI"の項目（60ページ）を参照。

AIS 2005	損傷内容	⇒ AIS98	⇐ AIS98	FCI
161007.4	**びまん性軸索損傷**（6時間を超える意識消失が外傷性の昏睡であり占拠性病変によるものではない）　詳細不明	160210.4	なし	5
161008.4	6〜24時間の意識消失（軽症びまん性軸索損傷）	160814.4	160814.4	5
161011.5	24時間を超える意識消失　詳細不明	160818.5	160818.5	5
161012.5	脳幹症状を伴わない（中等症びまん性軸索損傷）	160818.5	160818.5	1
161013.5	脳幹症状を伴う（重症びまん性軸索損傷）	160824.5	160824.5	1

> 脳幹症状：除脳状態；除皮質状態

---

[b] AIS2005で重症度に変更あり。
[i] "震盪損傷"の項目は，脳損傷について記述した最新の神経外傷の用語を反映している。AIS98では"意識消失の時間"と"意識レベル"の項目に相当する。今回の改訂で震盪損傷とびまん性軸索損傷という表現で大幅に異なる構成としたので，AIS2005とAIS98が一致するコードが最適な選択である。

顔　面
（目と耳を含む）

FACE (includes Eye and Ear)

AIS 2005	Injury Description	⇒ AIS98	⇐ AIS98	FCI
	WHOLE AREA			
	Use one of the following two descriptors when such vague information is the only information available. While these descriptors identify the occurrence of a facial injury, they do not specify its severity.			
200099.9	**Injuries to the Face** NFS	215099.9	215099.9	
200999.9	Died of facial injury without further substantiation of injuries or no autopsy confirmation of specific injuries	215999.9	215999.9	
	Use this category if penetrating injury does not involve internal structures. Assign to External body region for calculating an ISS. If underlying anatomical structures are involved, code documented diagnoses only ; do not use these generic descriptors.			
216000.1	**Penetrating injury** NFS	216000.1	216000.1	5
216002.1	minor ; superficial	216002.1	216002.1	5
216004.2	with tissue loss >25cm^2	216004.2	216004.2	5
216006.3	with blood loss >20% by volume	216006.3	216006.3	5
216008.4	massive destruction of whole face including both eyes[a]	None	None	1
	Assign AIS code 216008.4 to Face body region for calculating an ISS.			

---

[a] New descriptor in AIS 2005

顔面（目と耳を含む）

AIS 2005	損傷内容	⇒ AIS98	⇐ AIS98	FCI

全域

> 不確定な情報しか得られない場合には，以下の2つのコードのうちいずれかを選択する。しかし，これらのコードは，顔面損傷の存在を示すものであり，その重症度を明示したものではない。

200099.9	**顔面損傷**　詳細不明	215099.9	215099.9	
200999.9	他の明らかな損傷がないか，遺体解剖で特別な損傷がない顔面外傷の死亡例	215999.9	215999.9	

> もし穿通性損傷が内部構造を含まないなら，このカテゴリーを選択する。ISS計算においては，体表の部位を選択する。もし，解剖学的な構造物が損傷しているなら，診断されたもののみコードを選択し，以下のコードは選択しない。

216000.1	**穿通性損傷**　詳細不明	216000.1	216000.1	5
216002.1	小；表在性	216002.1	216002.1	5
216004.2	組織欠損が25cm^{2}を超える	216004.2	216004.2	5
216006.3	出血量が全血液量の20%を超える	216006.3	216006.3	5
216008.4	両眼を含んだ顔面全体の広範な高度損傷[a]	なし	なし	1

> 216008.4のAISコードは，ISS計算においては，顔面の部位を選択する。

---

[a] AIS 2005に加えられた新しいコード。

FACE (includes Eye and Ear)

AIS 2005	Injury Description	⇒ AIS98	⇐ AIS98	FCI
	Use the following section for blunt soft tissue injury to the face. Assign to External body region for calculating an ISS.			
210099.1	**Skin/subcutaneous/muscle** NFS	210099.1	210099.1	5
210202.1	abrasion	210202.1	210202.1	5
210402.1	contusion ; hematoma	210402.1	210402.1	5
210600.1	laceration NFS	210600.1	210600.1	5
210602.1	minor ; superficial	210602.1	210602.1	5
210604.2	major ; >10cm long <u>and</u> into subcutaneous tissue	210604.2	210604.2	5
210606.3	blood loss >20% by volume	210606.3	210606.3	5
210800.1	avulsion NFS	210800.1	210800.1	5
210802.1	minor ; superficial ; ≤25cm^2	210802.1	210802.1	5
210804.2	major ; >25cm^2	210804.2	210804.2	5
210806.3	blood loss >20% by volume	210806.3	210806.3	5

VESSELS

AIS 2005	Injury Description	⇒ AIS98	⇐ AIS98	FCI
220099.9	**Vascular Injury in Face** NFS[f]	None	None	
220200.1	External carotid artery branch (es) laceration NFS [includes facial, temporal, and internal maxillary]	220200.1	220200.1	5
220202.1	minor ; superficial	220202.1	220202.1	5
220204.3	major ; transection ; blood loss >20% by volume	220204.3	220204.3	5

---

[f] New descriptor in AIS 2005 that allows classification of trauma by body region, but does not allow assigning a severity code.

顔面（目と耳を含む）

AIS 2005	損傷内容	⇒ AIS98	⇐ AIS98	FCI
	顔面の鈍的軟部組織損傷は以下を選択する。ISS計算においては，体表の部位を選択する。			
210099.1	**皮膚／皮下組織／筋肉**　詳細不明	210099.1	210099.1	5
210202.1	擦過傷	210202.1	210202.1	5
210402.1	挫傷；血腫	210402.1	210402.1	5
210600.1	裂傷・裂創　詳細不明	210600.1	210600.1	5
210602.1	小；表在性	210602.1	210602.1	5
210604.2	大；長さが10cmを超え，かつ皮下組織に達する	210604.2	210604.2	5
210606.3	出血量が全血液量の20%を超える	210606.3	210606.3	5
210800.1	剥離　詳細不明	210800.1	210800.1	5
210802.1	小；表在性；25cm^{2}以下	210802.1	210802.1	5
210804.2	大；25cm^{2}を超える	210804.2	210804.2	5
210806.3	出血量が全血液量の20%を超える	210806.3	210806.3	5

血管

220099.9	**顔面の血管損傷**　詳細不明[f]	なし	なし	
220200.1	**外頸動脈の分枝の裂傷・裂創**　詳細不明 ［顔面動脈，側頭動脈，顎動脈を含む］	220200.1	220200.1	5
220202.1	小；表在性	220202.1	220202.1	5
220204.3	大；断裂；出血量が全血液量の20%を超える	220204.3	220204.3	5

---

[f] AIS2005に加えられた新しいコード。外傷の存在部位を示すことができる。ただし重症度はない。

FACE (includes Eye and Ear)

AIS 2005	Injury Description	⇒ AIS98	⇐ AIS98	FCI
	NERVES			
230299.1	**Optic Nerve** NFS	230299.1	230299.1	3
	Use this category for intraorbital portion only. For intracranial portion or if location is unknown, code under Cranial Nerves in Head.			
230202.2	contusion	230202.2	230202.2	3
230203.2	bilateral[c]	230202.2	None	2
230204.2	laceration	230204.2	230204.2	2
230205.3	bilateral[c]	230204.2[b]	None	2
230206.2	avulsion	230206.2	230206.2	2
230207.3	bilateral[c]	230206.2[b]	None	2
	INTERNAL ORGANS			
240299.1	**Ear** NFS	240299.1	240299.1	3
	Code ear amputation as skin avulsion according to its level of severity.			
240204.1	**Ear Canal** injury	240204.1	240204.1	5
240208.1	**Inner** or **Middle Ear** injury NFS	240208.1	240208.1	2
240207.2	bilateral[c]	240208.1[b]	None	2
240206.1	injury involving dizziness[a]	240208.1	None	4
240205.1	injury involving tinnitus[a]	240208.1	None	3
240212.1	**Ossicular chain (ear bone)** dislocation	240212.1	240212.1	2
240213.2	bilateral[c]	240212.1[b]	None	2
240216.1	**Tympanic membrane (eardrum)** rupture	240216.1	240216.1	3
240220.1	**Vestibular apparatus** injury	240220.1	240220.1	4

---

[a] New descriptor in AIS 2005
[b] Change in severity code in AIS 2005
[c] In previous editions of AIS, with few exceptions, each injury was coded separately. AIS 2005 introduces "bilateral". Some bilateral injuries may affect severity levels, and, therefore, the ISS for patients with these injuries.

顔面（目と耳を含む）

AIS 2005	損傷内容	⇒ AIS98	⇐ AIS98	FCI
	神 経			
230299.1	**視神経** 詳細不明	230299.1	230299.1	3
	眼窩内の損傷に限りこのカテゴリーを選択する。頭蓋内もしくは，損傷の局在が不明の場合は頭部の脳神経のコードを選択する。			
230202.2	挫傷	230202.2	230202.2	3
230203.2	両側[c]	230202.2	なし	2
230204.2	裂傷・裂創	230204.2	230204.2	2
230205.3	両側[c]	230204.2[b]	なし	2
230206.2	断裂	230206.2	230206.2	2
230207.3	両側[c]	230206.2[b]	なし	2
	内 臓			
240299.1	**耳** 詳細不明	240299.1	240299.1	3
	損傷の程度によって，皮膚の剥離として耳介の断裂をコード選択する。			
240204.1	**外耳道**損傷	240204.1	240204.1	5
240208.1	**内耳，中耳損傷** 詳細不明	240208.1	240208.1	2
240207.2	両側[c]	240208.1[b]	なし	2
240206.1	めまいを伴う損傷[a]	240208.1	なし	4
240205.1	耳鳴りを伴う損傷[a]	240208.1	なし	3
240212.1	**耳小骨**脱臼	240212.1	240212.1	2
240213.2	両側[c]	240212.1[b]	なし	2
240216.1	**鼓膜**破裂	240216.1	240216.1	3
240220.1	**前庭器官**損傷	240220.1	240220.1	4

[a] AIS2005に加えられた新しいコード。
[b] AIS2005で重症度に変更あり。
[c] 旧版のAISでは一部の例外を除き両側損傷はそれぞれ別にコード選択をしていた。AIS2005では，"両側"を導入した。いくつかの両側損傷は重症度が変化し，その結果，ISSが変わることがある。

FACE (includes Eye and Ear)

AIS 2005	Injury Description	⇒ AIS98	⇐ AIS98	FCI
240499.1	**Eye** NFS	240499.1	240499.1	3
240402.2	**Eye** avulsion ; enucleation	240402.2	240402.2	2
240403.3	bilateral[c]	240402.2[b]	None	2
240408.1	**Canaliculus (lacrimal/tear duct)** laceration	240408.1	240408.1	5
240599.1	**Choroid** NFS	240412.1	None	5
240502.1	rupture[e]	240412.1	240412.1	5
240504.1	peripheral – not involving macula	240412.1	None	5
240506.1	central – involving macula	240412.1	None	3
240508.1	detachment[a]	240412.1	None	5
240510.1	hemorrhage[a]	240412.1	None	5
240416.1	**Conjunctiva** injury	240416.1	240416.1	5
240699.1	**Cornea** NFS	240699.1	240699.1	3
240602.1	abrasion	240602.1	240602.1	5
240603.1	burn, thermal or chemical[a]	240699.1	None	5
240604.1	contusion[e]	240604.1	240604.1	5
240610.1	hyphema NFS[e]	240604.1	240604.1	5
240611.1	minor ; ≤50% of anterior chamber	240604.1	None	5
240612.1	major ; >50% of anterior chamber	240604.1	None	5
240620.1	laceration NFS[e]	240606.1	240606.1	3
240621.1	not involving central 3mm of cornea	240606.1	None	3
240622.1	without prolapse	240606.1	None	3
240623.1	with prolapse	240606.1	None	3
240624.1	involving central 3mm of cornea	240606.1	None	3
240625.1	without prolapse	240606.1	None	3
240626.1	with prolapse	240606.1	None	3
240799.1	Injury with retained **Intraocular Foreign Body**[a]	240499.1	None	3
240789.1	anterior chamber[a]	240499.1	None	3
240779.1	posterior chamber[a]	240499.1	None	3

[a] New descriptor in AIS 2005
[b] Change in severity code in AIS 2005
[c] In previous editions of AIS, with few exceptions, each injury was coded separately. AIS 2005 introduces "bilateral". Some bilateral injuries may affect severity levels and, therefore, the ISS for patients with those injuries.
[e] In AIS 98, this injury description had only one severity level. In AIS 2005, it has several.

顔面（目と耳を含む）

AIS 2005	損傷内容	⇒ AIS98	⇐ AIS98	FCI
240499.1	**目** 詳細不明	240499.1	240499.1	3
240402.2	**眼球**脱出；摘出	240402.2	240402.2	2
240403.3	両側[c]	240402.2[b]	なし	2
240408.1	**涙管**裂傷・裂創	240408.1	240408.1	5
240599.1	**脈絡膜**　詳細不明	240412.1	なし	5
240502.1	破裂[e]	240412.1	240412.1	5
240504.1	末梢 − 黄斑を含まない	240412.1	なし	5
240506.1	中心 − 黄斑を含む	240412.1	なし	3
240508.1	剥離[a]	240412.1	なし	5
240510.1	出血[a]	240412.1	なし	5
240416.1	**結膜**損傷	240416.1	240416.1	5
240699.1	**角膜**損傷　詳細不明	240699.1	240699.1	3
240602.1	擦過傷	240602.1	240602.1	5
240603.1	熱傷または化学熱傷[a]	240699.1	なし	5
240604.1	挫傷[e]	240604.1	240604.1	5
240610.1	前房出血　詳細不明[e]	240604.1	240604.1	5
240611.1	小；前眼房の50%以下	240604.1	なし	5
240612.1	大；前眼房の50%を超える	240604.1	なし	5
240620.1	裂傷・裂創　詳細不明[e]	240606.1	240606.1	3
240621.1	角膜の中心3mmを含まない	240606.1	なし	3
240622.1	脱出なし	240606.1	なし	3
240623.1	脱出あり	240606.1	なし	3
240624.1	角膜の中心3mmを含む	240606.1	なし	3
240625.1	脱出なし	240606.1	なし	3
240626.1	脱出あり	240606.1	なし	3
240799.1	**眼球内異物**遺残を伴う損傷[a]	240499.1	なし	3
240789.1	前眼房[a]	240499.1	なし	3
240779.1	後眼房[a]	240499.1	なし	3

[a] AIS2005に加えられた新しいコード。
[b] AIS2005で重症度に変更あり。
[c] 旧版のAISでは一部の例外を除き両側損傷はそれぞれ別にコード選択をしていた。AIS2005では，"両側"を導入した。いくつかの両側損傷は重症度が変化し，その結果，ISSが変わることがある。
[e] AIS98では，この損傷コードは1つだけであったが，AIS2005においては複数個ある。

FACE (includes Eye and Ear)

AIS 2005	Injury Description	⇒ AIS98	⇐ AIS98	FCI
	Eye (continued)			
240800.1	**Lens** NFS[a]	240499.1	None	5
240802.1	capsular rupture NFS[a]	240499.1	None	5
240804.1	anterior capsule[a]	240499.1	None	5
240806.1	posterior capsule[a]	240499.1	None	5
240808.1	both anterior and posterior capsules[a]	240499.1	None	5
240812.1	dislocation ; subluxation[a]	240499.1	None	5
240814.1	anterior segment[a]	240499.1	None	5
240816.1	posterior segment[a]	240499.1	None	5
240999.1	**Macula** NFS[a]	240499.1	None	5
240902.1	contusion ; edema[a]	240499.1	None	5
240904.2	hole[a]	240499.1	None	3
241099.1	**Retina** NFS[a]	241000.1	None	5
241000.1	laceration ; tear NFS[e]	241000.1	241000.1	3
241002.1	minor ; ≤90°	241000.1	None	5
241004.1	major ; >90°	241000.1	None	3
241006.2	detachment NFS[e]	241002.2	241002.2	5
241008.2	with macula attached	241002.2	None	5
241010.2	with macula detached	241002.2	None	3
241299.1	**Sclera [includes globe]** NFS	241200.1	None	5
241200.2	laceration ; rupture[e]	241202.2	241202.2	5
241201.2	anterior to ora serrata	241202.2	None	5
241202.2	without prolapse	241202.2	None	5
241203.2	with prolapse	241202.2	None	5
241204.2	posterior to ora serrata but anterior to equator	241202.2	None	5
241205.2	without prolapse	241202.2	None	5
241206.2	with prolapse	241202.2	None	5
241207.2	posterior to equator	241202.2	None	5
241208.2	without prolapse	241202.2	None	5
241209.2	with prolapse NFS	241202.2	None	3

---

[a] New descriptor in AIS 2005
[e] In AIS 98, this injury description had only one severity level. In AIS 2005, it has several.

AIS 2005	損傷内容	⇒ AIS98	⇐ AIS98	FCI
	目（続き）			
240800.1	**水晶体** 詳細不明[a]	240499.1	なし	5
240802.1	水晶体包破裂 詳細不明[a]	240499.1	なし	5
240804.1	前包[a]	240499.1	なし	5
240806.1	後包[a]	240499.1	なし	5
240808.1	前包と後包の両方[a]	240499.1	なし	5
240812.1	脱臼；不全脱臼[a]	240499.1	なし	5
240814.1	前方[a]	240499.1	なし	5
240816.1	後方[a]	240499.1	なし	5
240999.1	**黄斑** 詳細不明[a]	240499.1	なし	5
240902.1	挫傷；浮腫[a]	240499.1	なし	5
240904.2	穿孔[a]	240499.1	なし	3
241099.1	**網膜** 詳細不明[a]	241000.1	なし	5
241000.1	裂傷・裂創；詳細不明[e]	241000.1	241000.1	3
241002.1	小；90°以下	241000.1	なし	5
241004.1	大；90°を超える	241000.1	なし	3
241006.2	剝離 詳細不明[e]	241002.2	241002.2	5
241008.2	黄斑付着を伴う	241002.2	なし	5
241010.2	黄斑剝離を伴う	241002.2	なし	3
241299.1	**強膜**［眼球に達する］ 詳細不明	241200.1	なし	5
241200.2	裂傷・裂創；破裂[e]	241202.2	241202.2	5
241201.2	鋸状縁の前方	241202.2	なし	5
241202.2	脱出なし	241202.2	なし	5
241203.2	脱出あり	241202.2	なし	5
241204.2	鋸状縁の後方で赤道の前方	241202.2	なし	5
241205.2	脱出なし	241202.2	なし	5
241206.2	脱出あり	241202.2	なし	5
241207.2	赤道の後方	241202.2	なし	5
241208.2	脱出なし	241202.2	なし	5
241209.2	脱出あり 詳細不明	241202.2	なし	3

---

[a] AIS2005に加えられた新しいコード。
[e] AIS98では，この損傷コードは1つだけであったが，AIS2005においては複数個ある。

FACE (includes Eye and Ear)

AIS 2005	Injury Description	⇒ AIS98	⇐ AIS98	FCI
	Eye (continued)			
241499.1	Uvea injury	241499.1	241499.1	3
241699.1	Vitreous NFS[e]	241699.1	241699.1	3
241601.1	hemorrhage	241699.1	None	5
241602.1	retina visible	241699.1	None	5
241603.1	retina not visible	241699.1	None	5
241604.1	detachment	241699.1	None	5
243099.1	Mouth injury	243099.1	243099.1	5
243199.1	Palate NFS[a]	243099.1	None	5
243101.1	laceration[a]	243099.1	None	5
243102.2	fracture[a]	243099.1	None	5
243299.1	Gingiva (gum) NFS	243299.1	243299.1	5
243202.1	contusion	243202.1	243202.1	5
243204.1	laceration	243204.1	243204.1	5
243206.1	avulsion	243206.1	243206.1	5
243400.1	Tongue laceration NFS	243400.1	243400.1	5
243402.1	minor ; superficial	243402.1	243402.1	5
243404.2	deep ; extensive	243404.2	243404.2	3

JOINTS

AIS 2005	Injury Description	⇒ AIS98	⇐ AIS98	FCI
251699.1	Temporomandibular joint NFS	251699.1	251699.1	5
251604.2	dislocation	251604.2	251604.2	5

---

[a] New descriptor in AIS 2005
[e] In AIS 98, this injury description had only one severity level. In AIS 2005, it has several.

AIS 2005	損傷内容	⇒ AIS98	⇐ AIS98	FCI
	目（続き）			
241499.1	**ぶどう膜**損傷	241499.1	241499.1	3
241699.1	**硝子体**　詳細不明[e]	241699.1	241699.1	3
241601.1	出血	241699.1	なし	5
241602.1	網膜が見える	241699.1	なし	5
241603.1	網膜が見えない	241699.1	なし	5
241604.1	剥離	241699.1	なし	5
243099.1	**口**損傷	243099.1	243099.1	5
243199.1	**口蓋**　詳細不明[a]	243099.1	なし	5
243101.1	裂傷・裂創[a]	243099.1	なし	5
243102.2	骨折[a]	243099.1	なし	5
243299.1	**歯肉（歯茎）**　詳細不明	243299.1	243299.1	5
243202.1	挫傷	243202.1	243202.1	5
243204.1	裂傷・裂創	243204.1	243204.1	5
243206.1	剥離	243206.1	243206.1	5
243400.1	**舌裂傷・裂創**　詳細不明	243400.1	243400.1	5
243402.1	小；表在性	243402.1	243402.1	5
243404.2	深在性；広範囲	243404.2	243404.2	3
	関　節			
251699.1	**顎関節**　詳細不明	251699.1	251699.1	5
251604.2	脱臼	251604.2	251604.2	5

[a] AIS2005に加えられた新しいコード。
[e] AIS98では，この損傷コードは1つだけであったが，AIS2005においては複数個ある。

FACE (includes Eye and Ear)

AIS 2005	Injury Description	⇒ AIS98	⇐ AIS98	FCI
	SKELETAL			
250200.2	**Alveolar ridge** fracture with or without injury to teeth	250200.2	250200.2	5
	Do not code teeth separately when these occur simultaneously.			
250400.1	**Facial bone (s)** fracture NFS	250400.1	250400.1	5
250600.1	**Mandible** fracture NFS Code bilateral as single injury.	250600.1	250600.1	5
250602.1	closed but NFS as to site	250602.1	250602.1	5
250603.1	condyle[a]	250602.1	None	5
250604.1	coronoid[a]	250602.1	None	5
250605.1	angle[a]	250602.1	None	5
250606.1	symphysis/parasymphysis[a]	250602.1	None	5
250607.1	body	250604.1	250604.1	5
250608.1	ramus	250606.1	250606.1	5
250610.2	open/displaced/comminuted but NFS as to site	250610.2	250610.2	5
	Any or combination. Displacement must be significant.			
250611.2	condyle[a]	250610.2	None	5
250612.2	coronoid[a]	250610.2	None	5
250613.2	angle[a]	250610.2	None	5
250614.2	symphysis/parasymphysis[a]	250610.2	None	5
250615.2	body	250612.2	250612.2	5
250616.2	ramus	250614.2	250614.2	5

---

[a] New descriptor in AIS 2005

顔面（目と耳を含む）

AIS 2005	損傷内容	⇒ AIS98	⇐ AIS98	FCI
	骨　格			
250200.2	**歯槽骨**骨折，歯牙損傷の有無を問わない	250200.2	250200.2	5
	同時に生じた場合は，歯牙損傷のコードは選択しない。			
250400.1	**顔面骨**骨折　詳細不明	250400.1	250400.1	5
250600.1	**下顎骨**骨折　詳細不明	250600.1	250600.1	5
	両側性でも単一損傷としてコードを選択する。			
250602.1	非開放で部位が不明	250602.1	250602.1	5
250603.1	関節突起[a]	250602.1	なし	5
250604.1	筋突起[a]	250602.1	なし	5
250605.1	下顎角[a]	250602.1	なし	5
250606.1	オトガイ結合／その近傍[a]	250602.1	なし	5
250607.1	下顎体	250604.1	250604.1	5
250608.1	下顎枝	250606.1	250606.1	5
250610.2	開放／転位／粉砕で部位が不明	250610.2	250610.2	5
	いずれか1つ以上。転位が重要である。			
250611.2	関節突起[a]	250610.2	なし	5
250612.2	筋突起[a]	250610.2	なし	5
250613.2	下顎角[a]	250610.2	なし	5
250614.2	オトガイ結合／その近傍[a]	250610.2	なし	5
250615.2	下顎体	250612.2	250612.2	5
250616.2	下顎枝	250614.2	250614.2	5

[a] AIS2005に加えられた新しいコード。

FACE (includes Eye and Ear)

LeFort I	LeFort II	LeFort III
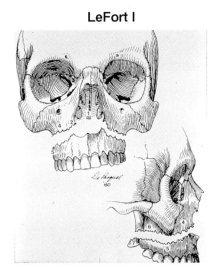	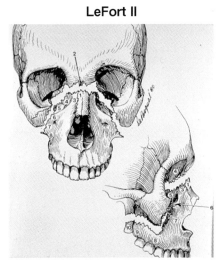	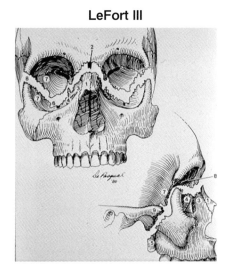

Copyright protected material used with permission of the author and the University of Iowa's Virtual Hospital, www.vh.org

顔面（目と耳を含む）

LeFort I

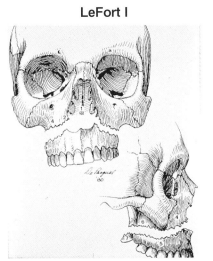

LeFort II

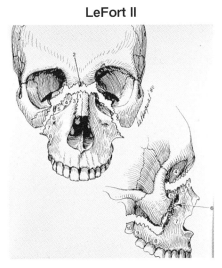

LeFort III

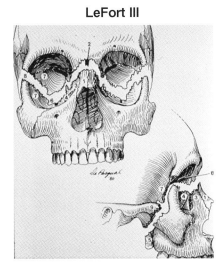

著者とアイオワ Virtual Hospital 大学 (www.vh.org) の許可を得て，著作権は保護されている。

FACE (includes Eye and Ear)

AIS 2005	Injury Description	⇒ AIS98	⇐ AIS98	FCI
250800.2	**Maxilla** fracture [including **maxillary sinus**]	250800.2	250800.2	5
	Code bilateral maxilla fractures as a single injury.			
250804.2	LeFort I	250804.2	250804.2	5
250806.2	LeFort II	250806.2	250806.2	5
250808.3	LeFort III	250808.3	250808.3	5
250810.4	blood loss >20% by volume	250810.4	250810.4	5

If a LeFort fracture is bilateral, code as single fracture to the more severe. LeFort II and III fractures, by definition, include nasal fractures ; the latter, therefore, are not coded separately. Read "LeFort Fractures" below for coding guidance.

LeFort Fractures

LeFort I - a transverse maxillary fracture through the lower maxilla including the maxillary alveolar process, portion of the maxillary sinus, the hard palate and the lower aspect of the pterygoid plates. Teeth are usually contained in the detached portion of the maxilla.

LeFort II - pyramidal fracture that passes through the nasal bone, lacrimal bone, floor of the orbit, infraorbital margin, across the upper portion of the zygomatic-maxillary suture line, maxillary sinus and pterygoid plate along the lateral wall of the maxilla into the pterygopalatine fossa. The fracture results in a floating maxilla and nose with a possible cribriform plate fracture.

LeFort III - complete separation of the facial bones from their cranial attachments [craniofacial dysjunction]. Fracture passes through the nasofrontal suture, the junction of the ethmoid and frontal bone, the superior orbital fissure, lateral wall of the orbit, zygomaticofrontal and temporal suture, with a high fracture of the pterygoid plate producing a dishface deformity.

AIS 2005	損傷内容	⇒ AIS98	⇐ AIS98	FCI
250800.2	**上顎骨**骨折［**上顎洞**を含む］	250800.2	250800.2	5
	両側性でも単一損傷としてコードを選択する。			
250804.2	LeFort Ⅰ型	250804.2	250804.2	5
250806.2	LeFort Ⅱ型	250806.2	250806.2	5
250808.3	LeFort Ⅲ型	250808.3	250808.3	5
250810.4	出血量が全血液量の20%を超える	250810.4	250810.4	5

> LeFort骨折が両側にあるときは，より重症であるほうだけを単一の損傷としてコード選択する。LeFort Ⅱ型とⅢ型は，鼻骨骨折を含むため，後者を別にコード選択しない。LeFort骨折は以下を参照。

LeFort骨折

LeFort Ⅰ-上顎歯槽突起，上顎洞，硬口蓋，翼状突起外側板の下側を通過する上顎下部を横切る上顎骨の水平方向の骨折。通常，歯牙は上顎の遊離側に含まれる。

LeFort Ⅱ-鼻骨，涙骨，眼窩底部，眼窩下縁を通り，頬骨上顎縫合，上顎の側壁に沿って，上顎洞，硬口蓋を通過し翼口蓋窩に達するピラミッド型の骨折。上顎と篩骨篩板骨折の可能性のある鼻骨の浮動状態を作り出す。

LeFort Ⅲ-顔面骨と頭蓋骨の完全分離［頭蓋顔面接合不全］。骨折線は鼻骨前頭骨縫合，篩骨前頭骨結合，眼窩上部，眼窩側壁，頬骨前頭骨縫合，頬骨側頭骨縫合を通り，翼状突起外側板の高度な骨折を伴い皿状顔面となる。

FACE (includes Eye and Ear)

AIS 2005	Injury Description	⇒ AIS98	⇐ AIS98	FCI
251099.1	**Nose** NFS	251099.1	251099.1	5
251000.1	fracture, closed or NFS	251002.1	251002.1	5
251002.2	open/displaced/comminuted	251004.2	251004.2	5
	Any or combination. Displacement must be significant.			
251004.1	ruptured mucosa/vessels (epistaxis)	251090.1	251090.1	5
	Use only in absence of nose or nasal septum fracture.			
251006.2	septum fracture	251000.1[b]	None	5
251200.2	**Orbit** fracture, closed or NFS	251202.2	251202.2	5
	Code orbital roof under skull base.			
251201.2	open but NFS as to site	251204.3[b]	251204.3[b]	5
251205.2	multiple fractures of same orbit, closed or NFS[a]	251202.2	None	5
251206.2	open[a]	251204.3[b]	None	5
251211.2	orbital rim, closed or NFS[a]	251202.2	None	5
251212.2	open NFS	251204.3[b]	None	5
251213.2	inferior orbital rim	251202.2	None	5
251214.2	open	251204.3[b]	None	5
251215.2	superior orbital rim	251202.2	None	5
251216.2	open	251204.3[b]	None	5
251221.2	orbital floor, closed or NFS[a]	251202.2	None	5
251222.2	open	251204.3[b]	None	5
251223.2	"blowout" fracture	251202.2	None	5
251224.2	open	251204.3[b]	None	5
251231.2	medial wall, closed or NFS[a]	251202.2	None	5
251232.2	open	251204.3[b]	None	5
251235.2	lateral wall, closed or NFS[a]	251202.2	None	5
251236.2	open	251204.3[b]	None	5

[a] New descriptor in AIS 2005
[b] Change in severity code in AIS 2005

顔面（目と耳を含む）

AIS 2005	損傷内容	⇒ AIS98	⇐ AIS98	FCI
251099.1	**鼻** 詳細不明	251099.1	251099.1	5
251000.1	骨折，非開放または詳細不明	251002.1	251002.1	5
251002.2	開放／転位／粉砕	251004.2	251004.2	5
	いずれか1つ以上。転位が重要である。			
251004.1	粘膜／血管の破裂（鼻出血）	251090.1	251090.1	5
	鼻骨もしくは鼻中隔骨折のないときにだけ選択する。			
251006.2	鼻中隔骨折	251000.1[b]	なし	5
251200.2	**眼窩**骨折，非開放または詳細不明	251202.2	251202.2	5
	眼窩上壁は，頭蓋底の項目でコード選択する。			
251201.2	開放で，部位は詳細不明	251204.3[b]	251204.3[b]	5
251205.2	同側眼窩の多発骨折，非開放または詳細不明[a]	251202.2	なし	5
251206.2	開放[a]	251204.3[b]	なし	5
251211.2	眼窩縁，非開放または詳細不明[a]	251202.2	なし	5
251212.2	開放　詳細不明	251204.3[b]	なし	5
251213.2	眼窩下縁	251202.2	なし	5
251214.2	開放	251204.3[b]	なし	5
251215.2	眼窩上縁	251202.2	なし	5
251216.2	開放	251204.3[b]	なし	5
251221.2	眼窩底，非開放または詳細不明[a]	251202.2	なし	5
251222.2	開放	251204.3[b]	なし	5
251223.2	"吹き抜け"骨折	251202.2	なし	5
251224.2	開放	251204.3[b]	なし	5
251231.2	内側壁，非開放または詳細不明[a]	251202.2	なし	5
251232.2	開放	251204.3[b]	なし	5
251235.2	外側壁，非開放または詳細不明[a]	251202.2	なし	5
251236.2	開放	251204.3[b]	なし	5

[a] AIS2005に加えられた新しいコード。
[b] AIS2005で重症度に変更あり。

FACE (includes Eye and Ear)

AIS 2005	Injury Description	⇒ AIS98	⇐ AIS98	FCI
251499.1	**Teeth**, any number but NFS as to injury	251499.1	251499.1	5
	See also Alveolar Ridge.			
251402.1	dislocation ; subluxation ; loosened	251402.1	251402.1	5
251404.1	fracture	251404.1	251404.1	5
251406.1	avulsion	251406.1	251406.1	5
251408.1	any combination of dislocation/fracture/avulsion	251499.1	None	5
251800.1	**Zygoma** fracture [Includes tripod and malar fractures]	251800.2[b]	251800.2[b]	5
251802.1	non-displaced [KN I][a]	251800.2[b]	None	5
251804.1	displaced NFS[a]	251800.2[b]	None	5
251806.1	arch [KN II][a]	251800.2[b]	None	5
251808.1	body[a]	251800.2[b]	None	5
251810.1	unrotated [KN III][a]	251800.2[b]	None	5
251812.1	rotated [KN IV, V][a]	251800.2[b]	None	5
251814.2	complex [KN VI][a]	251800.2	None	5
251900.3	**Panfacial** fracture[a]	None	None	3
251902.4	blood loss >20% by volume[a]	None	None	3

Multiple and complex fractures that may involve middle and lower face, upper and middle face or all three, but not LeFort fractures.

---

[a] New descriptor in AIS 2005
[b] Change in severity code in AIS 2005

顔面（目と耳を含む）

AIS 2005	損傷内容	⇒ AIS98	⇐ AIS98	FCI
251499.1	**歯牙**，本数は問わないが損傷として詳細不明	251499.1	251499.1	5
	歯槽骨の頁も参照			
251402.1	脱臼；亜脱臼；動揺	251402.1	251402.1	5
251404.1	破折	251404.1	251404.1	5
251406.1	脱落	251406.1	251406.1	5
251408.1	脱臼，破折，脱落いずれかの合併	251499.1	なし	5
251800.1	**頬骨**骨折［三脚骨折と頬骨体部骨折を含む］	251800.2[b]	251800.2[b]	5
251802.1	転位なし［KN Ⅰ］[a]	251800.2[b]	なし	5
251804.1	転位あり　詳細不明[a]	251800.2[b]	なし	5
251806.1	弓部［KN Ⅱ］[a]	251800.2[b]	なし	5
251808.1	体部[a]	251800.2[b]	なし	5
251810.1	非回旋［KN Ⅲ］[a]	251800.2[b]	なし	5
251812.1	回旋［KN Ⅳ, KN Ⅴ］[a]	251800.2[b]	なし	5
251814.2	複雑［KN Ⅵ］[a]	251800.2	なし	5
251900.3	**顔面の広汎**な骨折[a]	なし	なし	3
251902.4	出血量が全血液量の20％を超える[a]	なし	なし	3

> この2つのコードは，中部と下部顔面，上部と中部顔面，もしくは3部位すべての，多発かつ複雑な骨折を意味するが，LeFort骨折ではない。

顔面

---

[a] AIS2005に加えられた新しいコード。KN：Knight & North の分類。
[b] AIS2005で重症度に変更あり。

頸　部

NECK

AIS 2005	Injury Description	⇒ AIS98	⇐ AIS98	FCI

WHOLE AREA

> Use one of the following two descriptors when such vague information is the only information available. While these descriptors identify the occurrence of a neck injury, they do not specify its severity.

300099.9	Injuries to the Neck NFS	315099.9	315099.9	
300999.9	Died of neck injury without further substantiation of injuries or no autopsy confirmation of specific injuries	315999.9	315999.9	
311000.6	Decapitation	311000.6	311000.6	1

> Use this category if penetrating injury does not involve internal structures. Assign to External body region for calculating an ISS. If underlying anatomical structures are involved, code documented diagnoses only ; do not use these generic descriptors.

316000.1	Penetrating injury NFS	316000.1	316000.1	5
316002.1	minor ; superficial	316002.1	316002.1	5
316004.2	tissue loss $>25cm^{2j}$	316004.2	316004.2	5
316006.3	blood loss >20% by volume	316006.3	316006.3	5

> Use the following section for blunt soft tissue injuries to the Neck. Assign to External body region for calculating an ISS.

310099.1	Skin/subcutaneous tissue/muscle NFS	310099.1	310099.1	5
310202.1	abrasion	310202.1	310202.1	5
310402.1	contusion ; hematoma	310402.1	310402.1	5
310600.1	laceration NFS	310600.1	310600.1	5
310602.1	minor ; superficial	310602.1	310602.1	5
310604.2	major ; >10cm long <u>and</u> into subcutaneous tissue[j]	310604.2	310604.2	5
310606.3	blood loss >20% by volume	310606.3	310606.3	5
310800.1	avulsion NFS	310800.1	310800.1	5
310802.1	minor ; superficial ; $\leq 25cm^{2j}$	310802.1	310802.1	5
310804.2	major ; tissue loss $>25cm^{2j}$	310804.2	310804.2	5
310806.3	blood loss >20% by volume	310806.3	310806.3	5

---

[j] Change in size of injury in AIS 2005

頸　部

AIS 2005	損傷内容	⇒ AIS98	⇐ AIS98	FCI

全　域

> 詳細不明な情報しかない場合には，以下の2つの説明のいずれかを用いる。それらが頸部損傷を示していても重症度を表しているのではない。

300099.9	**頸部への損傷**　詳細不明	315099.9	315099.9	
300999.9	他の詳細な損傷や，他の損傷がないか剖検が行われていない頸部損傷による死亡	315999.9	315999.9	
311000.6	**断頭**	311000.6	311000.6	1

> 貫通創が体内の組織を損傷していない場合にこのカテゴリーを選択する。体表の領域はISSで計算する。解剖学的な組織が損傷されていれば，コードは診断のためだけに記録する；これらの一般的な記述を選択しない。

316000.1	**穿通性損傷**　詳細不明	316000.1	316000.1	5
316002.1	小；表在性	316002.1	316002.1	5
316004.2	組織欠損が25cm^{2}を超える[j]	316004.2	316004.2	5
316006.3	出血量が全血液量の20%を超える	316006.3	316006.3	5

> 頸部への鈍的軟部組織損傷の場合には以下を選択する。体表の領域はISSで計算する。

310099.1	**皮膚/皮下組織/筋肉**　詳細不明	310099.1	310099.1	5
310202.1	擦過傷	310202.1	310202.1	5
310402.1	挫傷；血腫	310402.1	310402.1	5
310600.1	裂傷・裂創　詳細不明	310600.1	310600.1	5
310602.1	小；表在性	310602.1	310602.1	5
310604.2	大；長さが10cmを超え，かつ皮下に達する[j]	310604.2	310604.2	5
310606.3	出血量が全血液量の20%を超える	310606.3	310606.3	5
310800.1	剥離　詳細不明	310800.1	310800.1	5
310802.1	小；表在性；25cm^{2}以下[j]	310802.1	310802.1	5
310804.2	大；組織欠損が25cm^{2}を超える[j]	310804.2	310804.2	5
310806.3	出血量が全血液量の20%を超える	310806.3	310806.3	5

---

[j] AIS 2005で損傷の範囲が変更になっている。

NECK

AIS 2005	Injury Description	⇒ AIS98	⇐ AIS98	FCI
	VESSELS			
320099.9	**Vascular Injury in Neck** NFS[f]	None	None	
320299.3	**Carotid artery [common, internal]** NFS	320299.3	320299.3	5
320202.3	intimal tear, no disruption	320202.3	320202.3	5
320204.4	neurological deficit (stroke) not head-injury related	320204.4	320204.4	1
320206.3	laceration ; perforation ; puncture NFS	320206.3	320206.3	5
320208.3	minor ; superficial ; incomplete circumferential involvement ; blood loss ≤20% by volume	320208.3	320208.3	5
320209.3	bilateral[c]	320208.3	None	5
320210.4	neurological deficit (stroke) not head-injury related	320210.4	320210.4	1
320211.4	bilateral[c]	320210.4	None	1
320212.4	major ; rupture ; transection ; segmental loss ; blood loss >20% by volume	320212.4	320212.4	5
320213.4	bilateral[c]	320212.4	None	5
320214.5	neurological deficit (stroke) not head-injury related	320214.5	320214.5	1
320215.5	bilateral[c]	320214.5	None	1
320216.3	with thrombosis (occlusion) secondary to trauma	320216.3	320216.3	5
320217.3	bilateral[c]	320216.3	None	5
320218.4	neurological deficit (stroke) not head-injury related	320218.4	320218.4	1
320219.4	bilateral[c]	320218.4	None	1
320220.3	thrombosis (occlusion) secondary to trauma from any lesion but laceration	320220.3	320220.3	5
320221.3	bilateral[c]	320220.3	None	5
320222.4	neurological deficit (stroke) not head-injury related	320222.4	320222.4	1
320223.4	bilateral[c]	320222.4	None	1

---

[c] In previous editions of AIS, each injury was coded separately. AIS 2005 introduces "bilateral" for certain injury descriptions. Some bilateral injuries may affect severity levels and, therefore, the ISS for patients with those injuries.

[f] New descriptor in AIS 2005 that allows classification of trauma by body region, but does not allow assigning a severity code.

AIS 2005	損傷内容	⇒ AIS98	⇐ AIS98	FCI
	血　管			
320099.9	頸部の血管損傷　詳細不明[f]	なし	なし	
320299.3	**頸動脈［総頸，内頸］　詳細不明**	320299.3	320299.3	5
320202.3	内膜剝離，断裂なし	320202.3	320202.3	5
320204.4	頭部外傷に関連のない神経脱落症状（脳卒中）	320204.4	320204.4	1
320206.3	裂傷・裂創；穿孔；穿刺　詳細不明	320206.3	320206.3	5
320208.3	小；表在性；非全周性；出血量が全血液量の20％以下	320208.3	320208.3	5
320209.3	両側性[c]	320208.3	なし	5
320210.4	頭部外傷に関連のない神経脱落症状（脳卒中）	320210.4	320210.4	1
320211.4	両側性[c]	320210.4	なし	1
320212.4	大；破裂；離断；部分欠損；出血量が全血液量の20％を超える	320212.4	320212.4	5
320213.4	両側性[c]	320212.4	なし	5
320214.5	頭部外傷に関連のない神経脱落症状（脳卒中）	320214.5	320214.5	1
320215.5	両側性[c]	320214.5	なし	1
320216.3	外傷に起因する血栓（閉塞）	320216.3	320216.3	5
320217.3	両側性[c]	320216.3	なし	5
320218.4	頭部外傷に関連のない神経脱落症状（脳卒中）	320218.4	320218.4	1
320219.4	両側性[c]	320218.4	なし	1
320220.3	裂傷・裂創以外の何らかの外傷に起因する血栓（閉塞）	320220.3	320220.3	5
320221.3	両側性[c]	320220.3	なし	5
320222.4	頭部外傷に関連のない神経脱落症状（脳卒中）	320222.4	320222.4	1
320223.4	両側性[c]	320222.4	なし	1

---

[c] 旧版の AIS では両側損傷はそれぞれ別にコード選択をしていた。AIS2005では，"両側"を導入した。いくつかの両側損傷は重症度が変化し，その結果 ISS が変わることがある。

[f] AIS 2005に加えられた新しいコード。外傷の存在部位を示すことができる。ただし重症度はない。

NECK

AIS 2005	Injury Description	⇒ AIS98	⇐ AIS98	FCI
320499.2	**Carotid artery [external]** NFS [includes **thyroid**]	320499.2	320499.2	5
320402.2	intimal tear, no disruption	320402.2	320402.2	5
320404.2	laceration ; perforation ; puncture NFS	320404.2	320404.2	5
320406.2	minor ; superficial ; incomplete circumferential involvement ; blood loss ≤20% by volume	320406.2	320406.2	5
320408.3	major ; rupture ; transection ; segmental loss ; blood loss >20% by volume	320408.3	320408.3	5
320410.2	with thrombosis ; (occlusion) secondary to trauma	320410.2	320410.2	5
320412.2	thrombosis (occlusion) secondary to trauma from any lesion but laceration	320412.2	320412.2	5
321099.2	**Vertebral artery** NFS	321099.2	321099.2	5
321002.2	intimal tear, no disruption	321002.2	321002.2	5
321004.3	neurological deficit (stroke) not head-injury related	321004.3	321004.3	2
321006.2	laceration ; perforation ; puncture NFS	321006.2	321006.2	5
321008.2	minor ; superficial ; incomplete circumferential involvement ; blood loss ≤20% by volume	321008.2	321008.2	5
321010.3	neurological deficit (stroke) not head-injury related	321010.3	321010.3	2
321012.3	major ; rupture ; transection ; blood loss > 20 % by volume	321012.3	321012.3	5
321014.4	neurological deficit (stroke) not head-injury related	321014.4	321014.4	2
321015.5	bilateral[c]	321014.4[b]	None	1
321016.4	with thrombosis (occlusion) secondary to trauma	321016.3[b]	321016.3[b]	5
321017.5	bilateral[c]	321016.3[b]	None	5
321018.3	thrombosis (occlusion) secondary to trauma from any lesion but laceration	321018.3	321018.3	5
321020.4	neurological deficit (stroke) not head-injury related	321020.4	321020.4	2
321021.5	bilateral[c]	321020.4[b]	None	1

---

[b] Change in severity code in AIS 2005

[c] In previous editions of AIS, each injury was coded separately. AIS 2005 introduces "bilateral" for certain injury descriptors. Some bilateral injuries may affect severity levels and, therefore, the ISS for patients with those injuries.

AIS 2005	損傷内容	⇒ AIS98	⇐ AIS98	FCI
320499.2	**頸動脈 [外頸]**　詳細不明 [甲状腺を含む]	320499.2	320499.2	5
320402.2	内膜剥離，断裂なし	320402.2	320402.2	5
320404.2	裂傷・裂創；穿孔；穿刺　詳細不明	320404.2	320404.2	5
320406.2	小；表在性；非全周性；出血量が全血液量の20%以下	320406.2	320406.2	5
320408.3	大；破裂；離断；部分欠損；出血量が全血液量の20%を超える	320408.3	320408.3	5
320410.2	外傷に起因する血栓（閉塞）を伴う	320410.2	320410.2	5
320412.2	裂傷・裂創以外の何らかの外傷に起因する血栓（閉塞）	320412.2	320412.2	5
321099.2	**椎骨動脈**　詳細不明	321099.2	321099.2	5
321002.2	内膜剥離，断裂なし	321002.2	321002.2	5
321004.3	頭部外傷に関連のない神経脱落症状（脳卒中）	321004.3	321004.3	2
321006.2	裂傷・裂創；穿孔；穿刺　詳細不明	321006.2	321006.2	5
321008.2	小；表在性；非全周性；出血量が全血液量の20%以下	321008.2	321008.2	5
321010.3	頭部外傷に関連のない神経脱落症状（脳卒中）	321010.3	321010.3	2
321012.3	大；破裂；離断；出血量が全血液量の20%を超える	321012.3	321012.3	5
321014.4	頭部外傷に関連のない神経脱落症状（脳卒中）	321014.4	321014.4	2
321015.5	両側性[c]	321014.4[b]	なし	1
321016.4	外傷に起因する血栓（閉塞）を伴う	321016.3[b]	321016.3[b]	5
321017.5	両側性[c]	321016.3[b]	なし	5
321018.3	裂傷・裂創以外の何らかの外傷に起因する血栓（閉塞）	321018.3	321018.3	5
321020.4	頭部外傷に関連のない神経脱落症状（脳卒中）	321020.4	321020.4	2
321021.5	両側性[c]	321020.4[b]	なし	1

[b] AIS 2005で重症度に変更あり。
[c] 旧版のAISでは両側損傷はそれぞれ別にコード選択をしていた。AIS2005では，"両側"を導入した。いくつかの両側損傷は重症度が変化し，その結果ISSが変わることがある。

NECK

AIS 2005	Injury Description	⇒ AIS98	⇐ AIS98	FCI
320699.1	**Jugular vein [external]** NFS	320699.1	320699.1	5
320602.1	laceration ; perforation ; puncture NFS	320602.1	320602.1	5
320604.1	minor ; superficial ; incomplete circumferential involvement ; blood loss ≤20% by volume	320604.1	320604.1	5
320606.3	major ; rupture ; transection ; segmental loss ; blood loss >20% by volume	320606.3	320606.3	5
320899.1	**Jugular vein [internal]** NFS	320899.1	320899.1	5
320802.2	laceration ; perforation ; puncture NFS	320802.2	320802.2	5
320804.2	minor ; superficial ; incomplete circumferential involvement ; blood loss ≤20% by volume	320804.2	320804.2	5
320806.3	major ; rupture ; transection ; blood loss > 20 % by volume	320806.3	320806.3	5

NERVES

330099.1	**Nerve Injury in Neck** NFS[a]	None	None	5
330299.2	**Phrenic nerve** injury	330299.2	330299.2	4
330298.4	bilateral[c]	330299.2[b]	None	2
330499.1	**Vagus nerve** injury	330499.1	330499.1	3
	See also Head, Thorax and Abdomen body regions.			

---

[a] New descriptor in AIS 2005

[b] Change in severity level in AIS 2005

[c] In previous editions of AIS, each injury was coded separately. AIS 2005 introduces "bilateral" for certain injury descriptions. Some bilateral injuries may affect severity levels and, therefore, the ISS for patients with these injuries.

AIS 2005	損傷内容	⇒ AIS98	⇐ AIS98	FCI
320699.1	**頸静脈［外頸］** 詳細不明	320699.1	320699.1	5
320602.1	裂傷・裂創；穿孔；穿刺 詳細不明	320602.1	320602.1	5
320604.1	小；表在性；非全周性；出血量が全血液量の20%以下	320604.1	320604.1	5
320606.3	大；破裂；離断；部分欠損；出血量が全血液量の20%を超える	320606.3	320606.3	5
320899.1	**頸静脈［内頸］** 詳細不明	320899.1	320899.1	5
320802.2	裂傷・裂創；穿孔；穿刺 詳細不明	320802.2	320802.2	5
320804.2	小；表在性；非全周性；出血量が全血液量の20%以下	320804.2	320804.2	5
320806.3	大；破裂；離断；出血量が全血液量の20%を超える	320806.3	320806.3	5

神 経

AIS 2005	損傷内容	⇒ AIS98	⇐ AIS98	FCI
330099.1	**頸部の神経損傷** 詳細不明[a]	なし	なし	5
330299.2	**横隔膜神経**損傷	330299.2	330299.2	4
330298.4	両側性[c]	330299.2[b]	なし	2
330499.1	**迷走神経**損傷	330499.1	330499.1	3
	頭部，胸部，腹部領域も参照。			

---

[a] AIS 2005に加えられた新しいコード。
[b] AIS 2005で重症度に変更あり。
[c] 旧版の AIS では両側損傷はそれぞれ別にコード選択をしていた。AIS2005では，"両側"を導入した。いくつかの両側損傷は重症度が変化し，その結果 ISS が変わることがある。

NECK

AIS 2005	Injury Description	⇒ AIS98	⇐ AIS98	FCI
	INTERNAL ORGANS			
340199.2	**Esophagus injury in Neck** NFS[k]	440899.2	None	5
	See also Thorax body region. Code to Neck if site NFS. If injury occurs at junction of neck and thorax (i.e., at sternal notch), assign to Neck.			
340102.2	contusion ; hematoma [OIS I]	440802.2	None	5
340103.3	ingestion injury NFS[a]	440899.2[b]	None	5
340104.3	partial thickness necrosis[a]	440899.2[b]	None	5
340105.4	full thickness necrosis[a]	440899.2[b]	None	5
340106.3	laceration ; tear NFS	440804.3	None	5
340107.3	no perforation ; partial thickness ; ≤50% circumference [OIS I, II]	440806.3	None	5
340108.4	perforation ; full thickness ; >50% circumference [OIS III]	440808.4	None	5
340109.5	avulsion ; rupture ; transection ; massive destruction [OIS IV, V]	440810.5	None	2
340299.2	**Larynx**, including **thyroid** and **cricoid cartilage**, NFS	340299.2	340299.2	5
340202.2	contusion ; hematoma	340202.2	340202.2	5
340204.2	laceration ; puncture NFS	340204.2	340204.2	5
340206.2	no perforation ; partial thickness ; mucosal tear	340206.2	340206.2	5
340208.3	perforation ; full thickness ; "fracture"	340208.3	340208.3	5
340210.4	vocal cord involvement	340210.4	340210.4	2
340212.5	avulsion ; rupture ; transection ; massive destruction ; crush	340212.5	340212.5	2
340699.2	**Pharynx or Retropharyngeal area**, NFS	340699.3[b]	340699.3[b]	5
340602.2	contusion ; hematoma NFS[e]	340602.3[b]	340602.3[b]	5
340603.2	minor ; ≤75% airway involvement	340602.3[b]	None	5
340605.3	major ; >75% airway involvement	340602.3	None	3
340604.2	laceration ; puncture NFS	340604.2	340604.2	5
340606.3	no perforation ; partial thickness ; mucosal tear	340606.3	340606.3	5
340608.4	perforation ; full thickness	340608.4	340608.4	5
340610.5	avulsion ; rupture ; transection ; massive destruction ; crush	340610.5	340610.5	1

---

[a] New descriptor in AIS 2005
[b] Change in severity code in AIS 2005
[e] In AIS 98, this injury description had only one severity level. In AIS 2005, it has several.
[k] Differentiation of esophageal and tracheal injuries between Neck and Thorax may affect severity levels and/or body regions and, therefore, the ISS for patients with those injuries.

AIS 2005	損傷内容	⇒ AIS98	⇐ AIS98	FCI

内 臓

AIS 2005	損傷内容	⇒ AIS98	⇐ AIS98	FCI
340199.2	**頸部食道** 詳細不明[k]	440899.2	なし	5

> 胸部領域も参照。詳細不明の部位であれば頸部とコードを選択する。損傷が頸部胸郭境界部で生じた場合（例：胸骨切痕）には頸部とする。

AIS 2005	損傷内容	⇒ AIS98	⇐ AIS98	FCI
340102.2	挫傷；血腫（OIS I）	440802.2	なし	5
340103.3	経口摂取による障害　詳細不明[a]	440899.2[b]	なし	5
340104.3	非全層性壊死[a]	440899.2[b]	なし	5
340105.4	全層性壊死[a]	440899.2[b]	なし	5
340106.3	裂傷・裂創；詳細不明	440804.3	なし	5
340107.3	穿孔なし；非全層性；周径の50％以下（OIS I, II）	440806.3	なし	5
340108.4	穿孔；全層性；周径の50％を超える（OIS III）	440808.4	なし	5
340109.5	剥離；破裂；離断；広範囲損傷（OIS IV, V）	440810.5	なし	2
340299.2	**喉頭**（**甲状腺**, **輪状軟骨**を含む）詳細不明	340299.2	340299.2	5
340202.2	挫傷；血腫	340202.2	340202.2	5
340204.2	裂傷・裂創；穿刺　詳細不明	340204.2	340204.2	5
340206.2	穿孔なし；非全層性；粘膜裂傷	340206.2	340206.2	5
340208.3	穿孔；全層性；"骨折"	340208.3	340208.3	5
340210.4	声帯損傷	340210.4	340210.4	2
340212.5	剥離；破裂；離断；広範囲損傷；挫滅	340212.5	340212.5	2
340699.2	**咽頭または後咽頭領域**　詳細不明	340699.3[b]	340699.3[b]	5
340602.2	挫傷；血腫　詳細不明[e]	340602.3[b]	340602.3[b]	5
340603.2	小；気道損傷の75％以下	340602.3[b]	なし	5
340605.3	大；気道損傷の75％を超える	340602.3	なし	3
340604.2	裂傷・裂創；穿刺　詳細不明	340604.2	340604.2	5
340606.3	穿孔なし；非全層性；粘膜裂傷	340606.3	340606.3	5
340608.4	穿孔；全層性	340608.4	340608.4	5
340610.5	剥離；破裂；離断；広範囲損傷；挫滅	340610.5	340610.5	1

---

[a] AIS2005に加えられた新しいコード。
[b] AIS2005で重症度に変更あり。
[e] AIS98ではこの損傷コードは1つだけであったが，AIS2005においては複数個ある。
[k] 食道や気管の損傷は，頸部と胸郭のいずれに分類されるかの違いにより重症度や領域にかかわるため，ISSにも影響を与える。

NECK

AIS 2005	Injury Description	⇒ AIS98	⇐ AIS98	FCI
341099.2	**Salivary gland** NFS	341099.2	341099.2	5
341002.3	ductal involvement ; transection	341002.3	341002.3	5
341499.1	**Thyroid gland** NFS	341499.1	341499.1	5
341402.1	contusion ; hematoma	341402.1	341402.1	5
341404.2	laceration	341404.2	341404.2	5
341699.2	**Trachea injury in Neck** NFS[k]	442699.3[b]	None	5

> See also Thorax body region. Code to Neck if site NFS. If injury occurs at junction of neck and thorax (i.e., at sternal notch), assign to Neck.

AIS 2005	Injury Description	⇒ AIS98	⇐ AIS98	FCI
341602.2	contusion ; hematoma	442602.3[b]	None	5
341604.2	laceration ; tear NFS	442604.3[b]	None	5
341606.2	no perforation ; partial thickness	442606.3[b]	None	5
341608.3	perforation ; full thickness ; "fracture"	442608.4[b]	None	5
341610.4	avulsion ; rupture ; transection ; massive destruction ; crush ; laryngeal-tracheal separation	442610.5[b]	None	2
341899.2	**Vocal cord** NFS [not due to intubation]	341899.2	341899.2	5
341802.2	unilateral	341802.2	341802.2	3
341804.3	bilateral	341804.3	341804.3	2

SKELETAL

AIS 2005	Injury Description	⇒ AIS98	⇐ AIS98	FCI
350200.2	**Hyoid** fracture	350200.2	350200.2	5

---

[b] Change in severity code in AIS 2005

[k] Differentiation of esophageal and tracheal injuries between Neck and Thorax may affect severity levels and/or body regions and, therefore, the ISS for patients with those injuries.

AIS 2005	損傷内容	⇒ AIS98	⇐ AIS98	FCI
341099.2	**唾液腺** 詳細不明	341099.2	341099.2	5
341002.3	導管損傷；離断	341002.3	341002.3	5
341499.1	**甲状腺** 詳細不明	341499.1	341499.1	5
341402.1	挫傷；血腫	341402.1	341402.1	5
341404.2	裂傷・裂創	341404.2	341404.2	5
341699.2	**頸部の気管損傷** 詳細不明[k]	442699.3[b]	なし	5

> 胸部領域も参照。詳細不明の部位であれば頸部とコードを選択する。損傷が頸部胸郭境界部で生じた場合（例：胸骨切痕）には頸部とする。

AIS 2005	損傷内容	⇒ AIS98	⇐ AIS98	FCI
341602.2	挫傷；血腫	442602.3[b]	なし	5
341604.2	裂傷・裂創；詳細不明	442604.3[b]	なし	5
341606.2	穿孔なし；非全層性	442606.3[b]	なし	5
341608.3	穿孔；全層性；"骨折"	442608.4[b]	なし	5
341610.4	剥離；破裂；離断；広範囲損傷；挫滅；喉頭と気管の解離	442610.5[b]	なし	2
341899.2	**声帯** 詳細不明［気管挿管が原因ではない］	341899.2	341899.2	5
341802.2	片側	341802.2	341802.2	3
341804.3	両側	341804.3	341804.3	2

骨　格

AIS 2005	損傷内容	⇒ AIS98	⇐ AIS98	FCI
350200.2	**舌骨**骨折	350200.2	350200.2	5

---

[b] AIS2005で重症度に変更あり。
[k] 食道や気管の損傷は，頸部と胸郭のいずれに分類されるかの違いにより重症度や領域にかかわるため，ISSにも影響を与える。

胸　部

THORAX

AIS 2005	Injury Description	⇒ AIS98	⇐ AIS98	FCI

WHOLE AREA

> Use one of the following two descriptors when such vague information is the only information available. While these descriptors identify the occurrence of a thoracic injury, they do not specify its severity.

400099.9	**Injuries to the Whole Thorax** NFS	415099.9	415099.9	
400999.9	Died of thoracic injury without further substantiation of injuries or no autopsy confirmation of specific injuries	415999.9	415999.9	
411000.2	**Breast** avulsion, **female**	411000.2	411000.2	5
413000.6	**Crush injury**	413000.6	413000.6	1

> Must involve massive bilateral destruction of skeletal, vascular, organ and tissue systems.

415000.4	**Open ("sucking") chest wound**	415000.4	415000.4	5
410102.2	**Pectoral muscle** tear ; laceration[a]	410099.1	None	5

> Use this category if penetrating injury does not involve internal structures. Assign to External body region for calculating an ISS. If underlying anatomical structures are involved, code documented diagnoses only ; do not use these generic descriptors.

416000.1	**Penetrating injury** NFS	416000.1	416000.1	5
416002.1	superficial ; minor ; into pleural cavity but not involving deeper structures	416002.1	416002.1	5
416004.2	with tissue loss $>100cm^2$	416004.2	416004.2	5
416006.3	with blood loss $>20\%$ by volume	416006.3	416006.3	5

---

[a] New descriptor in AIS 2005

胸　部

AIS 2005	損傷内容	⇒ AIS98	⇐ AIS98	FCI

全　域

> 不確定な情報しか得られない場合には，以下の2つのコードのいずれかを選択する。ただし，この胸部損傷の2つのコードを選択した場合には重症度は表さない。

AIS 2005	損傷内容	⇒ AIS98	⇐ AIS98	FCI
400099.9	胸部全体の損傷　詳細不明	415099.9	415099.9	
400999.9	具体的な損傷の詳細な記載がない，または剖検による損傷部位の特定がなされていない胸部損傷による死亡	415999.9	415999.9	
411000.2	乳房の剥離創，**女性**	411000.2	411000.2	5
413000.6	挫滅損傷	413000.6	413000.6	1

> 骨格，血管，臓器，組織系の広範な両側性高度損傷を伴わなくてはならない。

AIS 2005	損傷内容	⇒ AIS98	⇐ AIS98	FCI
415000.4	開放性胸壁損傷（吸い込み創）	415000.4	415000.4	5
410102.2	胸筋剥離；裂傷・裂創[a]	410099.1	なし	5

> 胸腔内に達していない穿通性損傷の場合，このコードを選択する。ISSを算出する際には「体表」の区分として取り扱う。下記に示す解剖学的損傷を伴う場合には，コードは診断としてのみ記録する；包括的な名称として用いてはならない。

AIS 2005	損傷内容	⇒ AIS98	⇐ AIS98	FCI
416000.1	穿通性損傷　詳細不明	416000.1	416000.1	5
416002.1	表在性；小；胸腔内に達するが深部組織の損傷は認めない	416002.1	416002.1	5
416004.2	組織欠損が100cm^{2}を超える	416004.2	416004.2	5
416006.3	出血量が全血液量の20%を超える	416006.3	416006.3	5

---

[a] AIS2005に加えられた新しいコード。

THORAX

AIS 2005	Injury Description	⇒ AIS98	⇐ AIS98	FCI
	Use the following section for blunt soft tissue injury to the thorax. Assign to External body region for calculating an ISS. If injury is described as "degloving", code as avulsion.			
410099.1	**Skin/subcutaneous/muscle** NFS	410099.1	410099.1	5
410202.1	abrasion	410202.1	410202.1	5
410402.1	contusion ; hematoma	410402.1	410402.1	5
410600.1	laceration NFS	410600.1	410600.1	5
410602.1	minor ; superficial	410602.1	410602.1	5
410604.2	major ; >20cm long <u>and</u> into subcutaneous tissue	410604.2	410604.2	5
410606.3	blood loss >20% by volume	410606.3	410606.3	5
410800.1	avulsion NFS	410800.1	410800.1	5
410802.1	minor ; superficial ; ≤100cm^2	410802.1	410802.1	5
410804.2	major ; >100cm^2	410804.2	410804.2	5
410806.3	blood loss >20% by volume	410806.3	410806.3	5

VESSELS

AIS 2005	Injury Description	⇒ AIS98	⇐ AIS98	FCI
	Vessel injuries are coded separately from other injuries to the chest, except for crush injury which includes all injuries to the chest.			
420099.9	**Vascular Injury in Thorax** NFS[f]	None	None	
420299.4	**Aorta, thoracic** NFS [*OIS IV or V* for entire category unless stated otherwise]	420299.4	420299.4	5
420202.4	intimal tear, no disruption	420202.4	420202.4	5
420204.5	with aortic valve involvement	420204.5	420204.5	5
420206.4	laceration ; perforation ; puncture NFS	420206.4	420206.4	5
420208.4	minor ; superficial ; incomplete circumferential involvement ; blood loss≤20% by volume	420208.4	420208.4	5
420210.5	major ; rupture ; transection ; segmental loss ; blood loss >20% by volume	420210.5	420210.5	5
420212.5	with aortic root or valve involvement	420212.5	420212.5	5
420216.5	with hemorrhage confined to mediastinum	420216.5	420216.5	5
420218.6	with hemorrhage not confined to mediastinum [*OIS VI*]	420218.6	420218.6	1

---

[f] New descriptor in AIS 2005 that allows classification of trauma by body region, but does not allow assigning a severity code.

AIS 2005	損傷内容	⇒ AIS98	⇐ AIS98	FCI
	胸部の鈍的組織損傷に対しては，下記のコードを選択する。ISS を算出する場合には「体表」の区分として取り扱う。デグロービング損傷の記載は剝離のコードを選択する。			
410099.1	**皮膚/皮下組織/筋肉**　詳細不明	410099.1	410099.1	5
410202.1	擦過傷	410202.1	410202.1	5
410402.1	挫傷；血腫	410402.1	410402.1	5
410600.1	裂傷・裂創　詳細不明	410600.1	410600.1	5
410602.1	小；表在性	410602.1	410602.1	5
410604.2	大；長さが20cmを超えかつ皮下組織に達する	410604.2	410604.2	5
410606.3	出血量が全血液量の20%を超える	410606.3	410606.3	5
410800.1	剝離　詳細不明	410800.1	410800.1	5
410802.1	小；表在性；100cm^{2}以下	410802.1	410802.1	5
410804.2	大；100cm^{2}を超える	410804.2	410804.2	5
410806.3	出血量が全血液量の20%を超える	410806.3	410806.3	5

血　管

血管損傷は，胸部損傷を伴う挫滅創を除き，胸部の他の損傷とは独立した損傷としてコードを選択する。

AIS 2005	損傷内容	⇒ AIS98	⇐ AIS98	FCI
420099.9	**胸部の血管損傷**　詳細不明[f]	なし	なし	
420299.4	**胸部大動脈**　詳細不明　［別の区分に入る場合を除き OIS IV, V］	420299.4	420299.4	5
420202.4	内膜剝離，断裂なし	420202.4	420202.4	5
420204.5	大動脈弁の損傷を伴う	420204.5	420204.5	5
420206.4	裂傷・裂創；穿孔；穿刺　詳細不明	420206.4	420206.4	5
420208.4	小；表在性；非全周性：出血量が全血液量の20%以下	420208.4	420208.4	5
420210.5	大；破裂；離断；部分欠損；出血量が全血液量の20%を超える	420210.5	420210.5	5
420212.5	大動脈基底部または大動脈弁の損傷を伴う	420212.5	420212.5	5
420216.5	縦隔内に限局した出血を伴う	420216.5	420216.5	5
420218.6	縦隔外への出血を伴う　［OIS VI］	420218.6	420218.6	1

---

[f] AIS2005に加えられた新しいコード。外傷の存在部位を示すことができる。ただし重症度はない。

THORAX

AIS 2005	Injury Description	⇒ AIS98	⇐ AIS98	FCI
420499.3	**Brachiocephalic (innominate) artery** NFS [*OIS III* for entire category]	420499.3	420499.3	5
420402.3	intimal tear, no disruption	420402.3	420402.3	5
420404.3	laceration ; perforation ; puncture NFS	420404.3	420404.3	5
420406.3	minor ; superficial ; incomplete circumferential involvement ; blood loss≤20% by volume	420406.3	420406.3	5
420408.4	major ; rupture ; transection ; segmental loss ; blood loss >20% by volume	420408.4	420408.4	5
420800.5	**Coronary artery** laceration or thrombosis to left main, right main or left anterior descending artery ; coronary sinus	420800.5	420800.5	2
421099.3	**Pulmonary artery** NFS [*OIS IV, V* for entire category]	421099.3	421099.3	5
421002.3	intimal tear, no disruption	421002.3	421002.3	5
421004.3	laceration ; perforation ; puncture NFS	421004.3	421004.3	5
421006.3	minor ; superficial ; incomplete circumferential involvement ; blood loss≤20% by volume	421006.3	421006.3	5
421008.5	major ; rupture ; transection ; segmental loss ; blood loss >20% by volume	421008.4[b]	421008.4[b]	5
421009.6	bilateral[c]	421008.4[b]	None	1
421499.3	**Subclavian artery** NFS [*OIS III* for entire category]	421499.3	421499.3	5
421402.3	intimal tear, no disruption	421402.3	421402.3	5
421404.3	laceration ; perforation ; puncture NFS	421404.3	421404.3	5
421406.3	minor ; superficial ; incomplete circumferential involvement ; blood loss≤20% by volume	421406.3	421406.3	5
421408.4	major ; rupture ; transection ; segmental loss ; blood loss >20% by volume	421408.4	421408.4	5
422099.2	**Other named arteries** e.g., **bronchial, esophageal, intercostal, internal mammary** NFS [*OIS I* for entire category]	422099.2	422099.2	5
422002.2	intimal tear, no disruption	422002.2	422002.2	5
422004.2	laceration ; perforation ; puncture NFS	422004.2	422004.2	5
422006.2	minor ; superficial ; incomplete circumferential involvement ; blood loss≤20% by volume	422006.2	422006.2	5
422008.3	major ; rupture ; transection ; segmental loss ; blood loss >20% by volume	422008.3	422008.3	5

[b] Change in severity in AIS 2005
[c] In previous editions of AIS, each injury was coded separately. AIS 2005 introduces "bilateral" for certain injury descriptions. Some bilateral injuries may affect severity levels and, therefore, the ISS for patients with those injuries.

AIS 2005	損傷内容	⇒ AIS98	⇐ AIS98	FCI
420499.3	**腕頭（無名）動脈** 詳細不明 ［OIS Ⅲに相当する］	420499.3	420499.3	5
420402.3	内膜剥離，断裂なし	420402.3	420402.3	5
420404.3	裂傷・裂創；穿孔；穿刺 詳細不明	420404.3	420404.3	5
420406.3	小；表在性；非全周性；出血量が全血液量の20%以下	420406.3	420406.3	5
420408.4	大；破裂；離断；部分欠損；出血量が全血液量の20%を超える	420408.4	420408.4	5
420800.5	**冠動脈** 左右の冠動脈本幹あるいは左前下行枝，冠静脈洞の裂傷・裂創あるいは血栓症	420800.5	420800.5	2
421099.3	**肺動脈** 詳細不明 ［OIS Ⅳ, Ⅴに相当する］	421099.3	421099.3	5
421002.3	内膜剥離，断裂なし	421002.3	421002.3	5
421004.3	裂傷・裂創；穿孔；穿刺 詳細不明	421004.3	421004.3	5
421006.3	小；表在性；非全周性；出血量が全血液量の20%以下	421006.3	421006.3	5
421008.5	大；破裂；離断；部分欠損；出血量が全血液量の20%を超える	421008.4[b]	421008.4[b]	5
421009.6	両側性[c]	421008.4[b]	なし	1
421499.3	**鎖骨下動脈** 詳細不明 ［OIS Ⅲに相当する］	421499.3	421499.3	5
421402.3	内膜剥離，断裂なし	421402.3	421402.3	5
421404.3	裂傷・裂創；穿孔；穿刺 詳細不明	421404.3	421404.3	5
421406.3	小；表在性；非全周性；出血量が全血液量の20%以下	421406.3	421406.3	5
421408.4	大；破裂；離断；部分欠損；出血量が全血液量の20%を超える	421408.4	421408.4	5
422099.2	**その他の動脈** 例：**気管支動脈，食道動脈，肋間動脈，内胸動脈** 詳細不明 ［OIS Ⅰに相当する］	422099.2	422099.2	5
422002.2	内膜剥離，断裂なし	422002.2	422002.2	5
422004.2	裂傷・裂創；穿孔；穿刺 詳細不明	422004.2	422004.2	5
422006.2	小；表在性；非全周性；出血量が全血液量の20%以下	422006.2	422006.2	5
422008.3	大；破裂；離断；部分欠損；出血量が全血液量の20%を超える	422008.3	422008.3	5

[b] AIS2005で重症度に変更あり。
[c] 旧版の AIS では両側損傷はそれぞれ別にコード選択をしていた。AIS2005では，"両側"を導入した。いくつかの両側損傷は重症度が変化し，その結果 ISS が変わることがある。

AIS 2005	Injury Description	⇒ AIS98	⇐ AIS98	FCI
420699.3	**Brachiocephalic (innominate) vein** NFS [*OIS II* for entire category]	420699.3	420699.3	5
420602.3	laceration ; perforation ; puncture NFS	420602.3	420602.3	5
420604.3	minor ; superficial ; incomplete circumferential involvement ; blood loss≤20% by volume	420604.3	420604.3	5
420606.4	major ; rupture ; transection ; segmental loss ; blood loss >20% by volume	420606.4	420606.4	5
420608.5	with air embolus right side	420608.5	420608.5	5
421299.3	**Pulmonary vein** NFS [*OIS IV, V* for entire category]	421299.3	421299.3	5
421202.3	laceration ; perforation ; puncture NFS	421202.3	421202.3	5
421204.3	minor ; superficial ; incomplete circumferential involvement ; blood loss≤20% by volume	421204.3	421204.3	5
421206.5	major ; rupture ; transection ; segmental loss ; blood loss >20% by volume	421206.4[b]	421206.4[b]	5
421207.6	bilateral[c]	421206.4[b]	None	1
421699.3	**Subclavian vein** NFS [*OIS II* for entire category]	421699.3	421699.3	5
421602.3	laceration ; perforation ; puncture NFS	421602.3	421602.3	5
421604.3	minor ; superficial ; incomplete circumferential involvement ; blood loss≤20% by volume	421604.3	421604.3	5
421606.4	major ; rupture ; transection ; segmental loss ; blood loss >20% by volume	421606.4	421606.4	5
421899.3	**Vena Cava, superior and thoracic portion of inferior**, NFS [*OIS IV, V* for entire category]	421899.3	421899.3	5
421802.3	laceration ; perforation ; puncture NFS	421802.3	421802.3	5
421804.3	minor ; superficial ; incomplete circumferential involvement ; blood loss≤20% by volume with or without thrombosis	421804.3	421804.3	5
421806.4	major ; rupture ; transection ; segmental loss ; blood loss >20% by volume	421806.4	421806.4	5
421808.5	with air embolus right side	421808.5	421808.5	5
422299.2	**Other named veins**, e.g., **azygos, bronchial, esophageal, hemiazygos, intercostal, internal jugular, internal mammary** [*OIS I* for entire category except **azygos and internal jugular**, *OIS II*]	422299.2	422299.2	5
422202.2	laceration ; perforation ; puncture NFS	422202.2	422202.2	5
422204.2	minor ; superficial ; incomplete circumferential involvement ; blood loss≤20% by volume	422204.2	422204.2	5

AIS 2005	損傷内容	⇒ AIS98	⇐ AIS98	FCI
420699.3	**腕頭（無名）静脈**　詳細不明　［すべて OIS II のカテゴリー］	420699.3	420699.3	5
420602.3	裂傷・裂創；穿孔；穿刺　詳細不明	420602.3	420602.3	5
420604.3	小；表在性；非全周性； 　　　　出血量が全血液量の20％以下	420604.3	420604.3	5
420606.4	大；破裂；離断；部分欠損；出血量が全血液量の20％ 　　　　を超える	420606.4	420606.4	5
420608.5	右心系に空気塞栓を伴う	420608.5	420608.5	5
421299.3	**肺静脈**　詳細不明　［すべて OIS IV, V のカテゴリー］	421299.3	421299.3	5
421202.3	裂傷・裂創；穿孔；穿刺　詳細不明	421202.3	421202.3	5
421204.3	小；表在性；非全周性； 　　　　出血量が全血液量の20％以下	421204.3	421204.3	5
421206.5	大；破裂；離断；部分欠損；出血量が全血液量の20％ 　　　　を超える	421206.4[b]	421206.4[b]	5
421207.6	両側[c]	421206.4[b]	なし	1
421699.3	**鎖骨下静脈**　詳細不明　［すべて OIS II のカテゴリー］	421699.3	421699.3	5
421602.3	裂傷・裂創；穿孔；穿刺　詳細不明	421602.3	421602.3	5
421604.3	小；表在性；非全周性； 　　　　出血量が全血液量の20％以下	421604.3	421604.3	5
421606.4	大；破裂；離断；部分欠損；出血量が全血液量の20％ 　　　　を超える	421606.4	421606.4	5
421899.3	**上大静脈，胸腔内下大静脈**　詳細不明　［すべて OIS IV, V の カテゴリー］	421899.3	421899.3	5
421802.3	裂傷・裂創；穿孔；穿刺　詳細不明	421802.3	421802.3	5
421804.3	小；表在性；非全周性； 　　　　出血量が全血液量の20％以下　血栓の有無を問わない	421804.3	421804.3	5
421806.4	大；破裂；離断；部分欠損；出血量が全血液量の20％ 　　　　を超える	421806.4	421806.4	5
421808.5	右心系に空気塞栓を伴う	421808.5	421808.5	5
422299.2	**その他の静脈**，例：**奇静脈，気管支静脈，食道静脈，半奇静脈， 肋間静脈，内頸静脈，内胸静脈**　［すべて OIS I のカテゴリー， 奇静脈と内頸静脈は OIS II］	422299.2	422299.2	5
422202.2	裂傷・裂創；穿孔；穿刺　詳細不明	422202.2	422202.2	5
422204.2	小；表在性；非全周性； 　　　　出血量が全血液量の20％以下	422204.2	422204.2	5

AIS 2005	Injury Description	⇒ AIS98	⇐ AIS98	FCI
422206.3	major ; rupture ; transection ; segmental loss ; blood loss >20% by volume	422206.3	422206.3	5

---

[b] Change in severity in AIS 2005
[c] In previous editions of AIS, each injury was coded separately. AIS 2005 introduces "bilateral" for certain injuries. Some bilateral injuries may affect severity levels and, therefore, the ISS for patients with those injuries.

AIS 2005	損傷内容	⇒ AIS98	⇐ AIS98	FCI
422206.3	大；破裂；離断；部分欠損；出血量が全血液量の20%を超える	422206.3	422206.3	5

---

[b] AIS2005で重症度に変更あり。
[c] 旧版の AIS では両側損傷はそれぞれ別にコード選択をしていた。AIS2005では，"両側"を導入した。いくつかの両側損傷は重症度が変化し，その結果 ISS が変わることがある。

AIS 2005	Injury Description	⇒ AIS98	⇐ AIS98	FCI
	NERVES			
430499.1	**Vagus nerve injury**
See also Head, Neck and Abdomen body regions.	430499.1	430499.1	5

CODING RULES : Thorax

Organ Injury Scales (OIS)

The organ injury grading system may be helpful in determining injury severity, but the grades should not be used as a substitute for clinical descriptions of injuries. For example, specific information recorded in the hospital chart about depth of laceration, vessel involvement or extent of penetration associated with an organ injury should take precedence over a surgeon's designation of a particular OIS grade for the injury. If no relevant detailed descriptive clinical information is available, however, it is reasonable to rely on the OIS grade recorded.

Multiple Trauma

Each documented diagnosis is assigned a separate AIS code. For example, if a patient sustains a left lung contusion, hemothorax and multiple rib fractures and all three diagnoses are substantiated, the appropriate codes are : lung contusion, unilateral NFS, 441406.2 ; hemothorax NFS, 442200.3 ; multiple rib fractures NFS, 450210.2.

Penetrating Injuries

An injury that penetrates the torso with both entry and exit wounds (i.e., through and through injury), but does not injure any internal anatomical structure is coded as a soft tissue injury under the Whole Area. If underlying structures or organs are injured, these are coded and not the soft tissue injury.

AIS 2005	損傷内容	⇒AIS98	⇐AIS98	FCI
	神 経			
430499.1	迷走神経損傷	430499.1	430499.1	5
	頭部，頸部，腹部の領域も参照。			

コード選択のルール：**胸部**

Organ Injury Score (OIS)

臓器損傷の重症度評価システムは外傷重症度の決定に有用である場合もあるが，外傷症例に対する臨床的記載の代用とすべきではない。例えば，裂傷・裂創の深さ，臓器損傷に合併した血管損傷や穿通の範囲などカルテに記載される特別な外傷の情報は，外科医が判断した詳細な OIS の記載より優先させるべきである。もし，臨床的な詳細情報が適切に記載されていなければ OIS の記載を用いるのが妥当である。

多発外傷

記載されたそれぞれの外傷診断に対して AIS コードを割り当てる。例えば左肺挫傷，血胸および多発肋骨骨折がある場合には，3つのすべての診断を記載する。適切なコードは片側の肺損傷　詳細不明，441406.2；血胸　詳細不明，442200.3；多発肋骨骨折　詳細不明，450210.2となる。

穿通性損傷

入口部と出口部の創が認められる体幹の穿通性損傷（例；貫通損傷）において解剖学的構造物損傷がなければ，全域の軟部組織損傷を選択する。もし，内部の構造物や臓器が損傷していればそれらのコードを付けて軟部組織損傷は選択しない。

AIS 2005	Injury Description	⇒ AIS98	⇐ AIS98	FCI
	INTERNAL ORGANS			
440099.9	**Bronchus injury** NFS[f]	None	None	
440199.3	**Bronchus, main stem,** NFS[l]	442699.3	442699.3	5
440102.3	contusion ; hematoma	442602.3	442602.3	5
440104.3	laceration ; tear NFS	442604.3	442604.3	5
440106.3	no perforation ; partial thickness	442606.3	442606.3	5
440108.4	perforation ; full thickness ; "fracture"	442608.4	442608.4[m]	5
440110.5	complex ; avulsion ; rupture ; transection ; with separation	442610.5	442610.5[n]	5
440299.1	**Bronchus, distal to main stem** NFS	440299.1	440299.1	5
440202.1	contusion ; hematoma	440202.1	440202.1	5
440204.2	laceration ; tear NFS	440204.2	440204.2	5
440206.2	no perforation ; partial thickness	440206.2	440206.2	5
440208.3	perforation ; full thickness ; "fracture"	440208.3	440208.3[o]	5
440210.4	complex ; avulsion ; rupture ; transection ; with separation	440210.4	440210.4[p]	5
440699.2	**Diaphragm** NFS	440699.2	440699.2	5
440602.2	contusion ; hematoma [OIS I]	440602.2	440602.2	5
440604.2	laceration NFS[e]	440604.3[b]	440604.3[b]	5
440606.3	≤10cm [OIS II, III]	440604.3	None	5
440608.4	>10cm ; with significant tissue loss [OIS IV, V]	440604.3[b]	None	5
440610.4	rupture with herniation	440606.4	440606.4	5

---

[b] Change in severity in AIS 2005

[e] In AIS 98, this injury description had only one severity level ; in AIS 2005, it has several.

[f] New descriptor in AIS 2005 that allows classification of trauma by body region, but does not allow assigning a severity code.

[l] Trachea and Main Stem Bronchus were combined as one descriptor in AIS 98. In AIS 2005, each is a separate category ; hence, the duplication of AIS 98 matching codes.

[m] Also matches with 442612.4 and 442614.4 in AIS 98

[n] Also matches with 442616.5 in AIS 98

[o] Also matches with 440212.3 and 440214.3 in AIS 98

[p] Also matches with 440216.4 in AIS 98

AIS 2005	損傷内容	⇒ AIS98	⇐ AIS98	FCI
	内 臓			
440099.9	気管支損傷　詳細不明[f]	なし	なし	
440199.3	**気管支，主気管支**　詳細不明[l]	442699.3	442699.3	5
440102.3	挫傷；血腫	442602.3	442602.3	5
440104.3	裂傷・裂創；断裂　詳細不明	442604.3	442604.3	5
440106.3	穿孔なし；非全層性	442606.3	442606.3	5
440108.4	穿孔；全層性；"骨折"	442608.4	442608.4[m]	5
440110.5	複雑；断裂；破裂；離断；断裂を伴う	442610.5	442610.5[n]	5
440299.1	**主気管支より末梢の気管支**　詳細不明	440299.1	440299.1	5
440202.1	挫傷；血腫	440202.1	440202.1	5
440204.2	裂傷・裂創；詳細不明	440204.2	440204.2	5
440206.2	穿孔なし；非全層性	440206.2	440206.2	5
440208.3	穿孔；全層性；"骨折"	440208.3	440208.3[o]	5
440210.4	複雑；断裂；破裂；離断；断裂を伴う	440210.4	440210.4[p]	5
440699.2	**横隔膜**　詳細不明	440699.2	440699.2	5
440602.2	挫傷；血腫　[OIS I]	440602.2	440602.2	5
440604.2	裂傷・裂創　詳細不明[e]	440604.3[b]	440604.3[b]	5
440606.3	10cm以下　[OIS II, III]	440604.3	なし	5
440608.4	10cmを超える；広範な組織欠損　[OIS IV, V]	440604.3[b]	なし	5
440610.4	ヘルニアを伴う破裂	440606.4	440606.4	5

[b] AIS2005で重症度に変更あり．
[e] AIS98ではこの損傷コードは1つだけであったが，AIS2005においては複数個ある．
[f] AIS2005に加えられた新しいコード．外傷の存在部位を示すことができる．ただし重症度はない．
[l] AIS98では気管と気管支は同一の記載．AIS2005ではそれぞれ別のカテゴリーであり，AIS98のコードを変換すると重複するコード．
[m] AIS98の442612.4と442614.4に一致するコード．
[n] AIS98の442616.5に一致するコード．
[o] AIS98の440212.3と440214.3に一致するコード．
[p] AIS98の440216.4に一致するコード．

THORAX

AIS 2005	Injury Description	⇒ AIS98	⇐ AIS98	FCI
440899.2	**Esophagus injury in Thorax** NFS	440899.2	440899.2	5
	See also Neck body region. Code to Neck if site NFS. If injury occurs at junction of neck and thorax (i.e., at sternal notch), assign to Neck.			
440802.2	contusion ; hematoma [OIS I]	440802.2	440802.2	5
440805.3	ingestion injury NFS[a]	440899.2[b]	None	5
440807.3	partial-thickness necrosis[a]	440899.2[b]	None	5
440809.4	full-thickness necrosis[a]	440899.2[b]	None	3
440804.3	laceration ; tear NFS	440804.3	440804.3	5
440806.3	no perforation ; partial thickness ; ≤50 % circumference [OIS I, II]	440806.3	440806.3	5
440808.4	perforation; full thickness; >50% circumference [OIS III]	440808.4	440808.4	5
440810.5	avulsion ; rupture ; transection ; massive destruction [OIS IV, V]	440810.5	440810.5	3
441099.1	**Heart (Myocardium) injury** NFS	441099.1	441099.1	5
441089.9	with cardiac arrest NFS[f]	None	None	
441002.1	contusion NFS	441002.1	441002.1	5
441004.1	minor [OIS I]	441004.1	441004.1	5
	Patients presenting with dysrhythmia, wall motion abnormality, other ECG changes not related to CAD.			
441006.4	major	441006.4	441006.4	5
	Must be substantiated e.g., by surgery, autopsy, EF <25% absent CAD.			
441008.3	laceration NFS	441008.3	441008.3	5
441010.3	no perforation ; no chamber involvement	441010.3	441010.3	5
441012.5	perforation, ventricular or atrial, with or without tamponade	441012.5	441012.5	5
441013.5	atrial rupture[a]	None	None	5
441014.6	ventricular rupture	441014.6	441014.6	1
441016.6	multiple lacerations ; > 50 % tissue loss of a chamber	441016.6	441016.6	1
441018.6	avulsion	441018.6	441018.6	1

---

[a] New descriptor in AIS 2005
[b] Change in severity in AIS 2005
[f] New descriptor in AIS 2005 that allows classification of trauma by body region but does not allow assigning a severity code.

胸　部

AIS 2005	損傷内容	⇒ AIS98	⇐ AIS98	FCI
440899.2	**胸部食道損傷**　詳細不明	440899.2	440899.2	5
	頸部の領域も確認する。損傷部位の詳細が不明であれば頸部食道のコードを選択する。損傷部が頸部・胸部の移行部（例：胸骨切痕部）であれば頸部食道のコードを選択する。			
440802.2	挫傷；血腫［OIS I］	440802.2	440802.2	5
440805.3	経口摂取による障害　詳細不明[a]	440899.2[b]	なし	5
440807.3	非全層性壊死[a]	440899.2[b]	なし	5
440809.4	全層性壊死[a]	440899.2[b]	なし	3
440804.3	裂傷・裂創；詳細不明	440804.3	440804.3	5
440806.3	穿孔なし；非全層性；周径の50％以下　［OIS I, II］	440806.3	440806.3	5
440808.4	穿孔；全層性；周径の50％を超える　［OIS III］	440808.4	440808.4	5
440810.5	剝離；破裂；離断；広範囲損傷　［OIS IV, V］	440810.5	440810.5	3
441099.1	**心臓（心筋）損傷**　詳細不明	441099.1	441099.1	5
441089.9	心停止を伴う　詳細不明[f]	なし	なし	
441002.1	挫傷　詳細不明	441002.1	441002.1	5
441004.1	小［OIS I］	441004.1	441004.1	5
	冠動脈疾患に関連しない，不整脈，壁運動異常および心電図変化。			
441006.4	大	441006.4	441006.4	5
	冠動脈疾患に関連しておらず，外科手術，剖検またはEF25％以下の所見を実証しなければならない。			
441008.3	裂傷・裂創　詳細不明	441008.3	441008.3	5
441010.3	穿孔なし；心室・心房損傷なし	441010.3	441010.3	5
441012.5	穿孔；心室・心房の穿孔を認め，タンポナーデの有無は問わない	441012.5	441012.5	5
441013.5	心房破裂[a]	なし	なし	5
441014.6	心室破裂	441014.6	441014.6	1
441016.6	多発裂傷・裂創；心室・心房の50％を超える組織欠損	441016.6	441016.6	1
441018.6	断裂	441018.6	441018.6	1

---

[a] AIS2005に加えられた新しいコード。
[b] AIS2005で重症度に変更あり。
[f] AIS2005に加えられた新しいコード。外傷の存在部位を示すことができる。ただし重症度はない。

THORAX

AIS 2005	Injury Description	⇒ AIS98	⇐ AIS98	FCI
440400.5	**Intracardiac chordae tendineae** laceration ; rupture	440400.5	440400.5	5
441300.5	**Intracardiac septum** laceration ; rupture	441300.5	441300.5	4
441200.5	**Intracardiac valve** laceration ; rupture	441200.5	441200.5	4
441499.3	**Lung** NFS	441499.3	441499.3	5
441420.3	blast injury (overpressure/explosive) NFS[a]	441499.3	None	5
441422.3	mild[a]	441499.3	None	5
441424.4	moderate ; uni/bilateral with pulmonary peripheral hemorrhage[a]	441499.3[b]	None	5
441426.5	severe ; bilateral with air embolus[a]	441499.3[b]	None	5
441402.3	contusion NFS	441402.3	441402.3	5

> Contusion should be coded only if there is history of chest trauma **and** a physician's diagnosis is documented by x-ray, CT, MRI, surgery or autopsy. Clinical pulmonary dysfunction (e.g., atelectasis or effusion) is insufficient evidence of a codeable injury.

AIS 2005	Injury Description	⇒ AIS98	⇐ AIS98	FCI
441406.2	unilateral NFS[e]	441406.3[b]	441406.3[b]	5
441407.2	minor ; <1 lobe	441406.3[b]	None	5
441408.3	major ; ≥1 lobe	441406.3	None	5
441410.3	bilateral NFS[e]	441410.4[b]	441410.4[b]	5
441411.3	minor ; <1 lobe	441410.4[b]	None	5
441412.4	major ; ≥1 lobe in at least one lung	441410.4	None	5
441414.3	laceration NFS	441414.3	441414.3	5
441430.3	unilateral NFS[e]	441430.3	441430.3	5
441431.3	minor ; <1 lobe	441430.3	None	5
441432.4	major ; ≥1 lobe	441430.3[b]	None	5
441450.4	bilateral NFS[e]	441450.4	441450.4	5
441551.4	minor ; <1 lobe	441450.4	None	5
441452.5	major ; ≥1 lobe in at least one lung	441450.4[b]	None	5

---

[a] New descriptor in AIS 2005
[b] Change in severity in AIS 2005
[e] In AIS 98, this injury description had only one severity level ; in AIS 2005, it has several.

胸　部

AIS 2005	損傷内容	⇒ AIS98	⇐ AIS98	FCI
440400.5	**心筋腱索**の裂傷・裂創；破裂	440400.5	440400.5	5
441300.5	**心室または心房中隔**の裂傷・裂創；破裂	441300.5	441300.5	4
441200.5	**心臓弁**の裂傷・裂創；破裂	441200.5	441200.5	4
441499.3	**肺**　詳細不明	441499.3	441499.3	5
441420.3	爆風傷（過度の圧力／爆発）　詳細不明[a]	441499.3	なし	5
441422.3	軽症[a]	441499.3	なし	5
441424.4	中等症；片側または両側の胸腔内出血を伴う[a]	441499.3[b]	なし	5
				5
441426.5	重症；両側の空気塞栓を伴う[a]	441499.3[b]	なし	
441402.3	挫傷　詳細不明	441402.3	441402.3	5

> 挫傷は胸部外傷の既往があり，かつ，X線，CT，MRI，手術または剖検により医師が肺損傷と診断した場合にのみコードを選択する。臨床的な肺機能障害（例：無気肺，胸水）はコード選択できる損傷としては十分ではない。

AIS 2005	損傷内容	⇒ AIS98	⇐ AIS98	FCI
441406.2	片側　詳細不明[e]	441406.3[b]	441406.3[b]	5
441407.2	小：一葉未満	441406.3[b]	なし	5
441408.3	大：一葉以上	441406.3	なし	5
441410.3	両側　詳細不明[e]	441410.4[b]	441410.4[b]	5
441411.3	小：一葉未満	441410.4[b]	なし	5
441412.4	大：少なくとも一側肺の一葉以上	441410.4	なし	5
441414.3	裂傷・裂創　詳細不明	441414.3	441414.3	5
441430.3	片側　詳細不明[e]	441430.3	441430.3	5
441431.3	小：一葉未満	441430.3	なし	5
441432.4	大：一葉以上	441430.3[b]	なし	5
441450.4	両側　詳細不明[e]	441450.4	441450.4	5
441551.4	小：一葉未満	441550.4	なし	5
441452.5	大：少なくとも一側肺の一葉以上	441450.4[b]	なし	5

---

[a] AIS2005に加えられた新しいコード。
[b] AIS2005で重症度に変更あり。
[e] AIS98ではこの損傷コードは1つだけであったが，AIS2005においては複数個ある。

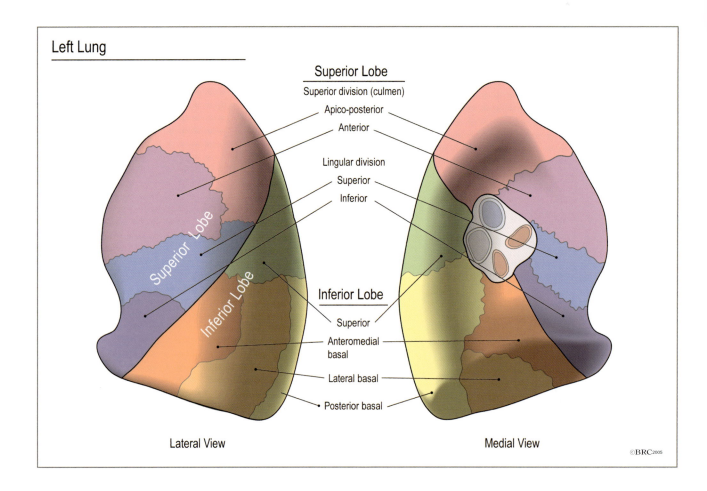

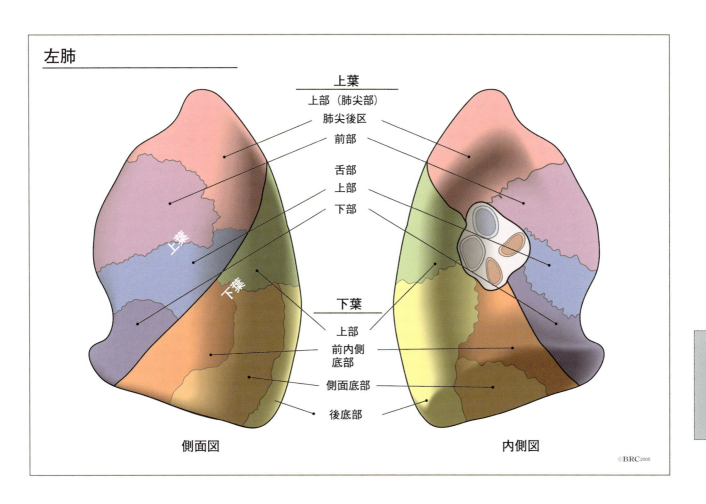

AIS 2005	Injury Description	⇒ AIS98	⇐ AIS98	FCI
	Lung (continued)			
419200.2	inhalation injury NFS (heat, particulate matter, noxious agents)	919200.2	919200.2	5
	Any one or combination of conditions may be present in the following injury descriptors.			
419201.2	absence of carbonaceous deposits, erythema, edema, bronchorrhea, obstruction	919201.2	919201.2	5
419202.3	minor or patchy areas of erythema, bronchorrhea, carbonaceous deposits in proximal or distal bronchi	919202.3	919202.3	5
419204.4	moderate degree of erythema, carbonaceous deposits, bronchorrhea with or without compromise of the bronchi	919204.4	919204.4	5
419206.5	severe inflammation with friability, copious carbonaceous deposits, bronchorrhea, bronchial obstruction, hypoxemia	919206.5	919206.5	5
419208.6	evidence of mucosal sloughing, necrosis, endoluminal obliteration	919208.6	919208.6	1
441699.2	**Pericardium** NFS	441699.2	441699.2	5
441602.2	laceration ; puncture	441602.2	441602.2	5
441603.3	hemopericardium NFS[a]	441699.2[b]	None	5
441604.3	without cardiac tamponade or heart injury[a]	441699.2[b]	None	5
441605.4	with cardiac tamponade but without heart injury	441604.3[b]	441604.3[b]	5
441606.5	herniation of heart through pericardium	441606.5	441606.5	5
441800.2	**Pleura** laceration	441800.2	441800.2	5

---

[a] New descriptors in AIS 2005
[b] Change in severity in AIS 2005

AIS 2005	損傷内容	⇒ AIS98	⇐ AIS98	FCI
	肺（続き）			
419200.2	吸入損傷　詳細不明（加熱，粒状物質，有害物質，腐食性物質）	919200.2	919200.2	5
	下記の外傷記述においていずれか1つ以上の状態があれば選択する。			
419201.2	すすの沈着，発赤，浮腫，気道分泌物，気管支閉塞の所見がない	919201.2	919201.2	5
419202.3	近位または遠位気管支への軽度または班状の発赤，気道分泌物，すすの沈着がある	919202.3	919202.3	5
419204.4	中等度の発赤，すすの沈着，気道分泌物（ただし，気管支損傷の有無を問わない）	919204.4	919204.4	5
419206.5	重度の炎症，多量のすすの沈着，多量の気道分泌物，気管支閉塞，低酸素血症	919206.5	919206.5	5
419208.6	粘膜の脱落，壊死，内腔の消失	919208.6	919208.6	1
441699.2	**心膜（心嚢）**　詳細不明	441699.2	441699.2	5
441602.2	裂傷・裂創；穿刺	441602.2	441602.2	5
441603.3	心膜（心嚢）・心膜血腫　詳細不明[a]	441699.2[b]	なし	5
441604.3	心タンポナーデや心損傷を伴わない[a]	441699.2[b]	なし	5
441605.4	心損傷を合併しない心タンポナーデ	441604.3[b]	441604.3[b]	5
441606.5	心嚢からの心ヘルニア	441606.5	441606.5	5
441800.2	**胸膜**　裂傷・裂創	441800.2	441800.2	5

[a] AIS2005に加えられた新しいコード。
[b] AIS2005で重症度に変更あり。

THORAX

AIS 2005	Injury Description	⇒ AIS98	⇐ AIS98	FCI
	Code the following types of thoracic trauma separate from and in addition to all documented thoracic injuries.			
442999.9	**Thoracic injury** NFS	442999.9	442999.9	
442200.3	**Hemothorax** NFS[q]	442202.3	442202.3	5
442201.4	major ; >1000cc blood loss on at least one side	442208.4	442208.4	5
442202.2	**Pneumothorax** NFS[q]	442202.3[b]	442202.3[b]	5
442203.4	major ; >50% collapse of lung documented on xray ; persistent air leak	442202.3[b]	None	5
442204.5	tension ; massive air leak	442210.5	442210.5	5
442205.3	**Hemopneumothorax** NFS	442202.3	442202.3	5
442206.4	major ; >1000cc blood loss on at least one side[a]	442202.3[b]	None	5
442207.5	**Air Embolus**	442212.5	442212.5	5
442208.2	**Hemomediastinum**	442206.4[b]	442206.4[b]	5
442209.2	**Pneumomediastinum**	442204.3[b]	442204.3[b]	5
442210.3	with cardiac tamponade[a]	442204.3	None	5
442402.2	**Thoracic duct** laceration	442402.2	442402.2	5
442502.2	**Thymus** laceration ; perforation[a]	None	None	5
442699.3	**Trachea injury in Thorax** NFS[l]	442699.3	442699.3	5
	See also Neck body region. Code to Neck if site NFS. If injury occurs at junction of neck and thorax (e.g., at sternal notch), assign to Neck.			
442602.3	contusion ; hematoma	442602.3	442602.3	5
442604.3	laceration NFS	442604.3	442604.3	5
442606.3	no perforation ; partial thickness	442606.3	442606.3	5
442608.4	perforation ; full thickness ; "fracture"	442608.4[m]	442608.4[m]	5
442610.5	avulsion ; rupture ; transection ; massive destruction ; crush ; laryngeal-tracheal separation	442610.5[n]	442610.5[n]	4

---

[a] New descriptor in AIS 2005
[b] Change in AIS 2005
[l] Trachea and Main Stem Bronchus were combined as one descriptor in AIS 98. In AIS 2005, each is a separate category ; hence, the duplication of AIS 98 matching codes.
[m] Also matches with 442612.4 or 442614.4 in AIS 98.
[n] Also matches with 442616.5 in AIS 98.
[q] Hemo/pneumothorax were combined as one descriptor in AIS 98. In AIS 2005, each is a separate category ; hence, the duplication of AIS 98 matching codes.

AIS 2005	損傷内容	⇒AIS98	⇐AIS98	FCI
	すべての胸部損傷の記載に加えて，以下の外傷を個別にコード選択する。			
442999.9	胸部損傷　詳細不明	442999.9	442999.9	
442200.3	血胸　詳細不明[q]	442202.3	442202.3	5
442201.4	大：少なくとも片側で1000mlを超える出血	442208.4	442208.4	5
442202.2	気胸　詳細不明[q]	442202.3[b]	442202.3[b]	5
442203.4	大：X線検査で50%を超える肺の虚脱；48時間以上持続する空気漏れ	442202.3[b]	なし	5
442204.5	緊張性：大量の空気漏れ	442210.5	442210.5	5
442205.3	血気胸　詳細不明	442202.3	442202.3	5
442206.4	大：少なくとも片側に1000mlを超える出血[a]	442202.3[b]	なし	5
442207.5	空気塞栓	442212.5	442212.5	5
442208.2	縦隔血腫	442206.4[b]	442206.4[b]	5
442209.2	縦隔気腫	442204.3[b]	442204.3[b]	5
442210.3	心タンポナーデを伴う[a]	442204.3	なし	5
442402.2	胸管　裂傷・裂創	442402.2	442402.2	5
442502.2	胸腺　裂傷・裂創；穿孔[a]	なし	なし	5
442699.3	胸部気管損傷　詳細不明[l]	442699.3	442699.3	5
	頸部の章も参照。部位が不明であれば頸部のコードを選択する。頸部・胸部の移行部（例：胸骨切痕）は頸部のコードを選択する。			
442602.3	挫傷；血腫	442602.3	442602.3	5
442604.3	裂傷・裂創　詳細不明	442604.3	442604.3	5
442606.3	穿孔なし；非全層性	442606.3	442606.3	5
442608.4	穿孔；全層性；"骨折"	442608.4[m]	442608.4[m]	5
442610.5	断裂；破裂；離断；広範な破壊；粉砕；咽頭と気管の分離	442610.5[n]	442610.5[n]	4

[a] AIS2005に加えられた新しいコード。
[b] AIS2005で重症度に変更あり。
[l] AIS98では気管と気管支は同一の記載。AIS2005ではそれぞれ別のカテゴリーであり，AIS98のコードを変換すると重複するコード。
[m] AIS98の442612.4と442614.4に一致するコード。
[n] AIS98の442616.5に一致するコード。
[q] AIS98では血/気胸は1つの記述にまとめられていた。AIS2005では別々にコードされる。

THORAX

AIS 2005	Injury Description	⇒ AIS98	⇐ AIS98	FCI

CODING RULES : Rib Fractures

The rib cage is treated as a single anatomical structure for coding fractures without flail and for bilateral flail. However, if a flail chest is documented on one side (unilateral) and fractured ribs without flail are documented on the other side, code as two separate injuries.

"Flail chest" is defined as three or more ribs fractured in more than one location (e.g., posterolateral and anterolateral) and/or resulting in paradoxical chest movement.

Multiple rib fractures, if documented but not further described, should be assigned 450210.2.

Costal cartilage fracture or tear is coded as a rib fracture.

For patients who die before any radiology is done and no autopsy is performed, a clinical diagnosis of multiple rib fractures made by detecting thoracic cage instability is acceptable for AIS coding. In such cases, use AIS code 450210.2. However, clinically diagnosed rib fractures in survivors are never coded ; these must be substantiated radiologically.

SKELETAL including thoracic wall involvement

AIS 2005	Injury Description	⇒ AIS98	⇐ AIS98	FCI
450299.1	**Rib Cage** NFS	450299.1	450299.1	5
450289.1	contusion	450202.1	450202.1	
	Read "Rib Fractures" for coding rules.			
450210.2	multiple rib fractures NFS	450210.2	450210.2	5
450200.1	fracture(s) without flail, any location unilateral or bilateral NFS	450212.1	450212.1	5
450201.1	one rib [OIS I]	450212.1	450212.1	5
450202.2	two ribs [OIS I]	450220.2	450220.2	5
450203.3	≥3 ribs [OIS II]	450230.3	450230.3	5
450209.3	fractures with flail, NFS	450260.3	450260.3	5
450211.3	unilateral flail chest NFS [OIS IV]	450260.3	450260.3	5
450212.3	3-5 flail ribs [OIS IV]	450260.3	None	5
450213.4	>5 flail ribs [OIS IV]	450260.3[b]	None	5
450214.5	bilateral flail chest [OIS V]	450266.5	450266.5	5
450899.1	**Sternum** NFS	450899.1	450899.1	5
450802.1	contusion	450802.1	450802.1	5
450804.2	fracture [OIS II, III]	450804.2	450804.2	5
451099.1	**Thoracic Wall** NFS[a]	None	None	5
451020.4	avulsion of chest wall tissues including rib cage [OIS IV for entire category][a]	None	None	5
451021.4	minor ; ≤15% of chest wall including rib cage[a]	None	None	5
451022.5	major ; >15% of chest wall including rib cage[a]	None	None	5

---

[a] New descriptor in AIS 2005
[b] Change in severity in AIS 2005

AIS 2005	損傷内容	⇒ AIS98	⇐ AIS98	FCI

コード選択のルール：**肋骨骨折**

肋骨は片側または両側の動揺性がない場合には1つの解剖学的構造物として取り扱う。しかし，片側にフレイルチェスト（胸郭動揺）が認められ，他方にフレイルチェストが認められない場合には別々に2つのコードを記載する。"フレイルチェスト"は隣り合う3本以上の肋骨にそれぞれ2カ所以上の骨折を認め（後側部と前側部），呼吸と逆の胸郭運動の有無は問わない状態と定義される。
多発肋骨骨折で詳細な記載がない場合には450210.2を選択する。
肋軟骨骨折や裂傷は肋骨骨折のコードを選択する。
死亡前のX線検査や剖検が施行されなかった場合，胸郭の不安定性から臨床所見より多発肋骨骨折と診断されていた場合にも，AISコードのコード選択は容認できる。そのような場合には450210.2のコードを用いる。しかし，生存例には臨床所見でのコード選択はできず，X線検査による診断を要する。

胸壁を構成する骨格

AIS 2005	損傷内容	⇒ AIS98	⇐ AIS98	FCI
450299.1	**肋骨** 詳細不明	450299.1	450299.1	5
450289.1	挫傷	450202.1	450202.1	
	肋骨骨折のコード選択のルールを参照。			
450210.2	多発肋骨骨折　詳細不明	450210.2	450210.2	5
450200.1	フレイルチェストを伴わない骨折，片側または両側　詳細不明	450212.1	450212.1	5
450201.1	1本の肋骨　[OIS I]	450212.1	450212.1	5
450202.2	2本の肋骨　[OIS I]	450220.2	450220.2	5
450203.3	3本以上の肋骨　[OIS II]	450230.3	450230.3	5
450209.3	フレイルチェストを伴う骨折　詳細不明	450260.3	450260.3	5
450211.3	片側性フレイルチェスト　詳細不明　[OIS IV]	450260.3	450260.3	5
450212.3	3～5本の動揺性骨折　[OIS IV]	450260.3	なし	5
450213.4	5本を超える動揺性骨折　[OIS IV]	450260.3[b]	なし	5
450214.5	両側のフレイルチェスト　[OIS V]	450266.5	450266.5	5
450899.1	**胸骨** 詳細不明	450899.1	450899.1	5
450802.1	挫傷	450802.1	450802.1	5
450804.2	骨折　[OIS II, III]	450804.2	450804.2	5
451099.1	**胸壁** 詳細不明[a]	なし	なし	5
451020.4	肋骨を含む胸壁の組織欠損　[OIS IVに相当する][a]	なし	なし	5
451021.4	小：肋骨を含む胸壁15%以下の欠損[a]	なし	なし	5
451022.5	大：肋骨を含む胸壁15%を超える欠損[a]	なし	なし	5

[a] AIS2005に加えられた新しいコード。
[b] AIS2005で重症度に変更あり。

腹　部

ABDOMEN

AIS 2005	Injury Description	⇒ AIS98	⇐ AIS98	FCI

WHOLE AREA

> Use one of the following two descriptors when such vague information is the only information available. While these descriptors identify the occurrence of an abdominal injury, they do not specify its severity.

500099.9	**Injuries to the Whole Abdomen** NFS	515099.9	515099.9	
500999.9	Died of abdominal injury without further substantiation of injuries or no autopsy confirmation of specific injuries	515999.9	515999.9	

> Use this category if penetrating injury does not involve internal structures. Assign to External body region for calculating an ISS. If underlying anatomical structures are involved, code documented diagnoses only ; do not use these generic descriptors.

516000.1	**Penetrating injury** NFS	516000.1	516000.1	5
516002.1	superficial ; minor ; into peritoneum but not involving underlying structures	516002.1	516002.1	5
516004.2	with tissue loss >100cm^2	516004.2	516004.2	5
516006.3	with blood loss >20% by volume	516006.3	516006.3	5
510100.2	**Rectus Abdominus** rupture NFS[a]	510099.1[b]	None	5
511000.6	**Torso** transection[a]	None	None	1

> Use the following section for blunt soft tissue injury to the abdomen. Assign to External body region for calculating an ISS. If injury is described as "degloving", code as avulsion.

510099.1	**Skin/Subcutaneous/Muscle [except rectus abdominus]** NFS	510099.1	510099.1	5
510202.1	abrasion	510202.1	510202.1	5
510402.1	contusion ; hematoma	510402.1	510402.1	5
510600.1	laceration NFS	510600.1	510600.1	5
510602.1	minor ; superficial	510602.1	510602.1	5
510604.2	major ; >20cm long <u>and</u> into subcutaneous tissue	510604.2	510604.2	5
510606.3	blood loss >20% by volume	510606.3	510606.3	5
510800.1	avulsion NFS	510800.1	510800.1	5
510802.1	minor ; superficial ; ≤100cm^2	510802.1	510802.1	5
510804.2	major ; >100cm^2	510804.2	510804.2	5
510806.3	blood loss >20% by volume	510806.3	510806.3	5

---

[a] New descriptor in AIS 2005
[b] Change in severity code in AIS 2005

腹　部

AIS 2005	損傷内容	⇒ AIS98	⇐ AIS98	FCI

> **全　域**
>
> 不確定な情報しか得られない場合には，以下の2つのコードのうちいずれかを選択する。これらのコードは腹部に損傷があることを示すものであるが，重症度を特定するものではない。

500099.9	**鈍的腹部損傷**　詳細不明	515099.9	515099.9	
500999.9	死亡（詳細な評価なし）；剖検なし	515999.9	515999.9	

> 深部組織の損傷を伴わない穿通性損傷には，以下のカテゴリーを選択する。ISS を算出する場合には，「腹部」ではなく「体表」の区分として取り扱う。深部組織の損傷を合併している場合には，記録されている診断名のみに対してコードを選択し，以下の包括的なコードは選択しない。

516000.1	**穿通性損傷**　詳細不明	516000.1	516000.1	5
516002.1	表在性；小；腹膜に達するが深部組織の損傷は伴わない	516002.1	516002.1	5
516004.2	組織欠損が100cm^{2}を超える	516004.2	516004.2	5
516006.3	出血量が全血液量の20%を超える	516006.3	516006.3	5
510100.2	**腹直筋断裂**　詳細不明[a]	510099.1[b]	なし	5
511000.6	**体幹部**離断[a]	なし	なし	1

> 腹部への軟部組織損傷には，以下のコードの中から適切なものを選択する。ただし，ISS を算出する場合には，「腹部」ではなく「体表」の区分として取り扱う。"デグロービング"と記載されている場合には，剥離のコードを選択する。

510099.1	**皮膚／皮下組織／筋肉［腹直筋を除く］**　詳細不明	510099.1	510099.1	5
510202.1	擦過傷	510202.1	510202.1	5
510402.1	挫傷；血腫	510402.1	510402.1	5
510600.1	裂傷・裂創　詳細不明	510600.1	510600.1	5
510602.1	小；表在性	510602.1	510602.1	5
510604.2	大；長さが20cmを超え，かつ皮下組織に達する	510604.2	510604.2	5
510606.3	出血量が全血液量の20%を超える	510606.3	510606.3	5
510800.1	剥離　詳細不明	510800.1	510800.1	5
510802.1	小；表在性；100cm^{2}以下	510802.1	510802.1	5
510804.2	大；100cm^{2}を超える	510804.2	510804.2	5
510806.3	出血量が全血液量の20%を超える	510806.3	510806.3	5

---

[a] AIS 2005に加えられた新しいコード。
[b] AIS 2005で重症度に変更あり。

ABDOMEN

AIS 2005	Injury Description	⇒ AIS98	⇐ AIS98	FCI

VESSELS

> Vessel injuries are coded separately from other injuries to the abdomen unless an organ injury descriptor includes the vessel injury. Branches of vessels are not coded unless they are named vessels and/or are listed within a specific vessel descriptor.

AIS 2005	Injury Description	⇒ AIS98	⇐ AIS98	FCI
520099.9	**Vascular Injury in Abdomen** NFS[f]	None	None	
520299.4	**Aorta, Abdominal** NFS	520299.4	520299.4	5
520202.4	intimal tear, no disruption	520202.4	520202.4	5
520204.4	laceration ; perforation ; puncture NFS	520204.4	520204.4	5
520206.4	minor ; superficial ; incomplete circumferential involvement ; blood loss ≤20% by volume	520206.4	520206.4	5
520208.5	major ; rupture ; transection ; segmental loss ; blood loss >20% by volume	520208.5	520208.5	5
520499.3	**Celiac Artery** NFS	520499.3	520499.3	5
520402.3	intimal tear ; no disruption	520402.3	520402.3	5
520404.3	laceration ; perforation ; puncture NFS	520404.3	520404.3	5
520406.4	minor ; superficial ; incomplete circumferential involvement ; blood loss ≤20% by volume	520406.4	520406.4	5
520408.5	major ; rupture ; transection ; segmental loss ; blood loss >20% by volume	520408.5	520408.5	5
520699.3	**Iliac Artery [common, internal, external]** and its named branches NFS	520699.3	520699.3	5
520698.4	bilateral[c] *for common iliac artery only*	520699.3[b]	None	5
520602.3	intimal tear, no disruption	520602.3	520602.3	5
520604.3	laceration ; perforation ; puncture NFS	520604.3	520604.3	5
520606.3	minor ; superficial ; incomplete circumferential involvement ; blood loss ≤20% by volume	520606.3	520606.3	5
520608.4	major ; rupture ; transection ; segmental loss ; blood loss >20% by volume	520608.4	520608.4	5

---

[b] Change in severity code in AIS 2005

[c] In previous editions of AIS, with few exceptions, each injury was coded separately. AIS 2005 introduces "bilateral". Some bilateral injuries may affect severity levels and, therefore, the ISS for patients with those injuries.

[f] New descriptor in AIS 2005 that allows classification of trauma by body region but does not allow assigning a severity code.

AIS 2005	損傷内容	⇒ AIS98	⇐ AIS98	FCI

血　管

> 血管損傷を含む臓器損傷のコードでない限り，血管損傷は他の腹部の損傷から独立した傷害としてコードを選択する。名前が付いている、あるいは特別にコードが存在しているもの以外は，血管分枝の損傷に対してコードは選択しない。

520099.9	腹部血管損傷　詳細不明[f]	なし	なし	
520299.4	**腹部大動脈**　詳細不明	520299.4	520299.4	5
520202.4	内膜剥離，断裂なし	520202.4	520202.4	5
520204.4	裂傷・裂創；穿孔；穿刺　詳細不明	520204.4	520204.4	5
520206.4	小；表在性；非全周性；出血量が全血液量の20%以下	520206.4	520206.4	5
520208.5	大；破裂；断裂；部分欠損；出血量が全血液量の20%を超える	520208.5	520208.5	5
520499.3	**腹腔動脈**　詳細不明	520499.3	520499.3	5
520402.3	内膜剥離，断裂なし	520402.3	520402.3	5
520404.3	裂傷・裂創；穿孔；穿刺　詳細不明	520404.3	520404.3	5
520406.4	小；表在性；非全周性；出血量が全血液量の20%以下	520406.4	520406.4	5
520408.5	大；破裂；断裂；部分欠損；出血量が全血液量の20%を超える	520408.5	520408.5	5
520699.3	**腸骨動脈［総，内，外］**（名前の付いた分枝血管を含む）　詳細不明	520699.3	520699.3	5
520698.4	両側[c]　総腸骨動脈に限る。	520699.3[b]	なし	5
520602.3	内膜剥離，断裂なし	520602.3	520602.3	5
520604.3	裂傷・裂創；穿孔；穿刺　詳細不明	520604.3	520604.3	5
520606.3	小；表在性；非全周性；出血量が全血液量の20%以下	520606.3	520606.3	5
520608.4	大；破裂；断裂；部分欠損；出血量が全血液量の20%を超える	520608.4	520608.4	5

---

[b] AIS 2005で重症度に変更あり。
[c] 旧版の AIS では一部の例外を除き両側損傷はそれぞれ別にコード選択をしていた。AIS 2005では，"両側"を導入した。いくつかの両側損傷は重症度が変化し，その結果 ISS が変わることがある。
[f] AIS 2005に加えられた新しいコード。外傷の存在部位を示すことができる。ただし重症度はない。

ABDOMEN

AIS 2005	Injury Description	⇒ AIS98	⇐ AIS98	FCI
521199.3	**Superior Mesenteric Artery** NFS[r]	521499.3	None	5
521102.3	intimal tear, no disruption	521402.3	None	5
521104.3	laceration ; perforation ; puncture NFS	521404.3	None	5
521106.3	minor ; superficial ; incomplete circumferential involvement ; blood loss ≤20% by volume	521406.3	None	5
521108.4	major ; rupture ; transection ; segmental loss ; blood loss >20% by volume	521408.4	None	5
521499.3	**Other named arteries** NFS [e.g., **hepatic, renal, splenic**]	521499.3	521499.3	5
521402.3	intimal tear, no disruption	521402.3	521402.3	5
521404.3	laceration ; perforation ; puncture NFS	521404.3	521404.3	5
521406.3	minor ; superficial ; incomplete circumferential involvement ; blood loss ≤20% by volume	521406.3	521406.3	5
521408.4	major ; rupture ; transection ; segmental loss ; blood loss >20% by volume	521408.4	521408.4	5
520899.3	**Iliac Vein [common]** NFS	520899.3	520899.3	5
520802.3	laceration ; perforation ; puncture NFS	520802.3	520802.3	5
520804.3	minor ; superficial ; incomplete circumferential involvement ; blood loss ≤20% by volume	520804.3	520804.3	5
520806.4	major ; rupture ; transection ; segmental loss ; blood loss >20% by volume	520806.4	520806.4	4
521099.2	**Iliac Vein [internal, external]** NFS	521099.2	521099.2	5
521002.2	laceration ; perforation ; puncture NFS	521002.2	521002.2	5
521004.2	minor ; superficial ; incomplete circumferential involvement ; blood loss ≤20% by volume	521004.2	521004.2	5
521006.3	major ; rupture ; transection ; segmental loss ; blood loss >20% by volume	521006.3	521006.3	4
521299.3	**Vena Cava, inferior** NFS	521299.3	521299.3	5
	See Liver for retrohepatic vena cava.			
521202.3	laceration ; perforation ; puncture NFS	521202.3	521202.3	5
521204.3	minor ; superficial ; incomplete circumferential involvement ; blood loss ≤20% by volume	521204.3	521204.3	5
521206.4	major ; rupture ; transection ; segmental loss ; blood loss >20% by volume	521206.4	521206.4	5

---

[r] The superior mesenteric artery was included in "other named arteries" in AIS 98. It is a separate injury descriptor in AIS 2005.

AIS 2005	損傷内容	⇒ AIS98	⇐ AIS98	FCI
521199.3	**上腸間膜動脈**　詳細不明[r]	521499.3	なし	5
521102.3	内膜剥離，断裂なし	521402.3	なし	5
521104.3	裂傷・裂創；穿孔；穿刺　詳細不明	521404.3	なし	5
521106.3	小；表在性；非全周性；出血量が全血液量の20%以下	521406.3	なし	5
521108.4	大；破裂；断裂；部分欠損；出血量が全血液量の20%を超える	521408.4	なし	5
521499.3	**その他の動脈**　詳細不明［例：**肝動脈，腎動脈，脾動脈**］	521499.3	521499.3	5
521402.3	内膜剥離，断裂なし	521402.3	521402.3	5
521404.3	裂傷・裂創；穿孔；穿刺　詳細不明	521404.3	521404.3	5
521406.3	小；表在性；非全周性；出血量が全血液量の20%以下	521406.3	521406.3	5
521408.4	大；破裂；断裂；部分欠損；出血量が全血液量の20%を超える	521408.4	521408.4	5
520899.3	**腸骨静脈［総］**　詳細不明	520899.3	520899.3	5
520802.3	裂傷・裂創；穿孔；穿刺　詳細不明	520802.3	520802.3	5
520804.3	小；表在性；非全周性；出血量が全血液量の20%以下	520804.3	520804.3	5
520806.4	大；破裂；断裂；部分欠損；全周性；出血量が全血液量の20%を超える	520806.4	520806.4	4
521099.2	**腸骨静脈［内，外］**　詳細不明	521099.2	521099.2	5
521002.2	裂傷・裂創；穿孔；穿刺　詳細不明	521002.2	521002.2	5
521004.2	小；表在性；非全周性；出血量が全血液量の20%以下	521004.2	521004.2	5
521006.3	大；破裂；断裂；部分欠損；出血量が全血液量の20%を超える	521006.3	521006.3	4
521299.3	**下大静脈**　詳細不明	521299.3	521299.3	5
	肝後面下大静脈は肝臓の項を参照。			
521202.3	裂傷・裂創；穿孔；穿刺　詳細不明	521202.3	521202.3	5
521204.3	小；表在性；非全周性；出血量が全血液量の20%以下	521204.3	521204.3	5
521206.4	大；破裂；断裂；部分欠損；出血量が全血液量の20%を超える	521206.4	521206.4	5

---

[r] 上腸間膜動脈は，AIS98では，その他の動脈に含まれていた。AIS 2005では独立したコードである。

ABDOMEN

AIS 2005	Injury Description	⇒ AIS98	⇐ AIS98	FCI
521699.3	**Other named veins** NFS [e.g., **portal, renal, splenic, superior mesenteric**]	521699.3	521699.3	5
521602.3	laceration ; perforation ; puncture NFS	521602.3	521602.3	5
521604.3	minor with or without thrombosis ; superficial ; incomplete circumferential involvement ; blood loss ≤20 % by volume	521604.3	521604.3	5
521606.4	major ; rupture ; transection ; segmental loss ; blood loss >20% by volume	521606.4	521606.4	5

NERVES

530499.1	**Vagus nerve injury**	530499.1	530499.1	5

See also Head, Neck and Thorax body regions.

AIS 2005	損傷内容	⇒ AIS98	⇐ AIS98	FCI
521699.3	その他の静脈　詳細不明［例：**門脈，腎静脈，脾静脈，上腸間膜静脈**］	521699.3	521699.3	5
521602.3	裂傷・裂創；穿孔；穿刺　詳細不明	521602.3	521602.3	5
521604.3	小；血栓の有無を問わない；表在性；非全周性；出血量が全血液量の 20%以下	521604.3	521604.3	5
521606.4	大；破裂；断裂；部分欠損；出血量が全血液量の 20%を超える	521606.4	521606.4	5

神　経

530499.1	迷走神経損傷	530499.1	530499.1	5

> 頭部，頸部および胸部の章も参照。

CODING RULES: Abdomen

Organ Injury Scales (OIS)

The organ injury grading system may be helpful in determining injury severity, but the grades should not be used as a substitute for clinical descriptions of injuries. For example, specific information recorded in the hospital chart about depth of laceration, vessel involvement or extent of penetration associated with an organ injury should take precedence over a surgeon's designation of a particular OIS grade for that injury. If no relevant detailed descriptive clinical information is available, however, it is reasonable to rely on the OIS grade recorded.

Organ Contusions, Lacerations

If an organ sustains both a contusion (i.e., perilesional) and a laceration that are directly related, code only the one of the two injuries that has the more severe AIS. If a contusion and a laceration are unrelated (i.e., located in different sites on/in the organ), code both injuries.

Duct Involvement

Duct involvement applies to gallbladder, liver and pancreas. Injuries to these organs, which share the same duct system, not infrequently involve injuries to the duct system of each organ. When only one ductal injury occurs, it should be assigned to either (not both) of the two involved organs. When separate ductal injuries (e.g., to the right hepatic duct and the pancreatic duct) occur, each should be assigned to the appropriate organ.

Penetrating Injury

An injury that penetrates the torso with both entry and exit wounds (i.e., through and through injury), but does not injure any internal anatomical structure is coded as a soft tissue injury under the Whole Area. If underlying structures or organs are injured, these are coded and not the soft tissue injury.

Injury Consequences

Abdominal compartment syndrome is a consequence of trauma, not an injury.

Fetal demise as a result of abdominal injury to a pregnant female is a consequence of trauma, not an injury itself.

コード選択のルール：腹部

Organ Injury Scales（OIS）

臓器損傷の重症度評価法は損傷の重症度を決定するのに役立つ可能性があるが，そのグレードを損傷に関する臨床的な記載内容の代用にすべきではない。例えば，臓器損傷に関連した裂傷・裂創の深さや，血管損傷の有無またはその損傷の程度が診療録に記載されている場合には，外科医が指示したOISのグレードよりも，それらの記載を優先すべきである。しかし，もしも適切な臨床情報に関する記載がない場合には，記録されているOISのグレードを参考にするのが合理的である。

臓器の挫傷，裂傷・裂創

挫傷とそれに直接関係する裂傷・裂創の双方をみとめる場合には，より重症度の高いAISのコードのみを選択する。挫傷と裂傷・裂創との間に関連性がない場合（例えば，同じ臓器ではあるが別の部位に存在する場合）には，両方の損傷のコードを選択する。

導管系（胆道系，膵管系）の損傷

「導管系の損傷の合併」は胆嚢，肝臓，膵臓に適用される。実際に1つの導管系を共有するこれらの臓器に損傷がある場合，しばしばそれぞれの臓器の導管系に損傷を伴う。1つの導管系の損傷の場合，その導管系が結ぶ2つの臓器のうちいずれか一方のコードを選択する。これに対し，別の2つの導管系に損傷が発生した場合（例えば，右肝管と膵管の損傷），両方の臓器のコードを選択する。

穿通性損傷

体幹部の穿通性損傷で，体幹内部の解剖学的構造が損なわれなかった場合（例えば，体幹皮膚から入り，そのまま皮膚から抜けた穿通性損傷），体表の区分の軟部組織損傷としてコードを選択する。もしも解剖学的構造の破綻や臓器損傷があった場合にはそれらについてのコードを選択し，軟部組織損傷のコードは選択しない。

続発する病態

腹部コンパートメント症候群は外傷の合併症であり，損傷ではない。

妊婦の腹部外傷による胎児死亡は，外傷の合併症であり，それ自体は損傷ではない。

ABDOMEN

AIS 2005	Injury Description	⇒ AIS98	⇐ AIS98	FCI
	INTERNAL ORGANS			
540299.1	**Adrenal Gland** NFS	540299.1	540299.1	5
540210.1	contusion ; hematoma NFS [OIS I]	540210.1	540210.1	5
540212.1	minor ; superficial [OIS I]	540212.1	540212.1	5
540214.2	major ; large [OIS I]	540214.2	540214.2	5
540220.1	laceration NFS	540220.1	540220.1	5
540222.1	minor ; superficial ; only cortex involvement ; <2cm [OIS II]	540222.1	540222.1	5
540224.2	major ; multiple lacerations ; extending into medulla ; ≥2cm [OIS III]	540224.2	540224.2	5
540226.3	massive ; avulsion ; complex ; rupture ; >50% parenchymal destruction [OIS IV, V]	540226.3	540226.3	5
540499.1	**Anus** NFS	540499.1	540499.1	5
540410.1	contusion ; hematoma	540410.1	540410.1	5
540420.2	laceration NFS	540420.2	540420.2	5
540422.2	no perforation ; partial thickness	540422.2	540422.2	5
540424.3	perforation ; full thickness	540424.3	540424.3	5
540426.4	massive ; avulsion ; complex ; rupture ; major tissue loss	540426.4	540426.4	2
540322.2	**Appendix** laceration ; perforation[a]	None	None	5
540699.2	**Bladder (urinary)** NFS	540699.2	540699.2	5
540610.2	contusion ; hematoma [OIS I]	540610.2	540610.2	5
540620.2	laceration NFS	540620.2	540620.2	5
540622.2	no perforation ; partial thickness [OIS I]	540622.3[b]	540622.3[b]	5
540623.2	extraperitoneal wall ≤2cm [OIS II][a]	540622.3[b]	None	5
540624.3	extraperitoneal wall >2cm ; intraperitoneal wall ≤2cm [OIS III][a]	540622.3	None	5
540625.3	intraperitoneal wall >2cm [OIS IV][a]	540624.4[b]	None	5
540626.4	massive ; avulsion ; complex, tissue loss ; involving urethral orifice (trigone) or bladder neck [OIS V]	540626.4	540626.4	2
540640.3	rupture NFS	540640.3	540640.3	5

Use "rupture" only when a more detailed descriptor is not available.

---

[a] New descriptor in AIS 2005
[b] Change in severity code in AIS 2005

AIS 2005	損傷内容	⇒ AIS98	⇐ AIS98	FCI
	内 臓			
540299.1	**副腎** 詳細不明	540299.1	540299.1	5
540210.1	挫傷；血腫　詳細不明 [OIS I]	540210.1	540210.1	5
540212.1	小；表在性 [OIS I]	540212.1	540212.1	5
540214.2	大；大きい [OIS I]	540214.2	540214.2	5
540220.1	裂傷・裂創　詳細不明	540220.1	540220.1	5
540222.1	小；表在性：皮質内にとどまる；2cm未満 [OIS II]	540222.1	540222.1	5
540224.2	大；多発性裂傷・裂創；髄質に及ぶ；2cm以上 [OIS III]	540224.2	540224.2	5
540226.3	広範囲；断裂；複雑；破裂；実質の破壊が50%を超える [OIS IV, V]	540226.3	540226.3	5
540499.1	**肛門** 詳細不明	540499.1	540499.1	5
540410.1	挫傷；血腫	540410.1	540410.1	5
540420.2	裂傷・裂創　詳細不明	540420.2	540420.2	5
540422.2	穿孔なし；非全層性	540422.2	540422.2	5
540424.3	穿孔あり；全層性	540424.3	540424.3	5
540426.4	広範囲；断裂；複雑；破裂；高度組織欠損	540426.4	540426.4	2
540322.2	**虫垂** 裂傷・裂創；穿孔[a]	なし	なし	5
540699.2	**膀胱** 詳細不明	540699.2	540699.2	5
540610.2	挫傷；血腫 [OIS I]	540610.2	540610.2	5
540620.2	裂傷・裂創　詳細不明	540620.2	540620.2	5
540622.2	穿孔なし；非全層性 [OIS I]	540622.3[b]	540622.3[b]	5
540623.2	腹膜外で2cm以下 [OIS II][a]	540622.3[b]	なし	5
540624.3	腹膜外で2cmを超える；腹膜内で2cm以下 [OIS III][a]	540622.3	なし	5
540625.3	腹膜内で2cmを超える [OIS IV][a]	540624.4[b]	なし	5
540626.4	広範囲；断裂；複雑；組織欠損；尿道口や膀胱頸部に及ぶ [OIS V]	540626.4	540626.4	2
540640.3	破裂　詳細不明	540640.3	540640.3	5

> より詳細な情報のない場合にのみ，このコードを選択する。

---

[a] AIS 2005に加えられた新しいコード。
[b] AIS 2005で重症度に変更あり。

ABDOMEN

AIS 2005	Injury Description	⇒ AIS98	⇐ AIS98	FCI
540899.2	**Colon (large bowel)** NFS	540899.2	540899.2	5
540810.2	contusion ; hematoma [*OIS I*]	540810.2	540810.2	5
540820.2	laceration NFS	540820.2	540820.2	5
540822.2	no perforation ; partial thickness ; < 50 % circumference [*OIS I, II*]	540822.2	540822.2	5
540824.3	perforation ; full thickness ; ≥50% circumference without transection ; multiple simple wounds [*OIS III*]	540824.3	540824.3	5
540826.4	massive ; avulsion ; complex ; tissue loss ; transection ; large areas of tissue devitalization or devascularization [*OIS IV, V*]	540826.4	540826.4	2
541099.2	**Duodenum** NFS	541099.2	541099.2	5
	If an injury occurs at the junction of the duodenum and jejunum, code to the jejunum.			
541010.2	contusion ; hematoma [*OIS I, II*]	541010.2	541010.2	5
541020.2	laceration NFS	541020.2	541020.2	5
541022.2	no perforation ; partial thickness ; serosal tear [*OIS I*]	541022.2	541022.2	5
541021.2	disruption <50% circumference [*OIS II*]	541022.2	541022.2	5
541023.3	disruption 50-100% circumference of D1 (superior or first part), D3 (transverse or third part) or D4 (ascending or fourth part) [*OIS III*]	541023.3	541023.3	5
541025.3	disruption 50-75 % circumference of D2 (descending or second part) [*OIS III*]	541023.3	541023.3	5
541024.4	disruption >75% circumference of D2 (descending or second part) ; involving ampulla or distal common bile duct [*OIS IV*]	541024.4	541024.4	5
541028.5	massive ; avulsion ; complex ; rupture ; tissue loss ; devascularization ; massive disruption of duodenopancreatic complex [*OIS V*]	541028.5	541028.5	3

AIS 2005	損傷内容	⇒ AIS98	⇐ AIS98	FCI
540899.2	**結腸（大腸）** 詳細不明	540899.2	540899.2	5
540810.2	挫傷；血腫 [OIS I]	540810.2	540810.2	5
540820.2	裂傷・裂創 詳細不明	540820.2	540820.2	5
540822.2	穿孔なし；非全層性；周径の50%未満 [OIS I, II]	540822.2	540822.2	5
540824.3	穿孔；全層性；周径の50%以上だが断裂には至らない；多発する単純裂創 [OIS III]	540824.3	540824.3	5
540826.4	広範囲；断裂；複雑；組織欠損；離断；広範囲の組織壊死または血行遮断 [OIS IV]	540826.4	540826.4	2
541099.2	**十二指腸** 詳細不明	541099.2	541099.2	5

> 十二指腸と空腸の接合部（十二指腸空腸曲）に損傷がある場合には，空腸のコードを選択する。

AIS 2005	損傷内容	⇒ AIS98	⇐ AIS98	FCI
541010.2	挫傷；血腫 [OIS I, II]	541010.2	541010.2	5
541020.2	裂傷・裂創 詳細不明	541020.2	541020.2	5
541022.2	穿孔なし；非全層性；漿膜裂傷 [OIS I]	541022.2	541022.2	5
541021.2	穿孔あり；周径の50%未満 [OIS II]	541022.2	541022.2	5
541023.3	D1（上部または第1部），D3（水平部または第3部）またはD4（上行部または第4部）の周径の50～100% [OIS III]	541023.3	541023.3	5
541025.3	D2（下行部または第2部）の周径の50～75% [OIS III]	541023.3	541023.3	5
541024.4	D2（下行部または第2部）の周径の75%を超える；膨大部または遠位総胆管の損傷を合併する [OIS IV]	541024.4	541024.4	5
541028.5	広範囲；断裂；複雑；破裂；組織欠損；血行遮断；十二指腸・膵臓結合部の高度損傷 [OIS V]	541028.5	541028.5	3

ABDOMEN

AIS 2005	Injury Description	⇒ AIS98	⇐ AIS98	FCI
541299.2	**Gallbladder** NFS	541299.2	541299.2	5
	Read coding rule below for "Duct Involvement".			
541210.2	contusion ; hematoma [OIS I]	541210.2	541210.2	5
541220.2	laceration ; perforation NFS [OIS II]	541220.2	541220.2	5
541222.2	minor ; superficial ; no cystic duct involvement [OIS II]	541222.2	541222.2	5
541224.3	massive ; avulsion ; complex ; rupture ; tissue loss ; cystic duct laceration or transection [OIS III]	541224.3	541224.3	5
541226.4	with common bile or hepatic duct laceration or transection [OIS IV, V]	541226.4	541226.4	5
541499.2	**Jejunum-Ileum (small bowel)** NFS	541499.2	541499.2	5
	If an injury occurs at the junction of the duodenum and jejunum, code to the jejunum.			
541410.2	contusion ; hematoma [OIS I]	541410.2	541410.2	5
541420.2	laceration NFS	541420.2	541420.2	5
541422.2	no perforation ; partial thickness ; < 50 % circumference [OIS I, II]	541422.2	541422.2	5
541424.3	perforation ; full thickness ; ≥50% circumference without transection ; multiple simple wounds [OIS III]	541424.3	541424.3	5
541426.4	massive ; avulsion ; complex ; tissue loss ; transection ; large areas of tissue devitalization or devascularization [OIS IV, V]	541426.4	541426.4	3

CODING RULE : **Duct Involvement**

Duct involvement applies to gallbladder, liver and pancreas. Injuries to these organs, which share the same duct system, not infrequently involve injuries to the duct system of each organ. When only one ductal injury occurs, it should be assigned to either (not both) of the two involved organs. When separate ductal injuries (e.g., to the right hepatic duct and the pancreatic duct) occur, each should be assigned to the appropriate organ.

AIS 2005	損傷内容	⇒ AIS98	⇐ AIS98	FCI
541299.2	**胆嚢**　詳細不明	541299.2	541299.2	5
	下記のコード選択のルール「管路の損傷」を参照。			
541210.2	挫傷；血腫［OIS I］	541210.2	541210.2	5
541220.2	裂傷・裂創；穿孔　詳細不明［OIS II］	541220.2	541220.2	5
541222.2	小；表在性；胆嚢管の損傷なし［OIS II］	541222.2	541222.2	5
541224.3	広範囲；断裂；複雑；破裂；組織欠損；胆嚢管の裂傷または断裂［OIS III］	541224.3	541224.3	5
541226.4	総胆管または肝管の裂傷・裂創または断裂を伴う［OIS IV, V］	541226.4	541226.4	5
541499.2	**空腸－回腸（小腸）**　詳細不明	541499.2	541499.2	5
	十二指腸と空腸の接合部（十二指腸空腸曲）に損傷がある場合には，空腸のコードを選択する。			
541410.2	挫傷；血腫［OIS I］	541410.2	541410.2	5
541420.2	裂傷・裂創　詳細不明	541420.2	541420.2	5
541422.2	穿孔なし；非全層性；周径の50％未満［OIS I, II］	541422.2	541422.2	5
541424.3	穿孔あり；全層性；周径の50％以上だが断裂には至らない；多数の単純裂傷［OIS III］	541424.3	541424.3	5
541426.4	広範囲；断裂；複雑；組織欠損；断裂；広範囲の組織壊死または血行遮断［OIS IV, V］	541426.4	541426.4	3

コード選択のルール：導管系損傷

導管系の損傷の合併は胆嚢，肝臓，膵臓に適用される。実際に1つの導管系を共有するこれらの臓器に損傷がある場合，しばしばそれぞれの臓器の導管系に損傷を伴う。1つの導管系の損傷の場合，その導管系に関係する2つの臓器のうちいずれか一方のコードを選択する。これに対し，別の2つの導管系に損傷が発生した場合（例えば，右肝管と膵管の損傷），両方の臓器のコードを選択する。

ABDOMEN

AIS 2005	Injury Description	⇒ AIS98	⇐ AIS98	FCI
541699.2	**Kidney** NFS	541699.2	541699.2	5
541610.2	contusion ; hematoma NFS	541610.2	541610.2	5
541612.2	subcapsular, nonexpanding ; confined to renal retroperitoneum ; minor ; superficial [OIS I, II]	541612.2	541612.2	5
541614.3	subcapsular, >50 % surface area or expanding ; major ; large [OIS III]	541614.3	541614.3	5
541620.2	laceration NFS	541620.2	541620.2	5
541622.2	≤1cm parenchymal depth of renal cortex, no urinary extravasation ; minor ; superficial [OIS II]	541622.2	541622.2	5
541624.3	>1cm parenchymal depth of renal cortex, no collecting system rupture or urinary extravasation ; moderate [OIS III]	541624.3	541624.3	5
541626.4	extending through renal cortex, medulla and collecting system ; main renal vessel injury with contained hemorrhage ; major [OIS IV]	541626.4	541626.4	5
541628.5	hilum avulsion ; total destruction of organ and its vascular system [OIS V]	541628.5	541628.5	5
541640.4	rupture	541640.4	541640.4	5

> Use "rupture" only when a more detailed descriptor is not available.

AIS 2005	損傷内容	⇒AIS98	⇐AIS98	FCI
541699.2	**腎臓**　詳細不明	541699.2	541699.2	5
541610.2	挫傷；血腫　詳細不明	541610.2	541610.2	5
541612.2	被膜下，後腹膜腔に限局；実質の裂傷なし；小；表在性［OIS Ⅰ, Ⅱ］	541612.2	541612.2	5
541614.3	被膜下；表面積の50％を超える，増大；大；広範囲［OIS Ⅲ］	541614.3	541614.3	5
541620.2	裂傷・裂創　詳細不明	541620.2	541620.2	5
541622.2	深さ1cm以下の腎皮質実質の損傷，溢尿なし；小；表在性；［OIS Ⅱ］	541622.2	541622.2	5
541624.3	深さ1cmを超える腎皮質実質の損傷，腎盂腎杯の破裂，溢尿なし；中等度；［OIS Ⅲ］	541624.3	541624.3	5
541626.4	腎皮質を貫通し，髄質，腎盂腎杯に達する損傷；腎茎部の主要血管損傷で出血を伴う；大［OIS Ⅳ］	541626.4	541626.4	5
541628.5	腎門部の断裂；腎組織および血管系の完全破壊［OIS Ⅴ］	541628.5	541628.5	5
541640.4	破裂	541640.4	541640.4	5

より詳細な情報がない場合に限り選択する。

ABDOMEN

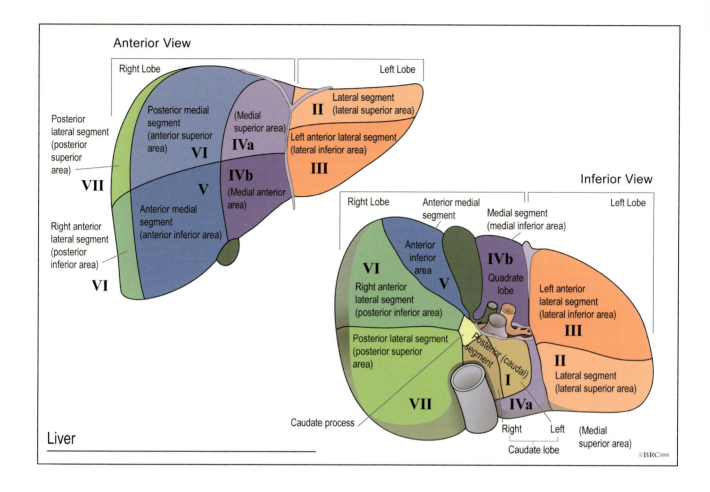

Liver

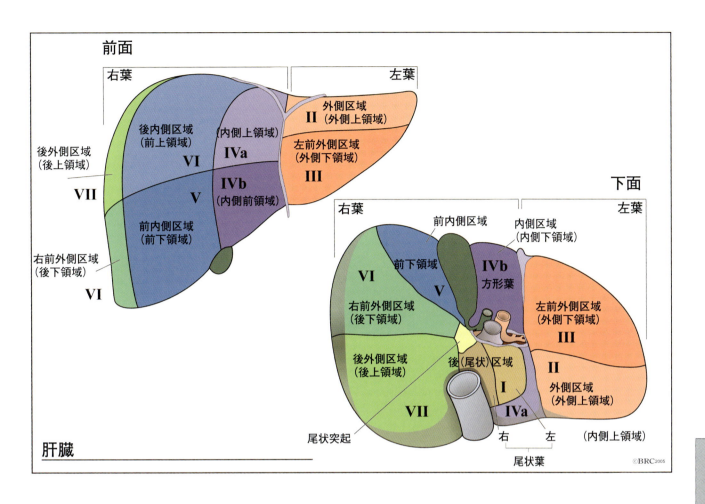

ABDOMEN

AIS 2005	Injury Description	⇒ AIS98	⇐ AIS98	FCI
541899.2	**Liver** NFS	541899.2	541899.2	5
	Read coding rule for "Duct Involvement" (page 99).			
541810.2	contusion ; hematoma NFS	541810.2	541810.2	5
541812.2	subcapsular, ≤50% surface area, or nonexpanding ; intraparenchymal ≤10cm in diameter ; minor ; superficial [OIS I, II]	541812.2	541812.2	5
541814.3	subcapsular, >50% surface area or expanding ; ruptured subcapsular or parenchymal ; intraparenchymal >10cm or expanding ; major [OIS III]	541814.3	541814.3	5
541820.2	laceration NFS	541820.2	541820.2	5
541822.2	simple capsular tears ; ≤3cm parenchymal depth ; ≤10cm long ; minor ; superficial [OIS II]	541822.2	541822.2	5
541824.3	>3cm parenchymal depth ; major duct involvement ; moderate [OIS III]	541824.3	541824.3	5
541826.4	parenchymal disruption≤75 % hepatic lobe ; multiple lacerations > 3cm deep ; "burst" injury ; major [OIS IV]	541826.4	541826.4	5
541828.5	parenchymal disruption of >75% of hepatic lobe or > 3 Couinard's segments within a single lobe ; or involving retrohepatic vena cava/central hepatic veins ; massive ; complex [OIS V]	541828.5	541828.5	5
541830.6	hepatic avulsion (total separation of all vascular attachments) [OIS VI]	541830.6	541830.6	1
541840.4	rupture	541840.4	541840.4	5
	Use "rupture" only when a more detailed descriptor is not available.			
542099.2	**Mesentery** NFS	542099.2	542099.2	5
542010.2	contusion ; hematoma	542010.2	542010.2	5
542020.2	laceration NFS	542020.2	542020.2	5
542022.2	minor ; superficial	542022.2	542022.2	5
542024.3	major	542024.3	542024.3	5
542026.4	massive ; avulsion ; complex ; tissue loss	542026.4	542026.4	5

AIS 2005	損傷内容	⇒ AIS98	⇐ AIS98	FCI
541899.2	**肝臓** 詳細不明	541899.2	541899.2	5
	管路損傷のコード選択のルールを参照（99ページ）。			
541810.2	挫傷；血腫 詳細不明	541810.2	541810.2	5
541812.2	被膜下，表面積の50％以下，限局性または直径10cm以下の実質損傷；小；表在性［OIS I, II］	541812.2	541812.2	5
541814.3	被膜下，表面積の50％を超える，増大；被膜下または実質の破裂；直径10cmを超える実質損傷；大［OIS III］	541814.3	541814.3	5
541820.2	裂傷・裂創 詳細不明	541820.2	541820.2	5
541822.2	単純な被膜損傷；実質の深さが3cm以下；長さ10cm以下；小；表在性［OIS II］	541822.2	541822.2	5
541824.3	実質の深さが3cmを超える；主要胆管の損傷；中等度［OIS III］	541824.3	541824.3	5
541826.4	肝葉の75％以下の実質破裂；深さ3cmを超える多発性裂傷・裂創；"破裂"損傷；大［OIS IV］	541826.4	541826.4	5
541828.5	肝葉の75％を超える実質破裂または一葉のうち4つ以上のクイノー肝区域にわたる実質損傷；肝後面下大静脈または肝静脈損傷を伴っている；広範囲；複雑［OIS V］	541828.5	541828.5	5
541830.6	肝断裂（すべての肝血管系の完全断裂）［OIS VI］	541830.6	541830.6	1
541840.4	破裂	541840.4	541840.4	5
	より詳細な情報がない場合にのみ"破裂"を選択する。			
542099.2	**腸間膜** 詳細不明	542099.2	542099.2	5
542010.2	挫傷；血腫	542010.2	542010.2	5
542020.2	裂傷・裂創 詳細不明	542020.2	542020.2	5
542022.2	小；表在性	542022.2	542022.2	5
542024.3	大	542024.3	542024.3	5
542026.4	広範囲；断裂；複雑；組織欠損	542026.4	542026.4	5

ABDOMEN

AIS 2005	Injury Description	⇒ AIS98	⇐ AIS98	FCI
542299.2	**Omentum** NFS	542299.2	542299.2	5
542210.2	contusion ; hematoma	542210.2	542210.2	5
542220.2	laceration NFS	542220.2	542220.2	5
542222.2	minor ; superficial	542222.2	542222.2	5
542224.3	major	542224.3	542224.3	5
542400.2	**Ovarian (Fallopian) tube** laceration	542400.2	542400.2	5
542699.1	**Ovary** NFS	542699.1	542699.1	5
542610.1	contusion ; hematoma [OIS I]	542610.1	542610.1	5
542620.1	laceration ; perforation NFS	542620.2[b]	542620.2[b]	5
542622.1	superficial ; ≤.5cm ; minor [OIS II]	542622.2[b]	542622.2[b]	5
542623.2	deep ; > .5cm [OIS III]	542624.3[b]	542624.3[b]	5
542624.2	complete parenchymal destruction ; massive ; avulsion ; complex [OIS IV, V]	542624.3[b]	542624.3[b]	5
542899.2	**Pancreas** NFS	542899.2	542899.2	5
	Read coding rule for "Duct Involvement" (page 99).			
542810.2	contusion ; hematoma NFS	542810.2	542810.2	5
542812.2	minor ; superficial ; no duct involvement [OIS I]	542812.2	542812.2	5
542814.3	major ; large ; extensive ; with duct involvement [OIS II]	542814.3	542814.3	5
542820.2	laceration NFS	542820.2	542820.2	5
542822.2	minor ; superficial ; no duct involvement [OIS I]	542822.2	542822.2	5
542824.3	moderate ; major vessel or major duct involvement ; distal transection [OIS III]	542824.3	542824.3	5
542826.4	if involving ampulla [OIS IV]	542826.4	542826.4	5
542828.4	major ; multiple lacerations ; proximal transection [OIS IV]	542828.4	542828.4	3
542830.4	if involving ampulla [OIS IV]	542830.4	542830.4	3
542832.5	massive ; avulsion ; complex ; tissue loss ; massive disruption of pancreatic head [OIS V]	542832.5	542832.5	3

---

[b] Change in severity in AIS 2005

AIS 2005	損傷内容	⇒ AIS98	⇐ AIS98	FCI
542299.2	**大網** 詳細不明	542299.2	542299.2	5
542210.2	挫傷；血腫	542210.2	542210.2	5
542220.2	裂傷・裂創 詳細不明	542220.2	542220.2	5
542222.2	小；表在性	542222.2	542222.2	5
542224.3	大	542224.3	542224.3	5
542400.2	**卵管（ファロピアン管）** 裂傷・裂創	542400.2	542400.2	5
542699.1	**卵巣** 詳細不明	542699.1	542699.1	5
542610.1	挫傷；血腫 [OIS I]	542610.1	542610.1	5
542620.1	裂傷・裂創；穿孔 詳細不明	542620.2[b]	542620.2[b]	5
542622.1	表在性；0.5cm以下；小 [OIS II]	542622.2[b]	542622.2[b]	5
542623.2	深在性；0.5cmを超える [OIS III]	542624.3[b]	542624.3[b]	5
542624.2	実質の完全破壊；広範囲；断裂；複雑 [OIS IV, V]	542624.3[b]	542624.3[b]	5
542899.2	**膵臓** 詳細不明	542899.2	542899.2	5
	管路損傷のコード選択のルールを参照（99ページ）。			
542810.2	挫傷；血腫 詳細不明	542810.2	542810.2	5
542812.2	小；表在性；膵管損傷なし [OIS I]	542812.2	542812.2	5
542814.3	大；大きい；広範囲；膵管損傷を伴う [OIS II]	542814.3	542814.3	5
542820.2	裂傷・裂創 詳細不明	542820.2	542820.2	5
542822.2	小；表在性；膵管損傷なし [OIS I]	542822.2	542822.2	5
542824.3	中；主要血管または主膵管の損傷を伴う；遠位側の離断 [OIS III]	542824.3	542824.3	5
542826.4	膨大部損傷を伴う [OIS IV]	542826.4	542826.4	5
542828.4	大；多発性裂傷；近位側の離断 [OIS IV]	542828.4	542828.4	3
542830.4	膨大部損傷を伴う [OIS IV]	542830.4	542830.4	3
542832.5	広範囲；断裂；複雑；組織欠損；膵頭部の高度損傷 [OIS V]	542832.5	542832.5	3

---

[b] AIS2005で重症度に変更あり。

ABDOMEN

AIS 2005	Injury Description	⇒ AIS98	⇐ AIS98	FCI
543099.1	**Penis** NFS	543099.1	543099.1	5
543010.1	contusion ; hematoma [OIS I]	543010.1	543010.1	5
543020.1	laceration ; perforation NFS	543020.1	543020.1	5
543022.1	minor ; superficial [OIS II, III]	543022.1	543022.1	5
543024.2	major [OIS IV]	543024.2	543024.2	3
543026.2	massive ; amputation ; avulsion ; complex ; [OIS V]	543026.3[b]	543026.3[b]	2
543299.1	**Perineum** NFS	543299.1	543299.1	5
543210.1	contusion ; hematoma	543210.1	543210.1	5
543220.1	laceration ; perforation NFS	543220.1	543220.1	5
543222.1	minor ; superficial	543222.1	543222.1	5
543224.2	major	543224.2	543224.2	5
543226.3	massive ; avulsion ; complex	543226.3	543226.3	2
543599.1	**Prostate** NFS[a]	None	None	5
543510.1	contusion ; hematoma[a]	None	None	5
543520.2	laceration NFS[a]	None	None	5
543522.3	involving urethra[a]	None	None	2
543699.2	**Rectum** NFS	543699.2	543699.2	5
543610.2	contusion ; hematoma [OIS I]	543610.2	543610.2	5
543620.2	laceration NFS	543620.2	543620.2	5
543622.2	no perforation ; partial thickness ; ≤50% of circumference [OIS I, II]	543622.2	543622.2	5
543624.3	full thickness ; >50% circumference [OIS III]	543624.3	543624.3	5
543625.4	extending into perineum [OIS IV]	543625.4	543625.4	2
543626.5	massive; avulsion; tissue loss; devascularization [OIS V]	543626.5	543626.5	2

[a] New descriptor in AIS 2005
[b] Change in severity code in AIS 2005

AIS 2005	損傷内容	⇒ AIS98	⇐ AIS98	FCI
543099.1	**陰茎** 詳細不明	543099.1	543099.1	5
543010.1	挫傷；血腫 [OIS I]	543010.1	543010.1	5
543020.1	裂傷・裂創；穿孔 詳細不明	543020.1	543020.1	5
543022.1	小；表在性 [OIS II, III]	543022.1	543022.1	5
543024.2	大 [OIS IV]	543024.2	543024.2	3
543026.2	広範囲；切断；断裂；複雑 [OIS V]	543026.3[b]	543026.3[b]	2
543299.1	**腹膜** 詳細不明	543299.1	543299.1	5
543210.1	挫傷；血腫	543210.1	543210.1	5
543220.1	裂傷・裂創；穿孔 詳細不明	543220.1	543220.1	5
543222.1	小；表在性	543222.1	543222.1	5
543224.2	大	543224.2	543224.2	5
543226.3	広範囲；断裂；複雑	543226.3	543226.3	2
543599.1	**前立腺** 詳細不明[a]	なし	なし	5
543510.1	挫傷；血腫[a]	なし	なし	5
543520.2	裂傷・裂創 詳細不明[a]	なし	なし	5
543522.3	尿道損傷を伴う[a]	なし	なし	2
543699.2	**直腸** 詳細不明	543699.2	543699.2	5
543610.2	挫傷；血腫 [OIS I]	543610.2	543610.2	5
543620.2	裂傷・裂創 詳細不明	543620.2	543620.2	5
543622.2	穿孔なし；非全層性；周径の50％以下 [OIS I, II]	543622.2	543622.2	5
543624.3	全層性；周径の50％を超える [OIS III]	543624.3	543624.3	5
543625.4	会陰部に達する [OIS IV]	543625.4	543625.4	2
543626.5	広範囲；断裂；組織欠損；血行遮断 [OIS V]	543626.5	543626.5	2

---

[a] AIS2005に加えられた新しいコード。
[b] AIS2005で重症度に変更あり。

ABDOMEN

AIS 2005	Injury Description	⇒ AIS98	⇐ AIS98	FCI
543800.2	**Retroperitoneum** hemorrhage or hematoma	543800.3[b]	543800.3[b]	5
	Code retroperitoneum hemorrhage or hematoma separate from and in addition to anatomically-described injuries unless an associated injury accounts for the blood loss into the retroperitoneal space. The following organs or structures, when injured, may cause retroperitoneal hemorrhage : pancreas, duodenum, kidney, aorta, vena cava, mesenteric vessel, pelvic or vertebral fractures.			
544099.1	**Scrotum** NFS	544099.1	544099.1	5
544010.1	contusion ; hematoma [*OIS I*]	544010.1	544010.1	5
544020.1	laceration ; perforation NFS	544020.1	544020.1	5
544022.1	minor ; superficial ; <25% diameter [*OIS II*]	544022.1	544022.1	5
544024.2	major ; amputation ; avulsion ; complex [*OIS III, IV,V*]	544024.2	544024.2	5
544299.2	**Spleen** NFS	544299.2	544299.2	5
544210.2	contusion ; hematoma NFS	544210.2	544210.2	5
544212.2	subcapsular, ≤50% surface area ; intraparenchymal, ≤5cm in diameter ; minor ; superficial [*OIS I, II*]	544212.2	544212.2	5
544214.3	subcapsular, >50% surface area or expanding ; ruptured subcapsular or parenchymal ; intraparenchymal >5cm in diameter or expanding ; major [*OIS III*]	544214.3	544214.3	5
544220.2	laceration NFS	544220.2	544220.2	5
544222.2	simple capsular tear ≤3cm parenchymal depth and no trabecular vessel involvement ; minor ; superficial [*OIS I, II*]	544222.2	544222.2	5
544224.3	no hilar or segmental parenchymal disruption or destruction ; >3cm parenchymal depth or involving trabecular vessels ; moderate [*OIS III*]	544224.3	544224.3	5
544226.4	involving segmental or hilar vessels producing major devascularization of >25% of spleen but no hilar injury ; major [*OIS IV*]	544226.4	544226.4	5
544228.5	hilar disruption producing total devascularization ; tissue loss ; avulsion ; massive [*OIS V*]	544228.5	544228.5	5
544240.3	rupture NFS	544240.3	544240.3	5
	Use "rupture" only when a more detailed description is not available.			

---

[b] Change in severity in AIS 2005

AIS 2005	損傷内容	⇒ AIS98	⇐ AIS98	FCI
543800.2	**後腹膜** 出血または血腫	543800.3[b]	543800.3[b]	5
	後腹膜腔内への出血の原因が関連した損傷によるものでない場合に限り，解剖学的に記述された損傷に加えてこのコードを選択する。次の臓器や構造物が損傷された場合，後腹膜出血を引き起こしうる：膵臓，十二指腸，腎臓，大動脈，大静脈，腸間膜血管，骨盤または脊椎の骨折。			
544099.1	**陰嚢** 詳細不明	544099.1	544099.1	5
544010.1	挫傷；血腫 [OIS I]	544010.1	544010.1	5
544020.1	裂傷・裂創；穿孔 詳細不明	544020.1	544020.1	5
544022.1	小；表在性；直径の25％未満 [OIS II]	544022.1	544022.1	5
544024.2	大；切断；断裂；複雑 [OIS III, IV, V]	544024.2	544024.2	5
544299.2	**脾臓** 詳細不明	544299.2	544299.2	5
544210.2	挫傷；血腫 詳細不明	544210.2	544210.2	5
544212.2	被膜下，表面積の50％以下；実質内，直径5cm以下；小；表在性 [OIS I, II]	544212.2	544212.2	5
544214.3	被膜下，表面積の50％を超える，増大；被膜下または実質の破裂；直径5cmを超える実質損傷；大 [OIS III]	544214.3	544214.3	5
544220.2	裂傷・裂創 詳細不明	544220.2	544220.2	5
544222.2	実質の深さ3cm以下の単純な被膜損傷で脾柱血管の損傷を伴わない；小；表在性 [OIS I, II]	544222.2	544222.2	5
544224.3	脾門部または区域性実質の破裂または破壊を伴わない；実質の深さ3cmを超える，または脾柱血管の損傷；中 [OIS III]	544224.3	544224.3	5
544226.4	脾門部離断を伴わないが脾臓の25％を超える血行遮断を生じるような区域性血管損傷または脾門部血管の損傷；大 [OIS IV]	544226.4	544226.4	5
544228.5	完全な血行遮断を生じる脾門部離断；組織欠損；断裂；広範囲 [OIS V]	544228.5	544228.5	5
544240.3	破裂 詳細不明	544240.3	544240.3	5
	より詳細な情報がない場合にのみ"破裂"を選択する。			

---

[b] AIS2005で重症度に変更あり。

ABDOMEN

AIS 2005	Injury Description	⇒ AIS98	⇐ AIS98	FCI
544499.2	**Stomach** NFS	544499.2	544499.2	5
544410.2	contusion ; hematoma [OIS I]	544410.2	544410.2	5
544414.3	ingestion injury[a]	544499.2[b]	None	5
544415.3	partial thickness necrosis[a]	544499.2[b]	None	5
544416.4	full thickness necrosis[a]	544499.2[b]	None	3
544420.2	laceration NFS	544420.2	544420.2	5
544422.2	no perforation ; partial thickness [OIS I]	544422.2	544422.2	5
544424.3	perforation ; full thickness [OIS II, III]	544424.3	544424.3	5
544426.4	avulsion ; complex ; rupture ; tissue loss ; massive ; devascularization [OIS IV, V]	544426.4	544426.4	3
544699.1	**Testes** NFS	544699.1	544699.1	5
544610.1	contusion ; hematoma [OIS I]	544610.1	544610.1	5
544620.1	laceration NFS	544620.1	544620.1	5
544622.1	minor ; superficial [OIS II, III]	544622.1	544622.1	5
544624.2	avulsion ; amputation ; complex ; massive [OIS IV, V]	544624.2	544624.2	5
544899.2	**Ureter** NFS	544899.2	544899.2	5
544810.2	contusion ; hematoma [OIS I]	544810.2	544810.2	5
544820.2	laceration NFS	544820.2	544820.2	5
544822.2	no perforation ; partial thickness [OIS II]	544822.2	544822.2	5
544824.3	perforation ; full thickness [OIS III]	544824.3	544824.3	5
544826.3	massive ; avulsion ; complex ; rupture ; tissue loss ; transection [OIS IV, V]	544826.3	544826.3	5
545099.2	**Urethra** NFS	545099.2	545099.2	5
545010.2	contusion ; hematoma [OIS I]	545010.2	545010.2	5
545020.2	laceration NFS	545020.2	545020.2	5
545022.2	no perforation ; partial thickness [OIS III]	545022.2	545022.2	5
545024.2	perforation ; full thickness ; urethral separation <2cm [OIS IV]	545024.3[b]	545024.3[b]	2
545026.2	avulsion ; complex ; tissue loss ; massive [OIS IV]	545026.3[b]	545026.3[b]	1
545028.3	posterior tissue loss ; transection ; urethral separation >2cm [OIS V]	545028.4[b]	545028.4[b]	1
545030.2	stretch injury [OIS II][a]	None	None	5

[a] New descriptor in AIS 2005
[b] Change in severity code in AIS 2005

AIS 2005	損傷内容	⇒ AIS98	⇐ AIS98	FCI
544499.2	**胃** 詳細不明	544499.2	544499.2	5
544410.2	挫傷；血腫 [OIS I]	544410.2	544410.2	5
544414.3	経口摂取による損傷[a]	544499.2[b]	なし	5
544415.3	部分壊死（非全層性）[a]	544499.2[b]	なし	5
544416.4	全層性壊死[a]	544499.2[b]	なし	3
544420.2	裂傷・裂創　詳細不明	544420.2	544420.2	5
544422.2	穿孔なし；非全層性 [OIS I]	544422.2	544422.2	5
544424.3	穿孔あり；全層性 [OIS II, III]	544424.3	544424.3	5
544426.4	断裂；複雑；破裂；組織欠損；広範囲；血行遮断 [OIS IV, V]	544426.4	544426.4	3
544699.1	**精巣** 詳細不明	544699.1	544699.1	5
544610.1	挫傷；血腫 [OIS I]	544610.1	544610.1	5
544620.1	裂傷・裂創　詳細不明	544620.1	544620.1	5
544622.1	小；表在性 [OIS II, III]	544622.1	544622.1	5
544624.2	断裂；切断；複雑；広範囲 [OIS IV, V]	544624.2	544624.2	5
544899.2	**尿管** 詳細不明	544899.2	544899.2	5
544810.2	挫傷；血腫 [OIS I]	544810.2	544810.2	5
544820.2	裂傷・裂創　詳細不明	544820.2	544820.2	5
544822.2	穿孔なし；非全層性 [OIS II]	544822.2	544822.2	5
544824.3	穿孔あり；全層性 [OIS III]	544824.3	544824.3	5
544826.3	広範囲；断裂；複雑；破裂；組織欠損；離断 [OIS IV, V]	544826.3	544826.3	5
545099.2	**尿道** 詳細不明	545099.2	545099.2	5
545010.2	挫傷；血腫 [OIS I]	545010.2	545010.2	5
545020.2	裂傷・裂創　詳細不明	545020.2	545020.2	5
545022.2	穿孔なし；非全層性 [OIS III]	545022.2	545022.2	5
545024.2	穿孔あり；全層性；2 cm未満の尿道裂孔 [OIS IV]	545024.3[b]	545024.3[b]	2
545026.2	断裂；複雑；組織欠損；広範囲 [OIS IV]	545026.3[b]	545026.3[b]	1
545028.3	後部尿道組織の欠損；離断；2 cmを超える尿道裂孔	545028.4[b]	545028.4[b]	1
545030.2	伸展損傷 [OIS II][a]	なし	なし	5

[a] AIS2005に加えられた新しいコード。
[b] AIS2005で重症度に変更あり。

ABDOMEN

AIS 2005	Injury Description	⇒ AIS98	⇐ AIS98	FCI
545299.1	**Uterus** NFS	545299.1	545299.1	5
545210.1	contusion ; hematoma	545210.2[b]	545210.2[b]	5
545220.2	laceration ; perforation NFS	545220.2	545220.2	5
545222.2	≤1cm ; minor ; superficial [OIS II]	545222.2	545222.2	5
545224.3	>1cm ; placental abruption ≤50% ; major ; deep [OIS III]	545230.3	545230.3	5
545226.4	involving uterine artery ; placental abruption >50% but not complete [OIS IV]	545240.3[b]	545240.3[b]	5
545228.5	uterine rupture ; avulsion ; devascularization ; complete placental abruption	545240.3[b]	545240.3[b]	5

> Note : Fetal demise as a result of abdominal injury to a pregnant female is a consequence of trauma, not an injury itself. Term of pregnancy, per se, is not a factor in determining AIS severity code.

AIS 2005	Injury Description	⇒ AIS98	⇐ AIS98	FCI
545499.1	**Vagina** NFS	545499.1	545499.1	5
545410.1	contusion ; hematoma [OIS I]	545410.1	545410.1	5
545420.1	laceration ; perforation NFS	545420.1	545420.1	5
545422.1	minor ; superficial ; mucosa only [OIS II]	545422.1	545422.1	5
545424.2	major ; deep into fat/muscle [OIS III]	545424.2	545424.2	5
545426.3	massive ; avulsion ; complex ; into cervix or peritoneum [OIS IV, V]	545426.3	545426.3	3
545699.1	**Vulva** NFS	545699.1	545699.1	5
545610.1	contusion ; hematoma	545610.1	545610.1	5
545620.1	laceration ; perforation NFS	545620.1	545620.1	5
545622.1	minor ; superficial ; skin only [OIS II]	545622.1	545622.1	5
545624.2	major ; deep into fat/muscle [OIS III]	545624.2	545624.2	5
545626.3	massive ; avulsion ; complex [OIS IV, V]	545626.3	545626.3	3

---

[b] Change in severity code in AIS 2005

AIS 2005	損傷内容	⇒ AIS98	⇐ AIS98	FCI
545299.1	**子宮**　詳細不明	545299.1	545299.1	5
545210.1	挫傷；血腫	545210.2[b]	545210.2[b]	5
545220.2	裂傷・裂創；穿孔　詳細不明	545220.2	545220.2	5
545222.2	1cm以下；小；表在性［OIS II］	545222.2	545222.2	5
545224.3	1cmを超える；50％以下の胎盤剥離；大；深在性［OIS III］	545230.3	545230.3	5
545226.4	子宮動脈の損傷を伴う；50％を超えるが完全ではない胎盤剥離［OIS IV］	545240.3[b]	545240.3[b]	5
545228.5	子宮破裂；断裂；血行遮断；完全な胎盤剥離	545240.3[b]	545240.3[b]	5

> メモ：妊娠女性への腹部外傷による胎児死亡は，外傷の結果であり，それ自身は外傷ではない。妊娠という用語自体は，AISの重症化を規定する因子ではない。

AIS 2005	損傷内容	⇒ AIS98	⇐ AIS98	FCI
545499.1	**腟**　詳細不明	545499.1	545499.1	5
545410.1	挫傷；血腫［OIS I］	545410.1	545410.1	5
545420.1	裂傷・裂創；穿孔　詳細不明	545420.1	545420.1	5
545422.1	小；表在性；粘膜損傷のみ［OIS II］	545422.1	545422.1	5
545424.2	大；脂肪組織または筋層にまで達する深在性［OIS III］	545424.2	545424.2	5
545426.3	広範囲；断裂；複雑；子宮頸部または腹膜にまで及ぶ［OIS IV, V］	545426.3	545426.3	3
545699.1	**外陰部**　詳細不明	545699.1	545699.1	5
545610.1	挫傷；血腫	545610.1	545610.1	5
545620.1	裂傷・裂創；穿孔　詳細不明	545620.1	545620.1	5
545622.1	小；表在性；皮膚損傷のみ［OIS II］	545622.1	545622.1	5
545624.2	大；脂肪組織または筋層にまで達する深在性［OIS III］	545624.2	545624.2	5
545626.3	広範囲；断裂；複雑［OIS IV, V］	545626.3	545626.3	3

[b] AIS2005で重症度に変更あり。

脊　椎

SPINE

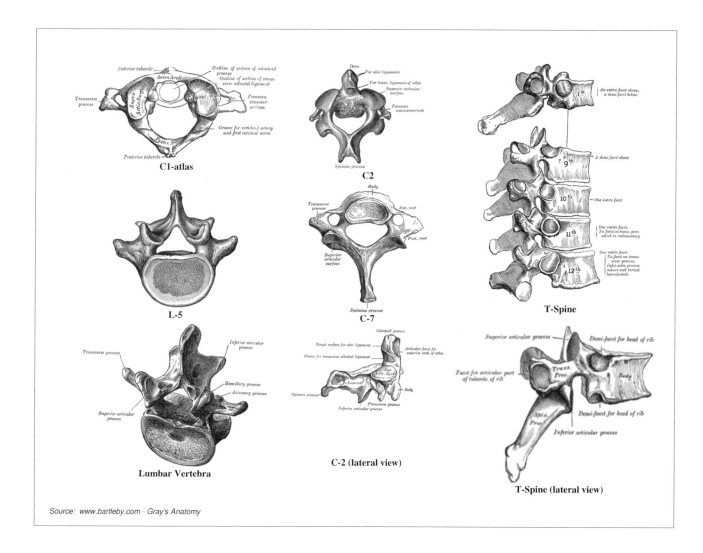

Source: www.bartleby.com - Gray's Anatomy

脊椎

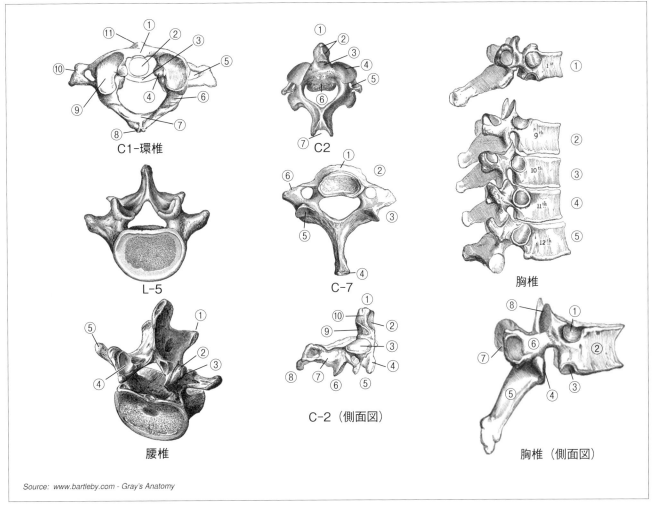

C1- 環椎
① 前弓
② 歯突起部の輪郭
③ 環椎横靱帯部の輪郭
④ 外側塊
⑤ 横突孔
⑥ 椎骨動脈と第一脊髄神経のための溝
⑦ 後弓
⑧ 後結節
⑨ 上関節窩
⑩ 横突起
⑪ 前結節

腰椎
① 下関節突起
② 乳頭突起
③ 副突起
④ 上関節突起
⑤ 横突起

C2
① 歯突起
② 翼状靱帯に対する面
③ 環椎横靱帯に対する面
④ 上関節面
⑤ 横突孔
⑥ 椎体
⑦ 棘突起

C-7
① 椎体
② 前根
③ 後根
④ 棘突起
⑤ 上関節面
⑥ 横突起

C-2（側面図）
① 歯突起
② 環椎輪に対する前関節面
③ 上関節面
④ 椎体
⑤ 横突起
⑥ 下関節突起
⑦ 椎弓根および椎弓板
⑧ 棘突起
⑨ 環椎横靱帯溝
⑩ 翼状靱帯に対する粗面

胸椎
① 上側全関節面；
　下側半関節面
② 上側半関節面
③ 全関節面
④ 全関節面
　（未発達の横突起に対する関節面なし）
⑤ 全関節面
　（横突起に対する関節面なし）
　（凸面で逆さまの外側方向）

胸椎（側面図）
① 肋骨頭に対する半関節面
② 椎体
③ 肋骨頭に対する半関節面
④ 下関節突起
⑤ 棘突起
⑥ 横突起
⑦ 肋骨結節の関節窩
⑧ 上関節突起

CODING RULES : Spine

Coexisting injuries to the spinal cord and to the vertebral column are coded as a single injury ; for example, cord contusion with paraplegia and associated fracture/dislocation is a single injury and is assigned only one AIS code. In such cases, the fracture/dislocation is not coded separately.

When a cord injury is continuous only the highest level is coded. When the cord is injured in more than one region and the injuries are separate and distinct, then all the injuries are coded.

Paralysis is coded according to its status at 24 hours post-injury. In cases where the patient dies within the first 24 hours, code the status of documented paralysis at the time of death.

"Spinal cord injury without radiological abnormality" [SCIWORA] was coined in 1982 to describe a syndrome of post-traumatic neurologic injury without evidence of fracture or ligamentous instability on plain radiographs or CT. With the advent of MRI, however, most patients who previously would have been diagnosed with SCIWORA have demonstrable radiographic findings. SCIWORA as a diagnosis is still used in some clinical settings. It should be coded as spinal cord contusion not further specified. This diagnosis is most commonly attributed to the cervical region rather than to either the thoracic or lumbar regions.

コード選択のルール：脊椎

同一部位の脊髄および脊椎に生じた損傷は1つの損傷としてコード選択をする。例：対麻痺を伴う脊髄挫傷と同部位の骨折／脱臼は単一の損傷として評価し，1つのコードとする。この場合，骨折／脱臼のコードは併記しない。

脊髄損傷が広範囲かつ連続している場合は，高位のコードを選択する。脊髄損傷が多部位（連続していない独立した複数損傷）の場合はすべての損傷をコード選択する。

麻痺は受傷後24時間の状態によりコード選択する。受傷後24時間以内に患者が死亡した場合は，死亡時の状態をコード選択する。

"Spinal cord injury without radiological abnormality"［SCIWORA］は，X線またはCT検査にて骨折や靱帯損傷所見を認めないものの，外傷に伴う神経損傷所見を呈する症候群として1982年に提唱された。MRI検査の出現により，かつてSCIWORAと診断されていた患者においても異常所見を指摘できるようになったが，現在もSCIWORAは臨床診断名として使われることがある（胸・腰部に比べ頸部に多い）。SCIWORAは脊髄挫傷としてコード選択する。

CERVICAL SPINE

AIS 2005	Injury Description	⇒ AIS98	⇐ AIS98	FCI
	Use one of the following two descriptors when such vague information is the only information available. While these descriptors identify the occurrence of an injury to the cervical spine, they do not specify its severity.			
600099.9	**Injuries to the Cervical Spine** NFS	615099.9	615099.9	
600999.9	Died of cervical spine injury without further substantiation of injuries or no autopsy confirmation of specific injuries.	615999.9	615999.9	
630299.2	**Brachial Plexus** injury NFS [includes trunks, divisions or cords]	630299.2	630299.2	2
630210.2	incomplete plexus injury NFS	630210.2	630210.2	2
630212.2	contusion ; stretch injury	630212.2	630212.2	2
630214.2	laceration	630214.2	630214.2	4
630216.2	avulsion	630216.2	630216.2	4
630220.3	complete plexus injury NFS	630220.2[b]	630220.2[b]	1
630221.4	bilateral[c]	630220.2[b]	None	1
630222.3	contusion ; stretch injury	630222.3	630222.3	1
630224.3	laceration	630224.3	630224.3	1
630226.3	avulsion	630226.3	630226.3	1
630227.4	bilateral[c]	630226.3[b]	None	1

---

[b] Change in severity code in AIS 2005

[c] In previous editions of AIS, with few exceptions, each injury was coded separately. AIS 2005 introduces "bilateral". Some bilateral injuries may affect severity levels and, therefore, the ISS for patients with those injuries.

頸　椎

AIS 2005	損傷内容	⇒ AIS98	⇐ AIS98	FCI
	不確定な情報しか得られない場合には，以下の2つのコードのうちいずれかを選択する。これらのコードは，頸椎に損傷が生じたことを記録する目的にのみ使用し，重症度の算出には用いない。			
600099.9	**頸椎損傷**　詳細不明	615099.9	615099.9	
600999.9	頸椎損傷による死亡（詳細不明）または剖検なし	615999.9	615999.9	
630299.2	**腕神経叢**損傷　詳細不明［神経幹，神経索，神経束を含む］	630299.2	630299.2	2
630210.2	不全型神経叢損傷　詳細不明	630210.2	630210.2	2
630212.2	挫傷；伸展損傷	630212.2	630212.2	2
630214.2	裂傷・裂創	630214.2	630214.2	4
630216.2	引き抜き損傷	630216.2	630216.2	4
630220.3	完全型神経叢損傷　詳細不明	630220.2[b]	630220.2[b]	1
630221.4	両側[c]	630220.2[b]	なし	1
630222.3	挫傷；伸展損傷	630222.3	630222.3	1
630224.3	裂傷・裂創	630224.3	630224.3	1
630226.3	引き抜き損傷	630226.3	630226.3	1
630227.4	両側[c]	630226.3[b]	なし	1

---

[b] AIS2005で重症度に変更あり。
[c] 旧版のAIS2005では一部の例外を除き両側損傷はそれぞれ別にコード選択をしていた。AIS2005では，"両側"を導入した。いくつかの両側損傷は重症度が変化し，その結果ISSが変わることがある。

脊椎

CERVICAL SPINE

AIS 2005	Injury Description	⇒ AIS98	⇐ AIS98	FCI
640200.3	**Cord** contusion NFS [includes the diagnosis of compression, or epidural or subdural hemorrhage within spinal canal documented by imaging studies or autopsy]	640200.3	640200.3	5
640201.3	with transient neurological signs (paresthesia), but NFS as to fracture/dislocation	640201.3	640201.3	5
640202.3	with no fracture or dislocation	640202.3	640202.3	5
640204.3	with fracture	640204.3	640204.3	5
640206.3	with dislocation	640206.3	640206.3	
640208.3	with both fracture and dislocation	640208.3	640208.3	5
640210.4	incomplete cord syndrome (preservation of some sensation or motor function; includes anterior cord, central cord, lateral cord (*Brown-Sequard*) syndromes), but NFS as to fracture/dislocation	640210.4	640210.4	1
640212.4	with no fracture or dislocation	640212.4	640212.4	1
640214.4	with fracture	640214.4	640214.4	1
640216.4	with dislocation	640216.4	640216.4	1
640218.4	with both fracture and dislocation	640218.4	640218.4	1
640220.5	complete cord syndrome (quadriplegia or paraplegia with no sensation)	640220.5	640220.5	1
640221.5	C-4 or below, but NFS as to fracture/dislocation or NFS as to site	640221.5	640221.5	1
640222.5	with no fracture or dislocation	640222.5	640222.5	1
640224.5	with fracture	640224.5	640224.5	1
640226.5	with dislocation	640226.5	640226.5	1
640228.5	with both fracture and dislocation	640228.5	640228.5	1
640229.6	C-3 or above, but NFS as to fracture/dislocation	640229.6	640229.6	1
640230.6	with no fracture or dislocation	640230.6	640230.6	1
640232.6	with fracture	640232.6	640232.6	1
640234.6	with dislocation	640234.6	640234.6	1
640236.6	with both fracture and dislocation	640236.6	640236.6	1

頸　椎

AIS 2005	損傷内容	⇒ AIS98	⇐ AIS98	FCI
640200.3	**頸髄**挫傷［画像診断法あるいは剖検により証明された脊柱管内の圧迫や硬膜外，硬膜下血腫の診断を含む］　詳細不明	640200.3	640200.3	5
640201.3	一過性の神経症状（知覚異常）を伴う　骨折・脱臼については不明	640201.3	640201.3	5
640202.3	骨折や脱臼を伴わない	640202.3	640202.3	5
640204.3	骨折を伴う	640204.3	640204.3	5
640206.3	脱臼を伴う	640206.3	640206.3	
640208.3	骨折かつ脱臼を伴う	640208.3	640208.3	5
640210.4	不全麻痺〔何らかの知覚あるいは運動機能の残存：前脊髄症候群，中心性脊髄症候群，外側脊髄症候群（Brown-Sequard症候群）〕を含む、骨折・脱臼については不明	640210.4	640210.4	1
640212.4	骨折や脱臼を伴わない	640212.4	640212.4	1
640214.4	骨折を伴う	640214.4	640214.4	1
640216.4	脱臼を伴う	640216.4	640216.4	1
640218.4	骨折かつ脱臼を伴う	640218.4	640218.4	1
640220.5	完全麻痺（知覚機能の消失した四肢麻痺または対麻痺）	640220.5	640220.5	1
640221.5	第4頸髄以下だが，骨折・脱臼については不明，もしくは部位については不明	640221.5	640221.5	1
640222.5	骨折や脱臼を伴わない	640222.5	640222.5	1
640224.5	骨折を伴う	640224.5	640224.5	1
640226.5	脱臼を伴う	640226.5	640226.5	1
640228.5	骨折かつ脱臼を伴う	640228.5	640228.5	1
640229.6	第3頸髄以上だが，骨折・脱臼については不明	640229.6	640229.6	1
640230.6	骨折や脱臼を伴わない	640230.6	640230.6	1
640232.6	骨折を伴う	640232.6	640232.6	1
640234.6	脱臼を伴う	640234.6	640234.6	1
640236.6	骨折かつ脱臼を伴う	640236.6	640236.6	1

脊椎

CERVICAL SPINE

AIS 2005	Injury Description	⇒ AIS98	⇐ AIS98	FCI
640240.5	**Cord** laceration NFS [includes penetrating injury, transection or crush]	640240.5	640240.5	2
640242.5	incomplete (preservation of some sensation or motor function), but NFS as to fracture/dislocation	640242.5	640242.5	2
640244.5	with no fracture or dislocation	640244.5	640244.5	2
640246.5	with fracture	640246.5	640246.5	2
640248.5	with dislocation	640248.5	640248.5	2
640250.5	with both fracture and dislocation	640250.5	640250.5	2
640260.5	complete cord syndrome NFS (quadriplegia or paraplegia with no sensation or motor function)	640260.5	640260.5	1
640261.5	C-4 or below, but NFS as to fracture/dislocation	640261.5	640261.5	1
640262.5	with no fracture or dislocation	640262.5	640262.5	1
640264.5	with fracture	640264.5	640264.5	1
640266.5	with dislocation	640266.5	640266.5	1
640268.5	with both fracture and dislocation	640268.5	640268.5	1
640269.6	C-3 or above, but NFS as to fracture/dislocation	640269.6	640269.6	1
640270.6	with no fracture or dislocation	640270.6	640270.6	1
640272.6	with fracture	640272.6	640272.6	1
640274.6	with dislocation	640274.6	640274.6	1
640276.6	with both fracture and dislocation	640276.6	640276.6	1
650299.2	**Disc** injury NFS	650299.2	650299.2	5
650200.2	herniation NFS	650200.2	650200.2	5
650202.2	no nerve root damage (radiculopathy)	650202.2	650202.2	5
650203.3	with nerve root damage (radiculopathy)	650203.3	650203.3	5
650205.3	rupture	650203.3	650203.3	
650204.2	**Dislocation** [subluxation], no fracture, no cord involvement NFS	650204.2	650204.2	5
	Code as one injury and assign to superior vertebra.			
650206.3	**atlanto-axial (odontoid)**	650206.3	650206.3	5
650208.2	**atlanto-occipital**	650208.2	650208.2	5
650209.2	**facet** NFS	650209.2	650209.2	5
650210.2	unilateral	650210.2	650210.2	5
650212.3	bilateral	650212.3	650212.3	5

頸　椎

AIS 2005	損傷内容	⇒ AIS98	⇐ AIS98	FCI
640240.5	**頸髄**裂傷・裂創［穿通性損傷，離断あるいは挫滅を含む］詳細不明	640240.5	640240.5	2
640242.5	不全麻痺（何らかの知覚あるいは運動機能の残存），骨折・脱臼については不明	640242.5	640242.5	2
640244.5	骨折や脱臼を伴わない	640244.5	640244.5	2
640246.5	骨折を伴う	640246.5	640246.5	2
640248.5	脱臼を伴う	640248.5	640248.5	2
640250.5	骨折かつ脱臼を伴う	640250.5	640250.5	2
640260.5	完全麻痺（知覚運動機能の消失した四肢麻痺または対麻痺）詳細不明	640260.5	640260.5	1
640261.5	第4頸髄以下だが，骨折・脱臼については不明	640261.5	640261.5	1
640262.5	骨折や脱臼を伴わない	640262.5	640262.5	1
640264.5	骨折を伴う	640264.5	640264.5	1
640266.5	脱臼を伴う	640266.5	640266.5	1
640268.5	骨折かつ脱臼を伴う	640268.5	640268.5	1
640269.6	第3頸髄以上だが，骨折・脱臼については不明	640269.6	640269.6	1
640270.6	骨折や脱臼を伴わない	640270.6	640270.6	1
640272.6	骨折を伴う	640272.6	640272.6	1
640274.6	脱臼を伴う	640274.6	640274.6	1
640276.6	骨折かつ脱臼を伴う	640276.6	640276.6	1
650299.2	**椎間板**損傷　詳細不明	650299.2	650299.2	5
650200.2	ヘルニア　詳細不明	650200.2	650200.2	5
650202.2	神経根損傷（神経根障害）を伴わない	650202.2	650202.2	5
650203.3	神経根損傷（神経根障害）を伴う	650203.3	650203.3	5
650205.3	破裂	650203.3	650203.3	
650204.2	頸椎脱臼［亜脱臼］骨折，頸髄損傷を伴わない　詳細不明	650204.2	650204.2	5
	上位頸椎の損傷として1つだけコードを選択する。			
650206.3	**環軸関節（歯突起）**	650206.3	650206.3	5
650208.2	**環椎後頭骨関節**	650208.2	650208.2	5
650209.2	**椎間関節**　詳細不明	650209.2	650209.2	5
650210.2	片側	650210.2	650210.2	5
650212.3	両側	650212.3	650212.3	5

脊椎

CERVICAL SPINE

AIS 2005	Injury Description	⇒ AIS98	⇐ AIS98	FCI
650216.2	Fracture with or without dislocation but no cord involvement NFS	650216.2	650216.2	5
	Code each vertebra separately. Note instructions at lamina, pedicle and vertebral body for coding fractures of the atlas (C1).			
650217.2	multiple fractures of same **vertebra**[a]	650216.2	None	5
	Exceptions: odontoid or major compression fracture which are coded additionally.			
650218.2	**spinous process**	650218.2	650218.2	5
650220.2	**transverse process**	650220.2	650220.2	5
650222.2	**facet**	650222.3[b]	650222.3[b]	5
650224.2	**lamina** code C1 posterior arch here	650224.3[b]	650224.3[b]	5
650226.2	**pedicle** code C1 lateral mass here	650226.3[b]	650226.3[b]	5
650228.3	**odontoid (dens)**	650228.3	650228.3	5
650230.2	**vertebral body** NFS ["burst" fracture] code C1 anterior arch here	650230.2	650230.2	5
650232.2	minor compression (≤20% loss of anterior height)	650232.2	650232.2	5
650234.3	major compression (>20% loss of anterior height)	650234.3	650234.3	5
640284.1	**Spinous ligament** injury	640284.1	640284.1	5
630260.2	**Nerve root**, single or multiple NFS	630260.2	630260.2	2
630202.2	contusion; stretch injury	630202.2	630202.2	2
630204.2	laceration NFS	630204.2	630204.2	2
630206.2	single nerve root	630206.2	630206.2	2
630208.3	multiple nerve roots	630208.3	630208.3	2
630262.2	avulsion NFS	630262.2	630262.2	2
630264.2	single nerve root	630264.2	630264.2	2
630266.3	multiple nerve roots	630266.3	630266.3	2
640278.1	Strain, acute, with no fracture or dislocation	640278.1	640278.1	5

---

[a] New descriptor in AIS 2005
[b] Change in severity code in AIS 2005

頸　椎

AIS 2005	損傷内容	⇒ AIS98	⇐ AIS98	FCI
650216.2	頸椎骨折（頸髄損傷は伴わないが脱臼の有無は問わない）詳細不明	650216.2	650216.2	5
	損傷が明らかな場合には以下のコードを選択する。環椎骨折に対するコード選択は下記の椎弓，椎弓根，椎体の説明を参照。			
650217.2	同一椎骨の多部位に及ぶ**骨折**[a]	650216.2	なし	5
	例外：歯突起骨折および椎体全面高の減少が20%を超える圧迫骨折は併せてコードを選択する。			
650218.2	**棘突起**	650218.2	650218.2	5
650220.2	**横突起**	650220.2	650220.2	5
650222.2	**関節突起**	650222.3[b]	650222.3[b]	5
650224.2	**椎弓**　環椎後弓骨折はこのコードを選択する。	650224.3[b]	650224.3[b]	5
650226.2	**椎弓根**　環椎外側塊骨折はこのコードを選択する。	650226.3[b]	650226.3[b]	5
650228.3	**歯突起（軸椎）**	650228.3	650228.3	5
650230.2	**椎体**　詳細不明［"破裂骨折"に使用］　環椎前弓骨折はこのコードを選択する。	650230.2	650230.2	5
650232.2	圧迫骨折　小（椎体前面高の減少が20%以下）	650232.2	650232.2	5
650234.3	圧迫骨折　大（椎体前面高の減少が20%を超える）	650234.3	650234.3	5
640284.1	**棘間靱帯**損傷	640284.1	640284.1	5
630260.2	**神経根**　単発あるいは多発　詳細不明	630260.2	630260.2	2
630202.2	挫傷；伸展損傷	630202.2	630202.2	2
630204.2	裂傷・裂創　詳細不明	630204.2	630204.2	2
630206.2	単一神経根	630206.2	630206.2	2
630208.3	複数神経根	630208.3	630208.3	2
630262.2	引き抜き損傷　詳細不明	630262.2	630262.2	2
630264.2	単一神経根	630264.2	630264.2	2
630266.3	複数神経根	630266.3	630266.3	2
640278.1	捻挫，急性，骨折や脱臼を伴わない	640278.1	640278.1	5

---

[a] AIS2005に加えられた新しいコード。
[b] AIS 2005で重症度に変更あり。

THORACIC SPINE

AIS 2005	Injury Description	⇒ AIS98	⇐ AIS98	FCI
	Use one of the following two descriptors when such vague information is the only information available. While these descriptors identify the occurrence of an injury to the thoracic spine, they do not specify its severity.			
620099.9	**Injuries to the Thoracic Spine** NFS	616099.9	616099.9	
620999.9	Died of thoracic spine injury without further substantiation of injuries or no autopsy confirmation of specific injuries.	616999.9	616999.9	
640400.3	**Cord** contusion [includes the diagnosis of compression, or epidural or subdural hemorrhage within spinal canal documented by imaging studies or autopsy]	640400.3	640400.3	5
640401.3	with transient neurological signs (paresthesia) but NFS as to fracture/dislocation	640401.3	640401.3	5
640402.3	with no fracture or dislocation	640402.3	640402.3	5
640404.3	with fracture	640404.3	640404.3	5
640406.3	with dislocation	640406.3	640406.3	5
640408.3	with both fracture and dislocation	640408.3	640408.3	1
640410.4	incomplete cord syndrome (preservation of some sensation or motor function ; includes anterior cord, central cord, lateral cord (*Brown-Sequard*) syndromes) but NFS as to fracture/dislocation	640410.4	640410.4	2
640412.4	with no fracture or dislocation	640412.4	640412.4	2
640414.4	with fracture	640414.4	640414.4	2
640416.4	with dislocation	640416.4	640416.4	2
640418.4	with both fracture and dislocation	640418.4	640418.4	2
640420.5	complete cord syndrome (paraplegia with no sensation) but NFS as to fracture/dislocation	640420.5	640420.5	1
640422.5	with no fracture or dislocation	640422.5	640422.5	1
640424.5	with fracture	640424.5	640424.5	1
640426.5	with dislocation	640426.5	640426.5	1
640428.5	with both fracture and dislocation	640428.5	640428.5	1

胸　椎

AIS 2005	損傷内容	⇒ AIS98	⇐ AIS98	FCI
	不確定な情報しか得られない場合には，以下の2つのコードのうちいずれかを選択する．これらコードは，胸椎に損傷が生じたことを記録する目的にのみ使用し，重症度の算出には用いない．			
620099.9	**胸椎損傷**　詳細不明	616099.9	616099.9	
620999.9	胸椎損傷による死亡（詳細不明）または剖検なし	616999.9	616999.9	
640400.3	**胸髄**挫傷［画像診断法あるいは剖検により証明された脊柱管内の圧迫や硬膜外，硬膜下血腫の診断を含む］	640400.3	640400.3	5
640401.3	一過性の神経症状（知覚異常）を伴うが骨折・脱臼については不明	640401.3	640401.3	5
640402.3	骨折や脱臼を伴わない	640402.3	640402.3	5
640404.3	骨折を伴う	640404.3	640404.3	5
640406.3	脱臼を伴う	640406.3	640406.3	5
640408.3	骨折かつ脱臼を伴う	640408.3	640408.3	1
640410.4	不全麻痺〔何らかの知覚あるいは運動機能の残存；前脊髄症候群，中心性脊髄症候群，外側脊髄症候群（Brown-Sequard症候群）〕を含む　骨折・脱臼については不明	640410.4	640410.4	2
640412.4	骨折や脱臼を伴わない	640412.4	640412.4	2
640414.4	骨折を伴う	640414.4	640414.4	2
640416.4	脱臼を伴う	640416.4	640416.4	2
640418.4	骨折かつ脱臼を伴う	640418.4	640418.4	2
640420.5	完全麻痺（知覚運動機能の消失した対麻痺）　骨折・脱臼については不明	640420.5	640420.5	1
640422.5	骨折や脱臼を伴わない	640422.5	640422.5	1
640424.5	骨折を伴う	640424.5	640424.5	1
640426.5	脱臼を伴う	640426.5	640426.5	1
640428.5	骨折かつ脱臼を伴う	640428.5	640428.5	1

脊椎

THORACIC SPINE

AIS 2005	Injury Description	⇒ AIS98	⇐ AIS98	FCI
640440.5	**Cord** laceration NFS [includes penetrating injury, transection or crush]	640440.5	640440.5	5
640442.5	incomplete (preservation of some sensation or motor function), but NFS as to fracture/dislocation	640442.5	640442.5	5
640444.5	with no fracture or dislocation	640444.5	640444.5	5
640446.5	with fracture	640446.5	640446.5	5
640448.5	with dislocation	640448.5	640448.5	5
640450.5	with both fracture and dislocation	640450.5	640450.5	5
640460.5	complete cord syndrome NFS (paraplegia with no sensation or motor function) but NFS as to fracture/dislocation	640460.5	640460.5	1
640462.5	with no fracture or dislocation	640462.5	640462.5	1
640464.5	with fracture	640464.5	640464.5	1
640466.5	with dislocation	640466.5	640466.5	1
640468.5	with both fracture and dislocation	640468.5	640468.5	1
650499.2	**Disc** injury NFS	650499.2	650499.2	5
650400.2	herniation NFS	650400.2	650400.2	5
650402.2	no nerve root damage (radiculopathy)	650402.2	650402.2	5
650403.3	with nerve root damage (radiculopathy)	650403.3	650403.3	5
650405.3	rupture	650403.3	650403.3	
650404.2	Dislocation [subluxation], no fracture, no cord involvement NFS	650404.2	650404.2	5
	Code as one injury and assign to superior vertebra.			
650409.2	**facet** NFS	650409.2	650409.2	5
650410.2	unilateral	650410.2	650410.2	5
650412.3	bilateral	650412.3	650412.3	5

胸 椎

AIS 2005	損傷内容	⇒ AIS98	⇐ AIS98	FCI
640440.5	**胸髄**裂傷・裂創［穿通性損傷，離断あるいは挫滅を含む］　詳細不明	640440.5	640440.5	5
640442.5	不全麻痺（何らかの知覚あるいは運動機能の残存）　骨折・脱臼については不明	640442.5	640442.5	5
640444.5	骨折や脱臼を伴わない	640444.5	640444.5	5
640446.5	骨折を伴う	640446.5	640446.5	5
640448.5	脱臼を伴う	640448.5	640448.5	5
640450.5	骨折かつ脱臼を伴う	640450.5	640450.5	5
640460.5	完全麻痺（知覚運動機能の消失した対麻痺）　骨折・脱臼については不明	640460.5	640460.5	1
640462.5	骨折や脱臼を伴わない	640462.5	640462.5	1
640464.5	骨折を伴う	640464.5	640464.5	1
640466.5	脱臼を伴う	640466.5	640466.5	1
640468.5	骨折かつ脱臼を伴う	640468.5	640468.5	1
650499.2	**椎間板**損傷　詳細不明	650499.2	650499.2	5
650400.2	ヘルニア　詳細不明	650400.2	650400.2	5
650402.2	神経根損傷（神経根障害）を伴わない	650402.2	650402.2	5
650403.3	神経根損傷（神経根障害）を伴う	650403.3	650403.3	5
650405.3	破裂	650403.3	650403.3	
650404.2	胸椎脱臼［亜脱臼］，骨折，胸髄損傷を伴わない　詳細不明	650404.2	650404.2	5
	上位胸椎の損傷として1つだけコードを選択する。			
650409.2	椎間関節　詳細不明	650409.2	650409.2	5
650410.2	片側	650410.2	650410.2	5
650412.3	両側	650412.3	650412.3	5

脊椎

THORACIC SPINE

AIS 2005	Injury Description	⇒ AIS98	⇐ AIS98	FCI
650416.2	Fracture with or without dislocation but no cord involvement NFS	650416.2	650416.2	5
	Code each vertebra separately.			
650417.2	multiple fractures of same **vertebra**[a]	650416.2	None	5
	Exception : major compression fracture which is coded additionally.			
650418.2	**spinous process**	650418.2	650418.2	5
650420.2	**transverse process**	650420.2	650420.2	5
650422.2	**facet**	650422.3[b]	650422.3[b]	5
650424.2	**lamina**	650424.3[b]	650424.3[b]	5
650426.2	**pedicle**	650426.3[b]	650426.3[b]	5
650430.2	**vertebral body** NFS ["burst fracture"]	650430.2	650430.2	5
650432.2	minor compression (≤20% loss of anterior height)	650432.2	650432.2	5
650434.3	major compression (>20% loss of anterior height)	650434.3	650434.3	5
640484.1	**Spinous ligament** injury	640484.1	640484.1	5
630499.2	**Nerve root**, single or multiple NFS	630499.2	630499.2	5
630402.2	contusion ; stretch injury	630402.2	630402.2	5
630404.2	laceration NFS	630404.2	630404.2	5
630406.2	single nerve root	630406.2	630406.2	5
630408.3	multiple nerve roots	630408.3	630408.3	3
630410.2	avulsion NFS	630410.2	630410.2	5
630412.2	single nerve root	630412.2	630412.2	5
630414.3	multiple nerve roots	630414.3	630414.3	3
640478.1	Strain, acute with no fracture or dislocation	640478.1	640478.1	5

---

[a] New descriptor in AIS 2005
[b] Change in severity code in AIS 2005

胸椎

AIS 2005	損傷内容	⇒ AIS98	⇐ AIS98	FCI
650416.2	胸椎骨折（胸髄損傷は伴わないが脱臼の有無は問わない）　詳細不明	650416.2	650416.2	5
	損傷が明らかな場合には以下のコードを選択する。			
650417.2	同一椎骨の多部位に及ぶ骨折[a]	650416.2	なし	5
	例外：椎体全面高の減少が20%を超える圧迫骨折は併せてコードを選択する。			
650418.2	棘突起	650418.2	650418.2	5
650420.2	横突起	650420.2	650420.2	5
650422.2	関節突起	650422.3[b]	650422.3[b]	5
650424.2	椎弓	650424.3[b]	650424.3[b]	5
650426.2	椎弓根	650426.3[b]	650426.3[b]	5
650430.2	椎体　詳細不明［"破裂骨折"に使用］	650430.2	650430.2	5
650432.2	圧迫骨折　小（椎体前面高の減少が20%以下）	650432.2	650432.2	5
650434.3	圧迫骨折　大（椎体前面高の減少が20%を超える）	650434.3	650434.3	5
640484.1	棘間靱帯損傷	640484.1	640484.1	5
630499.2	神経根，単発あるいは多発　詳細不明	630499.2	630499.2	5
630402.2	挫傷；伸展損傷	630402.2	630402.2	5
630404.2	裂傷・裂創　詳細不明	630404.2	630404.2	5
630406.2	単一神経根	630406.2	630406.2	5
630408.3	複数神経根	630408.3	630408.3	3
630410.2	引き抜き損傷　詳細不明	630410.2	630410.2	5
630412.2	単一神経根	630412.2	630412.2	5
630414.3	複数神経根	630414.3	630414.3	3
640478.1	捻挫，急性で骨折や脱臼を伴わない	640478.1	640478.1	5

脊椎

---

[a] AIS2005に加えられた新しいコード。
[b] AIS 2005で重症度に変更あり。

LUMBAR SPINE

AIS 2005	Injury Description	⇒ AIS98	⇐ AIS98	FCI
	Use one of the following two descriptors when such vague information is the only information available. While these descriptors identify the occurrence of an injury to the lumbar spine, they do not specify its severity.			
630099.9	**Injuries to the Lumbar Spine** NFS	617099.9	617099.9	
630999.9	Died of lumbar spine injury without further substantiation of injuries or no autopsy confirmation of specific injuries.	617999.9	617999.9	
630600.3	**Cauda equina** contusion NFS	630600.3	630600.3	5
630602.3	with transient neurological signs (paresthesia), but NFS as to fracture/dislocation	630602.3	630602.3	5
630604.3	with no fracture or dislocation	630604.3	630604.3	5
630606.3	with fracture	630606.3	630606.3	5
630608.3	with dislocation	630608.3	630608.3	5
630610.3	with both fracture and dislocation	630610.3	630610.3	5
630620.3	incomplete cauda equina syndrome, but NFS as to fracture/dislocation	630620.3	630620.3	5
630622.3	with no fracture or dislocation	630622.3	630622.3	5
630624.3	with fracture	630624.3	630624.3	5
630626.3	with dislocation	630626.3	630626.3	5
630628.3	with both fracture and dislocation	630628.3	630628.3	5
630630.4	complete cauda equina syndrome, but NFS as to fracture/dislocation	630630.4	630630.4	1
630632.4	with no fracture or dislocation	630632.4	630632.4	1
630634.4	with fracture	630634.4	630634.4	1
630636.4	with dislocation	630636.4	630636.4	1
630638.4	with both fracture and dislocation	630638.4	630638.4	1

腰　椎

AIS 2005	損傷内容	⇒ AIS98	⇐ AIS98	FCI
	不確定な情報しか得られない場合には，以下の2つのコードのうちいずれかを選択する。これらのコードは，腰椎に損傷が生じたことを記録する目的にのみ使用し，重症度の算出には用いない。			
630099.9	**腰椎損傷**　詳細不明	617099.9	617099.9	
630999.9	腰椎損傷による死亡（詳細不明）または剖検なし	617999.9	617999.9	
630600.3	**馬尾**挫傷　詳細不明	630600.3	630600.3	5
630602.3	一過性の神経症状（知覚異常）を伴う　骨折・脱臼については不明	630602.3	630602.3	5
630604.3	骨折や脱臼を伴わない	630604.3	630604.3	5
630606.3	骨折を伴う	630606.3	630606.3	5
630608.3	脱臼を伴う	630608.3	630608.3	5
630610.3	骨折かつ脱臼を伴う	630610.3	630610.3	5
630620.3	不完全馬尾症候群　骨折・脱臼については不明	630620.3	630620.3	5
630622.3	骨折や脱臼を伴わない	630622.3	630622.3	5
630624.3	骨折を伴う	630624.3	630624.3	5
630626.3	脱臼を伴う	630626.3	630626.3	5
630628.3	骨折かつ脱臼を伴う	630628.3	630628.3	5
630630.4	完全馬尾症候群　骨折・脱臼については不明	630630.4	630630.4	1
630632.4	骨折や脱臼を伴わない	630632.4	630632.4	1
630634.4	骨折を伴う	630634.4	630634.4	1
630636.4	脱臼を伴う	630636.4	630636.4	1
630638.4	骨折かつ脱臼を伴う	630638.4	630638.4	1

LUMBAR SPINE

AIS 2005	Injury Description	⇒ AIS98	⇐ AIS98	FCI
640600.3	**Cord** contusion [includes the diagnosis of compression, or epidural or subdural hemorrhage within spinal canal documented by imaging studies or autopsy]	640600.3	640600.3	5
640601.3	with transient neurological signs (paresthesia), but NFS as to fracture/dislocation	640601.3	640601.3	5
640602.3	with no fracture or dislocation	640602.3	640602.3	5
640604.3	with fracture	640604.3	640604.3	5
640606.3	with dislocation	640606.3	640606.3	5
640608.3	with both fracture and dislocation	640608.3	640608.3	5
640610.4	incomplete cord syndrome (preservation of some sensation or motor function; includes lateral cord (*Brown-Sequard*) syndrome) but NFS as to fracture/dislocation	640610.4	640610.4	5
640612.4	with no fracture or dislocation	640612.4	640612.4	5
640614.4	with fracture	640614.4	640614.4	5
640616.4	with dislocation	640616.4	640616.4	5
640618.4	with both fracture and dislocation	640618.4	640618.4	5
640620.5	complete cord syndrome (paraplegia with no sensation) but NFS as to fracture/dislocation	640620.5	640620.5	1
640622.5	with no fracture or dislocation	640622.5	640622.5	1
640624.5	with fracture	640624.5	640624.5	1
640626.5	with dislocation	640626.5	640626.5	1
640628.5	with both fracture and dislocation	640628.5	640628.5	1

腰　椎

AIS 2005	損傷内容	⇒ AIS98	⇐ AIS98	FCI
640600.3	**腰髄**挫傷［画像診断法あるいは剖検により証明された脊柱管内の圧迫や硬膜外，硬膜下血腫の診断を含む］	640600.3	640600.3	5
640601.3	一過性の神経症状（知覚異常）を伴う　骨折脱臼については不明	640601.3	640601.3	5
640602.3	骨折や脱臼を伴わない	640602.3	640602.3	5
640604.3	骨折を伴う	640604.3	640604.3	5
640606.3	脱臼を伴う	640606.3	640606.3	5
640608.3	骨折かつ脱臼を伴う	640608.3	640608.3	5
640610.4	不全麻痺〔何らかの知覚あるいは運動機能の残存；外側脊髄症候群（Brown-Sequard 症候群症候群）〕を含む　骨折・脱臼については不明	640610.4	640610.4	5
640612.4	骨折や脱臼を伴わない	640612.4	640612.4	5
640614.4	骨折を伴う	640614.4	640614.4	5
640616.4	脱臼を伴う	640616.4	640616.4	5
640618.4	骨折かつ脱臼を伴う	640618.4	640618.4	5
640620.5	完全麻痺（知覚運動機能の消失した対麻痺）　骨折・脱臼については不明	640620.5	640620.5	1
640622.5	骨折や脱臼を伴わない	640622.5	640622.5	1
640624.5	骨折を伴う	640624.5	640624.5	1
640626.5	脱臼を伴う	640626.5	640626.5	1
640628.5	骨折かつ脱臼を伴う	640628.5	640628.5	1

LUMBAR SPINE

AIS 2005	Injury Description	⇒ AIS98	⇐ AIS98	FCI
640640.5	**Cord** laceration NFS [includes penetrating injury, transection or crush]	640640.5	640640.5	5
640642.5	incomplete (preservation of some sensation or motor function), but NFS as to fracture/dislocation	640642.5	640642.5	5
640644.5	with no fracture or dislocation	640644.5	640644.5	5
640646.5	with fracture	640646.5	640646.5	5
640648.5	with dislocation	640648.5	640648.5	5
640650.5	with both fracture and dislocation	640650.5	640650.5	5
640660.5	complete cord syndrome NFS (paraplegia with no sensation or motor function) but NFS as to fracture/dislocation	640660.5	640660.5	1
640662.5	with no fracture or dislocation	640662.5	640662.5	1
640664.5	with fracture	640664.5	640664.5	1
640666.5	with dislocation	640666.5	640666.5	1
640668.5	with both fracture and dislocation	640668.5	640668.5	1
650699.2	**Disc** injury NFS	650699.2	650699.2	5
650600.2	herniation NFS	650600.2	650600.2	5
650602.2	no nerve root damage (radiculopathy)	650602.2	650602.2	5
650603.3	with nerve root damage (radiculopathy)	650603.3	650603.3	5
650605.3	rupture	650603.3	650603.3	5
650604.2	Dislocation [subluxation], no fracture, no cord involvement NFS	650604.2	650604.2	5
	Code as one injury and assign to superior vertebra.			
650609.2	**facet** NFS	650609.2	650609.2	5
650610.2	unilateral	650610.2	650610.2	5
650612.3	bilateral	650612.3	650612.3	5

腰 椎

AIS 2005	損傷内容	⇒ AIS98	⇐ AIS98	FCI
640640.5	**腰髄**裂傷・裂創［穿通性損傷，離断あるいは挫滅を含む］　詳細不明	640640.5	640640.5	5
640642.5	不全麻痺（何らかの知覚あるいは運動機能の残存）骨折・脱臼については不明	640642.5	640642.5	5
640644.5	骨折や脱臼を伴わない	640644.5	640644.5	5
640646.5	骨折を伴う	640646.5	640646.5	5
640648.5	脱臼を伴う	640648.5	640648.5	5
640650.5	骨折かつ脱臼を伴う	640650.5	640650.5	5
640660.5	完全麻痺（知覚運動機能の消失した対麻痺）骨折・脱臼については不明	640660.5	640660.5	1
640662.5	骨折や脱臼を伴わない	640662.5	640662.5	1
640664.5	骨折を伴う	640664.5	640664.5	1
640666.5	脱臼を伴う	640666.5	640666.5	1
640668.5	骨折かつ脱臼を伴う	640668.5	640668.5	1
650699.2	**椎間板**損傷　詳細不明	650699.2	650699.2	5
650600.2	ヘルニア　詳細不明	650600.2	650600.2	5
650602.2	神経根損傷（神経根障害）を伴わない	650602.2	650602.2	5
650603.3	神経根損傷（神経根障害）を伴う	650603.3	650603.3	5
650605.3	破裂	650603.3	650603.3	5
650604.2	腰椎脱臼［亜脱臼］，骨折や腰髄損傷を伴わない　詳細不明	650604.2	650604.2	5
	上位腰椎の損傷として1つだけコードを選択する。			
650609.2	**椎間関節**　詳細不明	650609.2	650609.2	5
650610.2	片側	650610.2	650610.2	5
650612.3	両側	650612.3	650612.3	5

LUMBAR SPINE

AIS 2005	Injury Description	⇒ AIS98	⇐ AIS98	FCI
650616.2	Fracture with or without dislocation but no cord involvement NFS	650616.2	650616.2	5
	Code each vertebra separately.			
650617.2	multiple fractures of same **vertebra**[a]	650616.2	None	5
	Exception: major compression fracture which is coded additionally.			
650618.2	**spinous process**	650618.2	650618.2	5
650620.2	**transverse process**	650620.2	650620.2	5
650622.2	**facet**	650622.3[b]	650622.3[b]	5
650624.2	**lamina**	650624.3[b]	650624.3[b]	5
650626.2	**pedicle**	650626.3[b]	650626.3[b]	5
650630.2	**vertebral body** NFS ["burst fracture"]	650630.2	650630.2	5
650632.2	minor compression (≤20% loss of anterior height)	650632.2	650632.2	5
650634.3	major compression (>20% loss of anterior height)	650634.3	650634.3	5
640684.1	**Spinous ligament** injury	640684.1	640684.1	5
630699.2	**Nerve root or sacral plexus**, single or multiple NFS	630699.2	630699.2	5
630660.2	contusion ; stretch injury	630660.2	630660.2	5
630662.2	laceration NFS	630662.2	630662.2	5
630664.2	single nerve root	630664.2	630664.2	5
630666.3	multiple nerve roots	630666.3	630666.3	4
630668.2	avulsion NFS	630668.2	630668.2	5
630612.2	single nerve root	630612.2	630612.2	5
630614.3	multiple nerve roots	630614.3	630614.3	4
640678.1	Strain, acute with no fracture or dislocation	640678.1	640678.1	5

腰椎

AIS 2005	損傷内容	⇒ AIS98	⇐ AIS98	FCI
650616.2	腰椎骨折（腰髄損傷は伴わないが脱臼の有無は問わない）　詳細不明	650616.2	650616.2	5
	損傷が明らかな場合には以下のコードを選択する。			
650617.2	同一**椎骨**の多部位に及ぶ骨折[a]	650616.2	None	5
	例外：椎体全面高の減少が20%を超える圧迫骨折は併せてコードを選択する。			
650618.2	棘突起	650618.2	650618.2	5
650620.2	横突起	650620.2	650620.2	5
650622.2	関節突起	650622.3[b]	650622.3[b]	5
650624.2	椎弓	650624.3[b]	650624.3[b]	5
650626.2	椎弓根	650626.3[b]	650626.3[b]	5
650630.2	椎体　詳細不明［"破裂骨折"］	650630.2	650630.2	5
650632.2	圧迫骨折　小（椎体前面高の減少が20%以下）	650632.2	650632.2	5
650634.3	圧迫骨折　大（椎体前面高の減少が20%を超える）	650634.3	650634.3	5
640684.1	**棘間靱帯**損傷	640684.1	640684.1	5
630699.2	**神経根あるいは仙骨神経叢**，単発あるいは多発　詳細不明	630699.2	630699.2	5
630660.2	挫傷；伸展損傷	630660.2	630660.2	5
630662.2	裂傷・裂創　詳細不明	630662.2	630662.2	5
630664.2	単一神経根	630664.2	630664.2	5
630666.3	複数神経根	630666.3	630666.3	4
630668.2	引き抜き損傷　詳細不明	630668.2	630668.2	5
630612.2	単一神経根	630612.2	630612.2	5
630614.3	複数神経根	630614.3	630614.3	4
640678.1	捻挫，急性で骨折や脱臼を伴わない	640678.1	640678.1	5

上　肢

UPPER EXTREMITY

AIS 2005	Injury Description	⇒ AIS98	⇐ AIS98	FCI
	WHOLE AREA			
	Use one of the following two descriptors when such vague information is the only information available. While these descriptors identify the occurrence of an upper extremity injury, they do not specify its severity.			
700099.9	**Injuries to the Whole Upper Extremity** NFS	715099.9	715099.9	
700999.9	Died of upper extremity injury without further substantiation of injuries or no autopsy confirmation of specific injuries	715999.9	715999.9	
711000.3	**Amputation [traumatic], partial or complete** between shoulder and hand, but NFS as to specific anatomical site[s]	711000.3	711000.3	2
	The above description does not apply to hands, thumbs or fingers.			
711001.4	at shoulder	711000.3[b]	None	1
711010.5	bilateral[c]	711000.3[b]	None	1
711002.4	at or above elbow, below shoulder	711000.3[b]	None	1
711012.5	bilateral[c]	711000.3[b]	None	1
711003.3	below elbow, at or above wrist	711000.3	None	1
711004.2	hand, partial or complete	711000.3[b]	None	2
711005.2	thumb	752402.2	None	2
711006.1	other fingers, single or multiple	752402.2[b]	752402.2[b]	4

---

[b] Change in severity code in AIS 2005

[c] In previous editions of AIS, with few exceptions, each injury was coded separately. AIS 2005 introduces "bilateral". Some bilateral injuries may affect severity levels and, therefore, the ISS for patients with those injuries.

[s] Differentiation of specific anatomical sites in this injury category was less detailed in AIS98 than in AIS 2005 ; hence the duplication of AIS98 matching codes.

上 肢

AIS 2005	損傷内容	⇒ AIS98	⇐ AIS98	FCI
	全 域			
	不確定な情報しか得られない場合には，以下の2つのコードのいずれかを選択する。これらのコードは上肢に外傷が存在することを示すが，重症度をもたない（訳者注：このコードがある場合は ISS などを計算できない）。			
700099.9	**上肢損傷** 詳細不明	715099.9	715099.9	
700999.9	上肢損傷で死亡 詳細な評価や損傷を特定しうる剖検なし	715999.9	715999.9	
711000.3	肩と手の間の**不完全または完全[外傷性]切断**，ただし具体的な場所は不明[s]	711000.3	711000.3	2
	上記のコードは手，手指，親指には適用しない。			
711001.4	肩で切断	711000.3[b]	なし	1
711010.5	両側[c]	711000.3[b]	なし	1
711002.4	肘と肩の間（肘を含む）	711000.3[b]	なし	1
711012.5	両側[c]	711000.3[b]	なし	1
711003.3	手関節と肘の間（手関節を含む）	711000.3	なし	1
711004.2	手，不完全または完全	711000.3[b]	なし	2
711005.2	母指	752402.2	なし	2
711006.1	他の手指，1指または複数指	752402.2[b]	752402.2[b]	4

---

[b] AIS2005で重傷度に変更あり。

[c] 旧版の AIS では一部の例外を除き両側損傷はそれぞれ別にコード選択をしていた。AIS2005では"両側"を導入した。いくつかの両側損傷は重症度が変化し，その結果 ISS が変わることがある。

[s] AIS98では切断の部位に関する記述が AIS2005に比べて少ない。したがって（訳者追加：711000.3から711004.2のコードに相当する）AIS98コードは同じものを使用している。

UPPER EXTREMITY

AIS 2005	Injury Description	⇒ AIS98	⇐ AIS98	FCI
	Use this category only if no specific injuries to the upper extremity are documented.			
712000.2	**Compartment syndrome** from trauma to soft tissue only, not involving fracture or massive destruction of bone or other anatomical structures, NFS	715000.2	715000.2	
712001.2	arm NFS	715000.2	None	5
712002.2	no muscle loss	715000.2	None	5
712003.3	with muscle loss	715000.2[b]	None	3
712004.2	forearm	715000.2	None	5
712005.2	no muscle loss	715000.2	None	5
712006.2	with muscle loss	715000.2	None	3
712007.2	hand	715000.2	None	4
712008.2	no muscle loss	715000.2	None	4
712009.2	with muscle loss	715000.2	None	4
713000.2	**Crush Injury** to limb between shoulder and wrist, but NFS as to specific anatomical site[s]	713000.3[b]	713000.3[b]	4
	Must involve massive destruction of skeletal, vascular, nervous and tissue systems. Do not use the above description for hands or fingers.			
713001.4	at shoulder	713000.3[b]	None	2
713002.4	at or above elbow, below shoulder	713000.3[b]	None	2
713003.3	below elbow, at or above wrist	713000.3	None	4
713004.2	hand, partial or complete	713000.3[b]	None	4
713005.2	thumb	752406.2	None	4
713006.1	non-thumb finger, single or multiple	752406.2[b]	752406.2[b]	4
	Assign degloving injuries to External body region for calculating an ISS.			
714000.2	**Degloving injury** NFS as to specific anatomical site[s]	None	None	4
714001.3	entire extremity	714006.3	714006.3	4
714002.2	arm or forearm, including elbow	714002.2	714002.2	5
714003.2	wrist or hand	714006.3[b]	714006.3[b]	4
714004.2	finger, single or multiple	714004.2	714004.2	4

---

[b] Change in severity code in AIS 2005

[s] The differentiation of specific anatomical sites in this injury category was less detailed in AIS98 than in AIS 2005 ; hence, the duplication of AIS98 matching codes.

AIS 2005	損傷内容	⇒ AIS98	⇐ AIS98	FCI
	下記のコードは，上肢の外傷について具体的な記述がない場合に選択する。			
712000.2	軟部組織損傷により生じた**コンパートメント症候群**，骨折や他の軟部組織以外の組織損傷を伴わない　詳細不明	715000.2	715000.2	
712001.2	上腕	715000.2	なし	5
712002.2	筋肉の欠損を伴わない	715000.2	なし	5
712003.3	筋肉の欠損を伴う	715000.2[b]	なし	3
712004.2	前腕	715000.2	なし	5
712005.2	筋肉の欠損を伴わない	715000.2	なし	5
712006.2	筋肉の欠損を伴う	715000.2	なし	3
712007.2	手	715000.2	なし	4
712008.2	筋肉の欠損を伴わない	715000.2	なし	4
712009.2	筋肉の欠損を伴う	715000.2	なし	4
713000.2	**挫滅損傷**　肩と手首の間の上肢，具体的な部位については詳細不明[s]	713000.3[b]	713000.3[b]	4
	骨，血管，神経，組織に広範囲の損傷を伴わなければならない。手や指の場合は上記コードを選択しない。			
713001.4	肩	713000.3[b]	なし	2
713002.4	肘と肩の間（肘を含む）	713000.3[b]	なし	2
713003.3	手関節と肘の間（手関節を含む）	713000.3	なし	4
713004.2	手，部分的または全体	713000.3[b]	なし	4
713005.2	母指	752406.2	なし	4
713006.1	母指以外の指で1指または複数指	752406.2[b]	752406.2[b]	4
	デグロービング損傷はISSを計算するときは体表で計算する。			
714000.2	**デグロービング損傷**　具体的な部位については詳細不明	なし	なし	4
714001.3	上肢全体	714006.3	714006.3	4
714002.2	上腕または前腕，肘を含む	714002.2	714002.2	5
714003.2	手関節または手	714006.3[b]	714006.3[b]	4
714004.2	指，1指または複数指	714004.2	714004.2	4

[b] AIS2005で重症度に変更あり。
[s] AIS98のこの損傷に関する部位の記述はAIS2005に比べて少ない。したがってAIS98コードは同じコードを使用している。

UPPER EXTREMITY

AIS 2005	Injury Description	⇒ AIS98	⇐ AIS98	FCI
	Use this category if penetrating injury does not involve bone or internal structures. Assign to External body region for calculating an ISS. If underlying anatomical structures are involved, code documented diagnoses only ; do not use these generic descriptors. Penetrating injury involving a bone is coded as open fracture to the specific bone.			
716000.1	**Penetrating injury** NFS as to specific anatomical site[s]	716000.1	716000.1	5
716002.1	superficial ; minor	716002.1	716002.1	5
716004.2	with tissue loss >25cm^2	716004.2	716004.2	3
716006.3	with blood loss >20% by volume	716006.3	716006.3	5
716010.1	**Penetrating injury** at shoulder, NFS as to severity	716000.1	None	5
716011.1	superficial ; minor	716002.1	None	5
716012.2	with tissue loss >25cm^2	716004.2	None	3
716013.3	with blood loss >20% by volume	716006.3	None	5
716014.1	**Penetrating injury** at or above elbow, below shoulder, NFS as to severity	716000.1	None	5
716015.1	superficial ; minor	716002.1	None	5
716016.2	with tissue loss >25cm^2	716004.2	None	2
716017.3	with blood loss >20% by volume	716006.3	None	5
716018.1	**Penetrating injury** below elbow, at or above wrist, NFS as to severity	716000.1	None	5
716019.1	superficial ; minor	716002.1	None	5
716020.2	with tissue loss >25cm^2	716004.2	None	3
716022.1	**Penetrating injury** hand, partial or complete, NFS as to severity	716000.1	None	5
716023.1	superficial ; minor	716002.1	None	5
716024.2	with tissue loss >25cm^2	716004.2	None	3
716026.1	**Penetrating injury** thumb, NFS as to severity	716000.1	None	5
716027.1	superficial ; minor	716002.1	None	5
716028.2	with tissue loss >25cm^2	716004.2	None	2
716030.1	**Penetrating injury** non-thumb finger, NFS as to severity	716000.1	None	5
716031.1	superficial ; minor	716002.1	None	5
716032.2	with tissue loss >25cm^2	716004.2	None	4

---

[s] Differentiation of specific anatomical sites of this injury description was less detailed in AIS98 than in AIS 2005 ; hence, the duplication of AIS98 matching codes.

上　肢

AIS 2005	損傷内容	⇒ AIS98	⇐ AIS98	FCI
	下記のコードは穿通性損傷が骨や臓器に及んでいない場合に選択する。ISSを計算するときは体表で計算する。もし創が骨や臓器に達する場合は，損傷した骨や臓器をコード選択する（訳者注：創をコード選択しない）。穿通性損傷が骨に及んでいる場合は，該当する骨の開放骨折をコード選択する。			
716000.1	**穿通性損傷**　具体的な部位については詳細不明[s]	716000.1	716000.1	5
716002.1	表在性；小	716002.1	716002.1	5
716004.2	25cm^{2}を超える組織欠損	716004.2	716004.2	3
716006.3	出血量が全血液量の20％を超える	716006.3	716006.3	5
716010.1	**穿通性損傷**　肩，重症度については詳細不明	716000.1	なし	5
716011.1	表在性；小	716002.1	なし	5
716012.2	25cm^{2}を超える組織欠損	716004.2	なし	3
716013.3	出血量が全血液量の20％を超える	716006.3	なし	5
716014.1	**穿通性損傷**　肘と肩の間（肘を含む）　重症度については詳細不明	716000.1	なし	5
716015.1	表在性；小	716002.1	なし	5
716016.2	25cm^{2}を超える組織欠損	716004.2	なし	2
716017.3	出血量が全血液量の20％を超える	716006.3	なし	5
716018.1	**穿通性損傷**　手関節と肘の間（手関節を含む），重症度については詳細不明	716000.1	なし	5
716019.1	表在性；小	716002.1	なし	5
716020.2	25cm^{2}を超える組織欠損	716004.2	なし	3
716022.1	**穿通性損傷**　手，部分的または全体，重症度については詳細不明	716000.1	なし	5
716023.1	表在性；小	716002.1	なし	5
716024.2	25cm^{2}を超える組織欠損	716004.2	なし	3
716026.1	**穿通性損傷**　母指　重症度については詳細不明	716000.1	なし	5
716027.1	表在性；小	716002.1	なし	5
716028.2	25cm^{2}を超える組織欠損	716004.2	なし	2
716030.1	**穿通性損傷**　指，1指または複数指　重症度については詳細不明	716000.1	なし	5
716031.1	表在性；小	716002.1	なし	5
716032.2	25cm^{2}を超える組織欠損	716004.2	なし	4

[s]　AIS98のこの損傷に関する部位の記述はAIS2005に比べて少ない。したがってAIS98コードは同じコードを使用している。

UPPER EXTREMITY

AIS 2005	Injury Description	⇒ AIS98	⇐ AIS98	FCI
	Use the following section for blunt soft tissue injury to the upper extremity. Assign to External body region for calculating an ISS.			
710099.1	**Skin/subcutaneous/muscle** NFS	710099.1	710099.1	5
710202.1	abrasion	710202.1	710202.1	5
710402.1	contusion ; hematoma	710402.1	710402.1	5
710600.1	laceration NFS	710600.1	710600.1	5
710602.1	minor ; superficial	710602.1	710602.1	5
710604.2	major ; >10cm long on hand or >20cm long on entire extremity and into subcutaneous tissue	710604.2	710604.2	5
710606.3	blood loss >20% by volume	710606.3	710606.3	5
710800.1	avulsion NFS	710800.1	710800.1	5
710802.1	minor ; superficial ; ≤25cm^2 on hand or ≤100cm^2 on entire extremity	710802.1	710802.1	5
710804.2	major ; tissue loss >25cm^2 on hand or >100cm^2 on entire extremity	710804.2	710804.2	4
710806.3	blood loss >20% by volume	710806.3	710806.3	5

AIS 2005	損傷内容	⇒ AIS98	⇐ AIS98	FCI
	下記のコードは上肢の鈍的損傷で選択する。ISS を計算するときは体表で計算する。			
710099.1	**皮膚／皮下／筋肉**　詳細不明	710099.1	710099.1	5
710202.1	擦過傷	710202.1	710202.1	5
710402.1	挫傷；血腫	710402.1	710402.1	5
710600.1	裂傷・裂創　詳細不明	710600.1	710600.1	5
710602.1	小；表在性	710602.1	710602.1	5
710604.2	大；手では10cm，手以外の上肢では長さが20cmを超え，かつ皮下組織に達する	710604.2	710604.2	5
710606.3	出血量が全血液量の20%を超える	710606.3	710606.3	5
710800.1	剥離　詳細不明	710800.1	710800.1	5
710802.1	小；表在性；手では25cm^{2}以下または上肢全体では100cm^{2}以下	710802.1	710802.1	5
710804.2	大；手では25cm^{2}または上肢全体では100cm^{2}を超える	710804.2	710804.2	4
710806.3	出血量が全血液量の20%を超える	710806.3	710806.3	5

AIS 2005	Injury Description	⇒ AIS98	⇐ AIS98	FCI
	VESSELS			
	Do not code upper extremity vessel injuries separately when they are directly involved in crush-type injuries or amputation of an upper extremity unless a vascular injury is higher in severity than the crush-type injury or amputation. Branches of vessels are not coded unless they are named vessels and/or are listed within a specific vessel descriptor.			
720099.9	**Vascular Injury in Upper Extremity NFS**[f]	None	None	
720299.2	**Axillary artery** NFS	720299.2	720299.2	5
720202.2	intimal tear, no disruption	720202.2	720202.2	5
720204.2	laceration ; perforation ; puncture NFS	720204.2	720204.2	5
720206.2	minor ; superficial ; incomplete circumferential involvement ; blood loss ≤20% by volume	720206.2	720206.2	5
720208.3	major ; rupture ; transection ; segmental loss ; blood loss >20% by volume	720208.3	720208.3	5
720499.2	**Axillary vein** NFS	720499.2	720499.2	5
720402.2	laceration ; perforation ; puncture NFS	720402.2	720402.2	5
720404.2	minor ; superficial ; incomplete circumferential involvement ; blood loss ≤20% by volume	720404.2	720404.2	5
720406.3	major ; rupture ; transection ; segmental loss ; blood loss >20% by volume	720406.3	720406.3	5
720699.2	**Brachial artery** NFS	720699.2	720699.2	5
720602.2	intimal tear, no disruption	720602.2	720602.2	5
720604.2	laceration ; puncture ; perforation NFS	720604.2	720604.2	5
720606.2	minor ; superficial ; incomplete circumferential involvement ; blood loss ≤20% by volume	720606.2	720606.2	5
720608.3	major ; rupture ; transection ; segmental loss ; blood loss >20% by volume	720608.3	720608.3	5

---

[f] New descriptor in AIS 2005 that allows classification of trauma by body region, but does not allow assigning a severity code.

AIS 2005	損傷内容	⇒ AIS98	⇐ AIS98	FCI

血 管

上肢の挫滅損傷や切断の場合は，血管損傷を別にコード選択しない。ただし，血管損傷の重症度のほうが挫滅損傷や切断の重症度より高い場合はコード選択する。主要な血管の枝はそれが名前をもち，かつ／またはその血管名が列挙されている場合に限り，コード選択をする。

AIS 2005	損傷内容	⇒ AIS98	⇐ AIS98	FCI
720099.9	上肢の血管損傷　詳細不明[f]	なし	なし	
720299.2	**腋窩動脈**　詳細不明	720299.2	720299.2	5
720202.2	内膜剥離，断裂なし	720202.2	720202.2	5
720204.2	裂傷・裂創；穿孔；穿刺　詳細不明	720204.2	720204.2	5
720206.2	小；表在性；非全周性；出血量が全血液量の20%以下	720206.2	720206.2	5
720208.3	大；破裂；断裂；部分欠損；出血量が全血液量の20%を超える	720208.3	720208.3	5
720499.2	**腋窩静脈**　詳細不明	720499.2	720499.2	5
720402.2	裂傷・裂創；穿孔；穿刺　詳細不明	720402.2	720402.2	5
720404.2	小；表在性；非全周性；出血量が全血液量の20%以下	720404.2	720404.2	5
720406.3	大；破裂；断裂；部分欠損；出血量が全血液量の20%を超える	720406.3	720406.3	5
720699.2	**上腕動脈**　詳細不明	720699.2	720699.2	5
720602.2	内膜剥離，断裂なし	720602.2	720602.2	5
720604.2	裂傷・裂創；穿孔；穿刺　詳細不明	720604.2	720604.2	5
720606.2	小；表在性；非全周性；出血量が全血液量の20%以下	720606.2	720606.2	5
720608.3	大；破裂；断裂；部分欠損；出血量が全血液量の20%を超える	720608.3	720608.3	5

---

[f] AIS2005に加えられた新しいコード。外傷の存在部位を示すことができる。ただし重症度はない。

UPPER EXTREMITY

AIS 2005	Injury Description	⇒ AIS98	⇐ AIS98	FCI
720899.1	**Brachial vein** NFS	720899.1	720899.1	5
720802.1	laceration ; perforation ; puncture NFS	720802.1	720802.1	5
720804.1	minor ; superficial ; incomplete circumferential involvement ; blood loss ≤20% by volume	720804.1	720804.1	5
720806.3	major ; rupture ; transection ; segmental loss ; blood loss >20% by volume	720806.3	720806.3	5
721099.1	**Other named arteries** NFS [e.g., **radial, ulnar**]	721099.1	721099.1	5
721002.1	intimal tear, no disruption	721002.1	721002.1	5
721004.1	laceration ; perforation ; puncture NFS	721004.1	721004.1	5
721006.1	minor ; superficial ; incomplete circumferential involvement ; blood loss ≤20% by volume	721006.1	721006.1	5
721008.3	major ; rupture ; transection ; segmental loss ; blood loss >20% by volume	721008.3	721008.3	5
721299.1	**Other named veins** NFS [e.g., **cephalic, basilic**]	721299.1	721299.1	5
721202.1	laceration ; perforation ; puncture NFS	721202.1	721202.1	5
721204.1	minor ; superficial ; incomplete circumferential involvement ;	721204.1	721204.1	5
721206.3	major ; rupture ; transection ; segmental loss ; blood loss >20% by volume	721206.3	721206.3	5

AIS 2005	損傷内容	⇒ AIS98	⇐ AIS98	FCI
720899.1	**上腕静脈**　詳細不明	720899.1	720899.1	5
720802.1	裂傷・裂創；穿孔；穿刺　詳細不明	720802.1	720802.1	5
720804.1	小；表在性；非全周性；出血量が全血液量の20%以下	720804.1	720804.1	5
720806.3	大；破裂；断裂；部分欠損；出血量が全血液量の20%を超える	720806.3	720806.3	5
721099.1	**その他の名前のある動脈**　［例：**橈骨，尺骨**］	721099.1	721099.1	5
721002.1	内膜剥離，断裂なし	721002.1	721002.1	5
721004.1	裂傷・裂創；穿孔；穿刺　詳細不明	721004.1	721004.1	5
721006.1	小；表在性；非全周性；出血量が全血液量の20%以下	721006.1	721006.1	5
721008.3	大；破裂；断裂；部分欠損；出血量が全血液量の20%を超える	721008.3	721008.3	5
721299.1	**その他の名前のある静脈**　［例：**橈側皮静脈，尺側皮静脈**］	721299.1	721299.1	5
721202.1	裂傷・裂創；穿孔；穿刺　詳細不明	721202.1	721202.1	5
721204.1	小；表在性；非全周性；	721204.1	721204.1	5
721206.3	大；破裂；断裂；部分欠損；出血量が全血液量の20%を超える	721206.3	721206.3	5

UPPER EXTREMITY

AIS 2005	Injury Description	⇒ AIS98	⇐ AIS98	FCI
	NERVES			
	A diagnosis of nerve palsy or neuropraxia should be coded as a contusion to the specific nerve.			
730099.9	**Nerve injury in upper extremity** NFS[f]	None	None	
730299.1	**Digital nerve** NFS	730299.1	730299.1	5
730202.1	contusion	730202.1	730202.1	5
730204.1	laceration	730204.1	730204.1	5
730499.1	**Median nerve** NFS[t]	730499.1	730499.1	5
730402.1	contusion	730410.1	730410.1	5
730404.2	laceration ; avulsion NFS	730420.1[b]	730420.1[b]	5
730406.2	with motor loss	730450.2	730450.2	4
730699.1	**Radial nerve** NFS[t]	730499.1	730499.1	5
730602.1	contusion	730410.1	730410.1	5
730604.2	laceration ; avulsion NFS	730420.1[b]	730420.1[b]	5
730606.2	with motor loss	730450.2	730450.2	4
730899.1	**Ulnar nerve** NFS[t]	730499.1	730499.1	5
730802.1	contusion	730410.1	730410.1	5
730804.2	laceration ; avulsion NFS	730420.1[b]	730420.1[b]	5
730806.2	with motor loss	730450.2	730450.2	4
	MUSCLES, TENDONS, LIGAMENTS			
740099.9	**Muscle, tendon or ligament injury** NFS[f]	None	None	
740600.1	**Joint capsule** ; rupture ; tear ; avulsion	740600.2[b]	740600.2[b]	5
740400.1	**Muscle** tear ; avulsion NFS	740400.2[b]	740400.2[b]	5
740401.1	partial disruption	740400.2[b]	None	5
740403.2	complete disruption	740400.2	740400.2	5
740402.1	contusion ; strain	740402.1	740402.1	5
740200.1	**Tendon** tear ; avulsion	740200.1	740200.1	4
740210.1	multiple tendons in hand	740210.1	740210.1	2
740220.1	multiple tendons other than hand	740220.1	740220.1	4

---

[b] Change in severity in AIS 2005

[f] New descriptor in AIS 2005 that allows classification of trauma by body region, but does not allow assigning a severity code.

[t] Median, radial and ulnar nerves were combined as one descriptor in AIS98. In AIS 2005, each is a separate injury descriptor ; hence, the duplication of AIS98 matching codes.

上　肢

AIS 2005	損傷内容	⇒ AIS98	⇐ AIS98	FCI

神　経

> 麻痺，神経遮断の診断があれば該当する神経の挫傷として
> コード選択する。

AIS 2005	損傷内容	⇒ AIS98	⇐ AIS98	FCI
730099.9	上肢の神経損傷　詳細不明[f]	なし	なし	
730299.1	指神経　詳細不明	730299.1	730299.1	5
730202.1	挫傷	730202.1	730202.1	5
730204.1	裂傷・裂創	730204.1	730204.1	5
730499.1	正中神経　詳細不明[t]	730499.1	730499.1	5
730402.1	挫傷	730410.1	730410.1	5
730404.2	裂傷・裂創；剝離　詳細不明	730420.1[b]	730420.1[b]	5
730406.2	運動麻痺を伴う	730450.2	730450.2	4
730699.1	橈骨神経　詳細不明[t]	730499.1	730499.1	5
730602.1	挫傷	730410.1	730410.1	5
730604.2	裂傷・裂創；剝離　詳細不明	730420.1[b]	730420.1[b]	5
730606.2	運動麻痺を伴う	730450.2	730450.2	4
730899.1	尺骨神経　詳細不明[t]	730499.1	730499.1	5
730802.1	挫傷	730410.1	730410.1	5
730804.2	裂傷・裂創；剝離　詳細不明	730420.1[b]	730420.1[b]	5
730806.2	運動麻痺を伴う	730450.2	730450.2	4

筋肉，腱，靱帯

AIS 2005	損傷内容	⇒ AIS98	⇐ AIS98	FCI
740099.9	筋肉，腱，靱帯の損傷　詳細不明[f]	なし	なし	
740600.1	関節包裂傷・裂創；破裂；断裂；剝離	740600.2[b]	740600.2[b]	5
740400.1	筋肉裂傷・裂創；剝離　詳細不明	740400.2[b]	740400.2[b]	5
740401.1	部分断裂	740400.2[b]	なし	5
740403.2	完全断裂	740400.2	740400.2	5
740402.1	挫傷；ストレイン（部分的過伸展損傷）	740402.1	740402.1	5
740200.1	腱断裂；剝離	740200.1	740200.1	4
740210.1	手の複数損傷	740210.1	740210.1	2
740220.1	手以外の複数損傷	740220.1	740220.1	4

---

[b] AIS2005で重症度に変更あり。
[f] AIS2005に加えられた新しいコード。外傷の存在部位を示すことができる。ただし重症度はない。
[t] AIS98では正中，橈骨，尺骨神経は同じコードであった。AIS2005ではそれぞれ別のコードをもつ。したがってAIS2005をAIS98に変換した場合，同じコードが割り当てられている。

UPPER EXTREMITY

AIS 2005	Injury Description	⇒ AIS98	⇐ AIS98	FCI
	JOINTS			
770099.9	**Upper extremity joint injury** NFS[f]	None	None	
770799.1	**Acromioclavicular joint** NFS	750299.1	750299.1	5
770789.1	open[a]	750299.1	None	5
770710.1	sprain	750220.1	750220.1	5
770720.1	subluxation	750230.2[b]	None	5
770730.2	dislocation	750230.2	750230.2	5
770731.2	open[a]	750230.2	None	5
772499.1	**Carpal (wrist) joint** NFS	751499.1	751499.1	5
772489.1	open[a]	751499.1	None	5
772410.1	sprain	751420.1	751420.1	5
772420.1	subluxation	751430.2[b]	None	5
772430.1	dislocation [carpal]	751430.2[b]	None	4
772431.1	open[a]	751430.2[b]	None	4
772230.1	dislocation [distal radioulnar]	751430.2[b]	None	4
772231.1	open[a]	751430.2[b]	None	4
772330.2	dislocation [radiocarpal]	751430.2	None	4
772331.2	open[a]	751430.2	None	4
772099.1	**Elbow joint** NFS	750699.1	750699.1	5
772089.1	open[a]	750699.1	None	5
772010.1	sprain	750620.1	750620.1	5
772020.1	subluxation	750630.1	None	5
772030.1	dislocation NFS	750630.1	750630.1	5
772031.1	open[a]	750630.1	None	5
772032.1	with radial head involvement [proximal radioulnar]	750630.1	750630.1	4
772033.2	open[a]	750630.1[b]	None	4

---

[a] New descriptor in AIS 2005
[b] Change in severity code in AIS 2005
[f] New descriptor in AIS 2005 that allows classification of trauma by body region, but does not allow assigning a severity code.

AIS 2005	損傷内容	⇒ AIS98	⇐ AIS98	FCI
	関 節			
770099.9	上肢　関節損傷　詳細不明[f]	なし	なし	
770799.1	**肩鎖関節**　詳細不明	750299.1	750299.1	5
770789.1	開放[a]	750299.1	なし	5
770710.1	捻挫	750220.1	750220.1	5
770720.1	亜脱臼	750230.2[b]	なし	5
770730.2	脱臼	750230.2	750230.2	5
770731.2	開放[a]	750230.2	なし	5
772499.1	**手関節**　詳細不明	751499.1	751499.1	5
772489.1	開放[a]	751499.1	なし	5
772410.1	捻挫	751420.1	751420.1	5
772420.1	亜脱臼	751430.2[b]	なし	5
772430.1	脱臼［手根］	751430.2[b]	なし	4
772431.1	開放[a]	751430.2[b]	なし	4
772230.1	脱臼［遠位橈尺骨］	751430.2[b]	なし	4
772231.1	開放[a]	751430.2[b]	なし	4
772330.2	脱臼［橈骨手根］	751430.2	なし	4
772331.2	開放[a]	751430.2	なし	4
772099.1	**肘関節**　詳細不明	750699.1	750699.1	5
772089.1	開放[a]	750699.1	なし	5
772010.1	捻挫	750620.1	750620.1	5
772020.1	亜脱臼	750630.1	なし	5
772030.1	脱臼　詳細不明	750630.1	750630.1	5
772031.1	開放[a]	750630.1	なし	5
772032.1	橈骨頭に達する［近位橈尺骨］	750630.1	750630.1	4
772033.2	開放[a]	750630.1[b]	なし	4

[a] AIS2005に加えられた新しいコード。
[b] AIS2005で重症度に変更あり。
[f] AIS2005に加えられた新しいコード。外傷の存在部位を示すことができる。ただし重症度はない。

UPPER EXTREMITY

AIS 2005	Injury Description	⇒ AIS98	⇐ AIS98	FCI
772599.1	**Metacarpophalangeal or Interphalangeal joint** NFS[s]	750499.1	750499.1	5
772589.1	open[a]	750499.1	None	5
772540.1	**Thumb** NFS	750499.1	750499.1	5
772541.1	open[a]	750499.1	None	5
772510.1	sprain	750402.1	750402.1	5
772520.1	dislocation/subluxation	750404.1	750404.1	5
772521.1	open[a]	750404.1	None	5
772550.1	**Non-thumb phalange** NFS	750499.1	750499.1	5
772551.1	open[a]	750499.1	None	5
772560.1	sprain	750402.1	750402.1	5
772570.1	dislocation/subluxation	750404.1	750404.1	5
772571.1	open[a]	750404.1	None	5
771099.1	**Shoulder (glenohumeral) joint** NFS	751099.1	771099.1	5
771089.1	open[a]	751099.1	None	5
771010.1	sprain	751020.1	751020.1	5
771020.1	subluxation	751030.2[b]	None	5
771030.2	dislocation	751030.2	751030.2	5
771031.2	open[a]	751030.2	None	5
770599.1	**Sternoclavicular joint** NFS	751299.1	751299.1	5
770589.1	open[a]	751299.1	None	5
770510.1	sprain	751220.1	751220.1	5
770520.1	subluxation	751230.2[b]	None	5
770530.2	dislocation	751230.2	751230.2	5
770531.2	open[a]	751230.2	None	5

[a] New descriptor in AIS 2005
[b] Change in severity code in AIS 2005
[s] Differentiation of specific anatomical site for this injury descriptor was less detailed in AIS98 than in AIS 2005 ; hence, the duplication of AIS98 matching codes.

AIS 2005	損傷内容	⇒ AIS98	⇐ AIS98	FCI
772599.1	**中手指節関節または指節間関節** 詳細不明[s]	750499.1	750499.1	5
772589.1	開放	750499.1	なし	5
772540.1	**母指** 詳細不明	750499.1	750499.1	5
772541.1	開放[a]	750499.1	なし	5
772510.1	捻挫	750402.1	750402.1	5
772520.1	脱臼／亜脱臼	750404.1	750404.1	5
772521.1	開放[a]	750404.1	なし	5
772550.1	**非母指**	750499.1	750499.1	5
772551.1	開放[a]	750499.1	なし	5
772560.1	捻挫	750402.1	750402.1	5
772570.1	脱臼／亜脱臼	750404.1	750404.1	5
772571.1	開放[a]	750404.1	なし	5
771099.1	**肩関節** 詳細不明	751099.1	771099.1	5
771089.1	開放[a]	751099.1	なし	5
771010.1	捻挫	751020.1	751020.1	5
771020.1	亜脱臼	751030.2[b]	なし	5
771030.2	脱臼	751030.2	751030.2	5
771031.2	開放[a]	751030.2	なし	5
770599.1	**胸鎖関節** 詳細不明	751299.1	751299.1	5
770589.1	開放[a]	751299.1	なし	5
770510.1	捻挫	751220.1	751220.1	5
770520.1	亜脱臼	751230.2[b]	なし	5
770530.2	脱臼	751230.2	751230.2	5
770531.2	開放[a]	751230.2	なし	5

[a] AIS2005に加えられた新しいコード。
[b] AIS2005で重症度に変更あり。
[s] AIS98のこの損傷に関する部位の記述はAIS2005に比べて少ない。したがってAIS98コードは同じコードを使用している。

AIS 2005	Injury Description	⇒ AIS98	⇐ AIS98	FCI

SKELETAL

Classification of Long Bone Fractures

Long bone fractures are classified as to their location on the bone (i.e., proximal, shaft [diaphyseal] or distal). Proximal and distal fractures are further classified by the extent of articular (joint) involvement, and shaft fractures are classified by their degree of complexity. For long bone shaft fractures, "complex" means multifragmentary. Other clinical descriptors are: spiral, segmental, irregular or comminuted. Selected anatomical drawings and a sample of specific long bone fractures are included to aid the AIS user in becoming familiar with these classification changes and with contemporary orthopedic trauma terminology. The Introduction to the AIS dictionary includes further notes describing the changes.

CODING RULE : Upper Extremities

For patients who die before any radiology is done and no autopsy is performed, a clinical diagnosis of a fracture made by detecting obvious instability of an extremity is acceptable for AIS coding. In such cases, the least severe AIS code should be assigned. (Example : forearm fracture NFS, 751900.2, if neither ulna nor radius is named. Alternatively, radius fracture NFS, 752800.2 or ulna fracture NFS, 753200.2, if known.

Use one of the following seven descriptors if specific anatomical information is unknown.

750099.9	**Upper Extremity** fracture NFS[f]	None	None	
751800.2	**Arm** fracture NFS	751800.2	751800.2	5
751801.2	open	751800.2	None	5
751900.2	**Forearm** fracture NFS	751900.2	751900.2	5
751901.2	open	751900.2	None	5
752000.2	**Hand** fracture NFS	752500.2	752500.2	5
752001.2	open	752500.2	None	5

---

[f] New descriptor in AIS 2005 that allows classification of trauma by body region, but does not allow assigning a severity code.

上　肢

AIS 2005	損傷内容	⇒ AIS98	⇐ AIS98	FCI

骨　格

長管骨骨折の分類

長管骨骨折は骨折のある部位により分類されている（例：近位，骨幹部，遠位）。近位および遠位の骨折はさらに軟骨（関節）の損傷程度により分類されている。また骨幹部も複雑度に応じてさらに分類されている。長管骨骨幹部骨折において，「複雑」とは骨片が複数あることをいう。臨床的に用いられるその他の用語には螺旋状，部分的，不整，粉砕がある。AISのユーザーがこれらの分類の変更に慣れ，かつ整形外科学的用語に慣れるよう，解剖学的図譜や具体的な長管骨骨折の例を取り入れてある。本手引書の序説にこれらの変更についてさらに詳しく記述している。

コード選択のルール：上肢

画像検査なしに死亡し，剖検もされない患者について，上肢の明らかな動揺を認めれば，それを臨床的に骨折と診断し，コード選択を行ってもよい。そのような場合は重症度のもっとも低いコードを選択すること。（例：橈骨または尺骨の記載がない場合　前腕骨折 詳細不明，751900.2橈骨，尺骨の区別があれば，橈骨骨折　詳細不明，752800.2または　尺骨骨折　詳細不明，753200.2）

具体的な解剖学的情報がわからなければ，下記のいずれかのコードを選択する。

AIS 2005	損傷内容		⇒ AIS98	⇐ AIS98	FCI
750099.9	**上肢の骨折**	詳細不明[f]	なし	なし	
751800.2	**上腕の骨折**	詳細不明	751800.2	751800.2	5
751801.2		開放	751800.2	なし	5
751900.2	**前腕の骨折**	詳細不明	751900.2	751900.2	5
751901.2		開放	751900.2	なし	5
752000.2	**手の骨折**	詳細不明	752500.2	752500.2	5
752001.2		開放	752500.2	なし	5

---

[f] AIS2005に加えられた新しいコード。外傷の存在部位を示すことができる。ただし重症度はない。

UPPER EXTREMITY

AIS 2005	Injury Description	⇒ AIS98	⇐ AIS98	FCI
750500.2	**Clavicle** fracture NFS	752200.2	752200.2	5
750501.2	open	752200.2	752200.2	5
750511.2	**Proximal clavicle** fracture	752200.2	None	5
750512.2	open	752200.2	None	5
750621.2	**Clavicle shaft** fracture	752200.2	None	5
750622.2	open	752200.2	None	5
750651.2	simple	752200.2	None	5
750652.2	open	752200.2	None	5
750661.2	wedge ; "butterfly" fragment	752200.2	None	5
750662.2	open	752200.2	None	5
750671.2	comminuted ; segmental	752200.2	None	5
750672.2	open	752200.2	None	5
750731.2	**Distal (lateral end) clavicle** fracture	752200.2	None	5
750732.2	open	752200.2	None	5
750751.2	extra-articular	752200.2	None	5
750752.2	open	752200.2	None	5
750761.2	intra-articular	752200.2	None	5
750762.2	open	752200.2	None	5
750900.2	**Scapula** fracture NFS	753000.2	753000.2	5
750901.2	open	753000.2	None	5
750951.2	body	753000.2	None	5
750952.2	open	753000.2	None	5
750961.2	neck with or without body	753000.2	None	5
750962.2	open	753000.2	None	4
750971.2	glenoid with or without neck or body	753000.2	None	4
750972.2	open	753000.2	None	5

AIS 2005	損傷内容	⇒ AIS98	⇐ AIS98	FCI
750500.2	**鎖骨**骨折　詳細不明	752200.2	752200.2	5
750501.2	開放	752200.2	752200.2	5
750511.2	**近位部**骨折	752200.2	なし	5
750512.2	開放	752200.2	なし	5
750621.2	**骨幹部**骨折	752200.2	なし	5
750622.2	開放	752200.2	なし	5
750651.2	単純	752200.2	なし	5
750652.2	開放	752200.2	なし	5
750661.2	楔状骨折；"蝶形"破片	752200.2	なし	5
750662.2	開放	752200.2	なし	5
750671.2	粉砕骨折；分節骨折	752200.2	なし	5
750672.2	開放	752200.2	なし	5
750731.2	**遠位（外側端）部**骨折	752200.2	なし	5
750732.2	開放	752200.2	なし	5
750751.2	関節外	752200.2	なし	5
750752.2	開放	752200.2	なし	5
750761.2	関節内	752200.2	なし	5
750762.2	開放	752200.2	なし	5
750900.2	**肩甲骨**骨折　詳細不明	753000.2	753000.2	5
750901.2	開放	753000.2	なし	5
750951.2	体部	753000.2	なし	5
750952.2	開放	753000.2	なし	5
750961.2	頸部　体部を伴うもしくは伴わない	753000.2	なし	5
750962.2	開放	753000.2	なし	4
750971.2	関節窩　体部や頸部を伴うもしくは伴わない	753000.2	なし	4
750972.2	開放	753000.2	なし	5

UPPER EXTREMITY

BONE:
Humerus

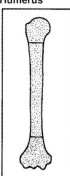

LOCATION:
Proximal segment

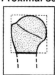

TYPES:
Extra-articular,
Unifocal

Partial articular,
Bifocal

Articular

LOCATION:
Shaft [diaphyseal] segment

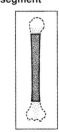

TYPES:
Simple

Wedge

Complex

LOCATION:
Distal segment

TYPES:
Extra-articular →

Partial articular →

Complete articular →

Examples:

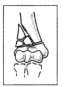

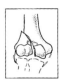

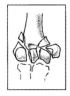

骨：
上腕骨

部位：
近位部

型：
関節外
単極

部分関節内
双極

関節

部位：
体(骨幹)部

型：
単純

楔状

粉砕

部位：
遠位部

型：
関節外

部分関節内

完全関節内

例：

上肢

UPPER EXTREMITY

AIS 2005	Injury Description	⇒ AIS98	⇐ AIS98	FCI
751100.2	**Humerus** fracture NFS	752600.2	752600.2	5
751101.2	open	752604.3[b]	752604.3[b]	5
751111.2	**Proximal humerus** NFS	752600.2	None	4
751112.2	open	752604.3[b]	None	4
751151.2	extra-articular ; unifocal [either one of the tuberosities or the metaphysis] ; single fracture line	752600.2	None	5
751152.2	open	752604.3[b]	None	5
751161.2	extra-articular ; bifocal [either one of the tuberosities and the metaphysis] ; ≥2 fracture lines	752600.2	None	5
751162.3	open	752604.3	None	5
751171.2	articular ; head or anatomical neck	752600.2	None	4
751172.3	open	752604.3	None	4
751221.2	**Humerus shaft** fracture	752600.2	None	5
751222.2	open	752604.3[b]	None	5
751251.2	simple ; oblique ; transverse	752600.2	None	5
751252.2	open	752604.3[b]	None	5
751261.2	wedge ; "butterfly" segment	752600.2	None	5
751262.3	open	752604.3	None	5
751271.2	complex ; comminuted ; segmental	752604.3[b]	None	5
751272.3	open	752604.3	None	5
751331.2	**Distal humerus** fracture	752600.2	None	5
751332.2	open	752604.3[b]	None	5
751351.2	extra-articular ; supracondylar	752600.2	None	5
751352.2	open	752604.3[b]	None	5
751361.2	partial articular ; capitular	752600.2	None	5
751362.3	open	752604.3	None	5
751371.2	complete articular ; T-shaped ; Y-shaped ; T-condylar	752600.2	None	3
751372.3	open	752604.3	None	3

---

[b] Change in severity in AIS 2005

上　肢

AIS 2005	損傷内容	⇒ AIS98	⇐ AIS98	FCI
751100.2	**上腕骨**骨折　詳細不明	752600.2	752600.2	5
751101.2	開放	752604.3[b]	752604.3[b]	5
751111.2	**近位部**骨折　詳細不明	752600.2	なし	4
751112.2	開放	752604.3[b]	なし	4
751151.2	関節外；単極［大結節または小結節または骨幹端］；単純骨折線	752600.2	なし	5
751152.2	開放	752604.3[b]	なし	5
751161.2	関節外；双極［大結節または小結節と骨幹端］；2つ以上の骨折線	752600.2	なし	5
751162.3	開放	752604.3	なし	5
751171.2	関節；骨頭または解剖頸	752600.2	なし	4
751172.3	開放	752604.3	なし	4
751221.2	**骨幹部**骨折	752600.2	なし	5
751222.2	開放	752604.3[b]	なし	5
751251.2	単純；斜；横	752600.2	なし	5
751252.2	開放	752604.3[b]	なし	5
751261.2	楔状；"蝶形"破片	752600.2	なし	5
751262.3	開放	752604.3	なし	5
751271.2	複雑；粉砕；分節	752604.3[b]	なし	5
751272.3	開放	752604.3	なし	5
751331.2	**遠位部**骨折	752600.2	なし	5
751332.2	開放	752604.3[b]	なし	5
751351.2	関節外；顆上	752600.2	なし	5
751352.2	開放	752604.3[b]	なし	5
751361.2	部分関節内；小頭	752600.2	なし	5
751362.3	開放	752604.3	なし	5
751371.2	完全関節内；T字型；Y字型；顆部骨折	752600.2	なし	3
751372.3	開放	752604.3	なし	3

[b] AIS2005で重症度に変更あり。

UPPER EXTREMITY

BONE: Radius/Ulna

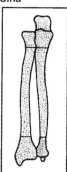

LOCATION: Proximal segment

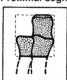

TYPES:
Extra-articular

Partial articular

Complete Articular

LOCATION: Shaft [diaphyseal] segment

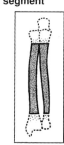

TYPES:
Simple

Wedge

Complex

LOCATION: Distal segment

TYPES:
Extra-articular →

Partial articular →

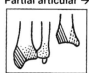

Complete articular →

Examples:

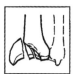

骨：
橈骨／
尺骨

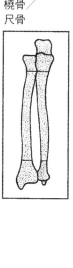

部位：
近位部

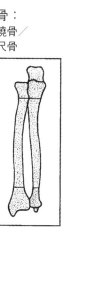

型：
関節外

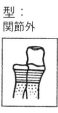

部分関節内

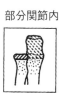

完全関節内

部位：
体（骨幹）部

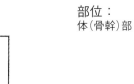

型：
単純

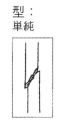

楔状

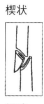

粉砕

部位：
遠位部

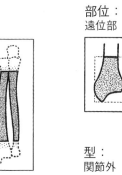

型：
関節外

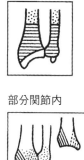

部分関節内

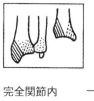

完全関節内

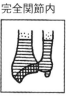

例：

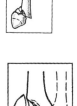

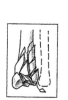

UPPER EXTREMITY

AIS 2005	Injury Description	⇒ AIS98	⇐ AIS98	FCI
752800.2	**Radius** fracture NFS	752800.2	752800.2	5
752801.2	open	752804.3[b]	752804.3[b]	5
752111.2	**Proximal radius** fracture	752800.2	None	4
752112.2	open	752804.3[b]	None	4
752151.2	extra-articular ; radial neck	752800.2	None	4
752152.2	open	752804.3[b]	None	4
752161.2	partial articular ; radial head	752800.2	None	4
752162.3	open	752804.3	None	4
752171.2	complete articular	752800.2	None	4
752172.3	open	752804.3	None	4
752211.2	**Radius shaft** fracture	752800.2	None	5
752212.2	open	752804.3[b]	None	5
752251.2	simple ; oblique ; transverse	752800.2	None	5
752252.2	open	752804.3[b]	None	5
752261.2	wedge ; "butterfly" fragment	752800.2	None	5
752262.3	open	752804.3	None	5
752271.2	complex ; comminuted ; segmental	752804.3[b]	None	4
752272.3	open	752804.3	None	4
752311.2	**Distal Radius** fracture	752800.2	None	5
752312.2	open	752804.3[b]	None	5
752351.2	extra-articular [includes styloid]	752800.2	None	5
752352.2	open	752804.3[b]	None	5
752361.2	partial articular ; *Colles*	752800.2	None	4
752362.3	open	752804.3	None	4
752371.2	complete articular ; T-shaped ; Y-shaped ; T-condylar ; *Barton*	752800.2	None	4
752372.3	open	752804.3	None	4

[b] Change in severity code in AIS 2005

AIS 2005	損傷内容	⇒ AIS98	⇐ AIS98	FCI
752800.2	**橈骨**骨折　詳細不明	752800.2	752800.2	5
752801.2	開放	752804.3[b]	752804.3[b]	5
752111.2	**近位部（端）**骨折	752800.2	なし	4
752112.2	開放	752804.3[b]	なし	4
752151.2	関節外；橈骨頸	752800.2	なし	4
752152.2	開放	752804.3[b]	なし	4
752161.2	部分関節内；橈骨頭	752800.2	なし	4
752162.3	開放	752804.3	なし	4
752171.2	完全関節内	752800.2	なし	4
752172.3	開放	752804.3	なし	4
752211.2	**骨幹部**骨折	752800.2	なし	5
752212.2	開放	752804.3[b]	なし	5
752251.2	単純；斜走；横断	752800.2	なし	5
752252.2	開放	752804.3[b]	なし	5
752261.2	楔状；"蝶形"破片	752800.2	なし	5
752262.3	開放	752804.3	なし	5
752271.2	複合；粉砕；分節	752804.3[b]	なし	4
752272.3	開放	752804.3	なし	4
752311.2	**遠位部（端）**骨折	752800.2	なし	5
752312.2	開放	752804.3[b]	なし	5
752351.2	関節外［茎状突起を含む］	752800.2	なし	5
752352.2	開放	752804.3[b]	なし	5
752361.2	部分関節内；*Colles*	752800.2	なし	4
752362.3	開放	752804.3	なし	4
752371.2	完全関節内；T字型；Y字型；顆部骨折；*Barton*	752800.2	なし	4
752372.3	開放	752804.3	なし	4

[b] AIS2005で重症度に変更あり。

UPPER EXTREMITY

BONE: Radius/Ulna

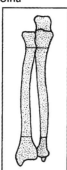

LOCATION: Proximal segment

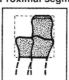

LOCATION: Shaft [diaphyseal] segment

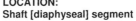
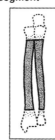

LOCATION: Distal segment

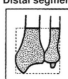

TYPES: Extra-articular

TYPES: Simple

TYPES: Extra-articular →

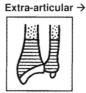

Examples:

Partial articular

Wedge

Partial articular →

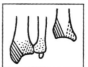

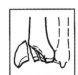

Complete Articular

Complex

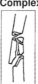

Complete articular →

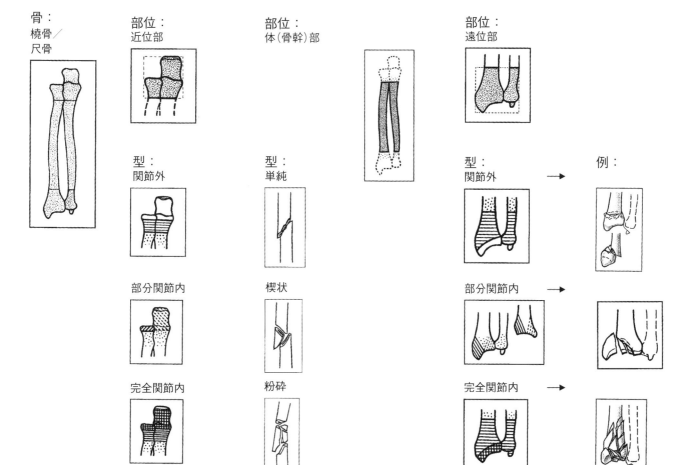

UPPER EXTREMITY

AIS 2005	Injury Description	⇒ AIS98	⇐ AIS98	FCI
753200.2	**Ulna** fracture NFS	753200.2	753200.2	4
753201.2	open	753204.3[b]	753204.3[b]	4
752113.2	**Proximal Ulna** fracture [olecranon]	753200.2	None	4
752114.2	open	753204.3[b]	None	4
752153.2	extra-articular	753200.2	None	4
752154.2	open	753204.3[b]	None	4
752163.2	partial articular	753200.2	None	3
752164.3	open	753204.3	None	3
752173.2	complete articular	753200.2	None	3
752174.3	open	753204.3	None	3
752213.2	**Ulna Shaft** fracture	753200.2	753200.2	5
752214.2	open	753204.3[b]	753204.3[b]	5
752253.2	simple ; oblique ; transverse	753200.2	None	5
752254.2	open	753204.3[b]	None	5
752263.2	wedge ; "butterfly" fragment	753200.2	None	5
752264.3	open	753204.3	None	5
752273.2	complex ; comminuted ; segmental	753204.3[b]	None	5
752274.3	open	753204.3	None	5
752313.2	**Distal Ulna** fracture	753200.2	None	5
752314.2	open	753204.3[b]	None	5
752353.2	extra-articular [includes styloid]	753200.2	None	5
752354.2	open	753204.3[b]	None	5
752363.2	partial articular	753200.2	None	5
752364.3	open	753204.3	None	5
752373.2	complete articular	753200.2	None	5
752374.3	open	753204.3	None	5

---

[b] Change in severity code in AIS 2005

上　肢

AIS 2005	損傷内容	⇒ AIS98	⇐ AIS98	FCI
753200.2	**尺骨**骨折　詳細不明	753200.2	753200.2	4
753201.2	開放	753204.3[b]	753204.3[b]	4
752113.2	**近位部**骨折［肘頭］	753200.2	なし	4
752114.2	開放	753204.3[b]	なし	4
752153.2	関節外	753200.2	なし	4
752154.2	開放	753204.3[b]	なし	4
752163.2	部分関節内	753200.2	なし	3
752164.3	開放	753204.3	なし	3
752173.2	完全関節内	753200.2	なし	3
752174.3	開放	753204.3	なし	3
752213.2	**骨幹部**骨折	753200.2	753200.2	5
752214.2	開放	753204.3[b]	753204.3[b]	5
752253.2	単純；斜走；横断	753200.2	なし	5
752254.2	開放	753204.3[b]	なし	5
752263.2	楔状；"蝶形"分節	753200.2	なし	5
752264.3	開放	753204.3	なし	5
752273.2	複合；粉砕；分節	753204.3[b]	なし	5
752274.3	開放	753204.3	なし	5
752313.2	**遠位部**骨折	753200.2	なし	5
752314.2	開放	753204.3[b]	なし	5
752353.2	関節外［茎状突起を含む］	753200.2	なし	5
752354.2	開放	753204.3[b]	なし	5
752363.2	部分関節内	753200.2	なし	5
752364.3	開放	753204.3	なし	5
752373.2	完全関節内	753200.2	なし	5
752374.3	開放	753204.3	なし	5

[b] AIS2005で重症度に変更あり。

UPPER EXTREMITY

Bones of the Hand

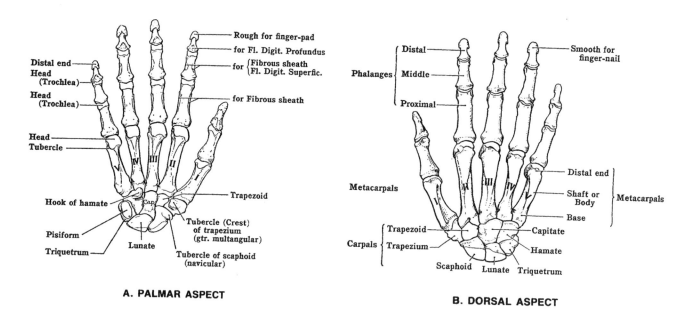

手の骨

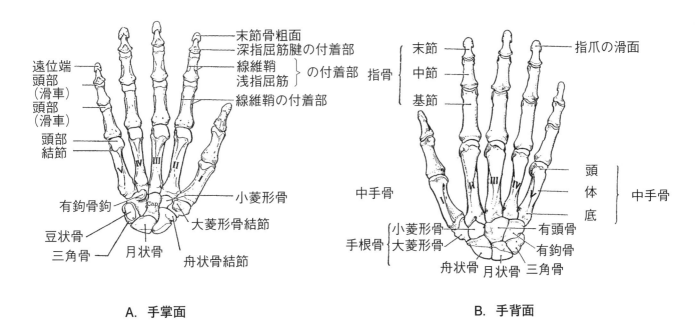

A. 手掌面　　　　　　　　B. 手背面

UPPER EXTREMITY

AIS 2005	Injury Description	⇒ AIS98	⇐ AIS98	FCI
752400.2	**Carpus** fracture NFS[u]	752002.2	752002.2	5
752401.2	open	752002.2	None	5
752451.2	scaphoid only	752002.2	None	5
752452.2	open	752002.2	None	5
752461.2	bone other than scaphoid	752002.2	None	5
752462.2	open	752002.2	None	5
752471.2	≥2 carpal bones	752002.2	None	5
752472.2	open	752002.2	None	5
752500.2	**Metacarpus** fracture NFS[u]	752002.2	752002.2	5
752501.2	open	752002.2	None	5
752511.2	**Thumb**[v]	752002.2	None	5
752512.2	open	752002.2	None	5
752551.2	extra-articular or shaft	752002.2	None	5
752552.2	open	752002.2	None	5
752561.2	partial articular	752002.2	None	5
752562.2	open	752002.2	None	5
752571.2	complete articular	752002.2	None	5
752572.2	open	752002.2	None	5
752521.2	**One of Lateral Four Fingers**[v]	752002.2	None	5
752522.2	open	752002.2	None	5
752553.2	extra-articular or shaft	752002.2	None	5
752554.2	open	752002.2	None	5
752563.2	partial articular	752002.2	None	5
752564.2	open	752002.2	None	5
752573.2	complete articular	752002.2	None	5
752574.2	open	752002.2	None	5

[u] Carpus and metacarpus were combined as one descriptor in AIS98. In AIS 2005, each is a separate injury category; hence the duplication of AIS98 matching codes.

[v] Thumb and non-thumb fingers were combined as one descriptor in AIS98. In AIS 2005, each is a separate injury category; hence, the duplication of AIS98 matching codes.

上　肢

AIS 2005	損傷内容	⇒ AIS98	⇐ AIS98	FCI
752400.2	**手根骨**骨折　詳細不明[u]	752002.2	752002.2	5
752401.2	開放	752002.2	なし	5
752451.2	舟状骨のみ	752002.2	なし	5
752452.2	開放	752002.2	なし	5
752461.2	舟状骨以外	752002.2	なし	5
752462.2	開放	752002.2	なし	5
752471.2	2つ以上の手根骨	752002.2	なし	5
752472.2	開放	752002.2	なし	5
752500.2	**中手骨**骨折　詳細不明[u]	752002.2	752002.2	5
752501.2	開放	752002.2	なし	5
752511.2	**母指（第1指）**[v]	752002.2	なし	5
752512.2	開放	752002.2	なし	5
752551.2	関節外または骨幹部	752002.2	なし	5
752552.2	開放	752002.2	なし	5
752561.2	部分関節内	752002.2	なし	5
752562.2	開放	752002.2	なし	5
752571.2	完全関節内	752002.2	なし	5
752572.2	開放	752002.2	なし	5
752521.2	**第2〜5指の1つ**[v]	752002.2	なし	5
752522.2	開放	752002.2	なし	5
752553.2	関節外または骨幹部	752002.2	なし	5
752554.2	開放	752002.2	なし	5
752563.2	部分関節内	752002.2	なし	5
752564.2	開放	752002.2	なし	5
752573.2	完全関節内	752002.2	なし	5
752574.2	開放	752002.2	なし	5

[u] 手根骨と中手骨はAIS98では同一のコードであったが，AIS2005では，それぞれ独立した損傷カテゴリーとなっている；したがってAIS98のコードでは重複がある。

[v] 親指と親指以外の指はAIS98では同一のコードであったが，AIS2005では，それぞれ独立した損傷カテゴリーとなっている；したがってAIS98のコードでは重複がある。

UPPER EXTREMITY

AIS 2005	Injury Description	⇒ AIS98	⇐ AIS98	FCI
752600.1	**Phalange** fracture NFS[v]	752404.1	752404.1	5
752601.1	open	752404.1	None	5
752611.1	**Thumb**[v]	752404.1	752404.1	5
752612.1	open	752404.1	None	5
752651.1	extra-articular or shaft	752404.1	None	5
752652.1	open	752404.1	None	5
752661.1	partial articular	752404.1	None	5
752662.1	open	752404.1	None	5
752671.1	complete articular	752404.1	None	5
752672.1	open	752404.1	None	5
752621.1	**One of Lateral Four Fingers**[v]	752404.1	752404.1	5
752622.1	open	752404.1	None	5
752653.1	extra-articular or shaft	752404.1	None	5
752654.1	open	752404.1	None	5
752663.1	partial articular	752404.1	None	5
752664.1	open	752404.1	None	5
752673.1	complete articular	752404.1	None	5
752674.1	open	752404.1	None	5

[v] Thumb and non-thumb finger were combined as one descriptor in AIS98. In AIS 2005, each is a separate injury category ; hence, the duplication of AIS98 matching codes.

AIS 2005	損傷内容	⇒ AIS98	⇐ AIS98	FCI
752600.1	**指骨**骨折詳細不明[v]	752404.1	752404.1	5
752601.1	開放	752404.1	なし	5
752611.1	**母指（第1指）**[v]	752404.1	752404.1	5
752612.1	開放	752404.1	なし	5
752651.1	関節外または骨幹部	752404.1	なし	5
752652.1	開放	752404.1	なし	5
752661.1	部分関節内	752404.1	なし	5
752662.1	開放	752404.1	なし	5
752671.1	完全関節内	752404.1	なし	5
752672.1	開放	752404.1	なし	5
752621.1	**第2〜5指の1つ**[v]	752404.1	752404.1	5
752622.1	開放	752404.1	なし	5
752653.1	関節外または骨幹部	752404.1	なし	5
752654.1	開放	752404.1	なし	5
752663.1	部分関節内	752404.1	なし	5
752664.1	開放	752404.1	なし	5
752673.1	完全関節内	752404.1	なし	5
752674.1	開放	752404.1	なし	5

---

[v] 親指と親指以外の指はAIS98では同一のコードであったが，AIS2005では，それぞれ独立した損傷カテゴリーとなっている；したがって，AIS98のコードでは重複がある。

下肢・骨盤・殿部

LOWER EXTREMITY, PELVIS and BUTTOCKS

AIS 2005	Injury Description	⇒ AIS98	⇐ AIS98	FCI
	WHOLE AREA			
	Use one of the following two descriptors when such vague information is the only information available. While these descriptors identify the occurrence of a lower extremity injury, they do not specify its severity.			
800099.9	**Injuries to the Whole Lower Extremity** NFS	815099.9	815099.9	
800999.9	Died of lower extremity injury without further substantiation of injuries or no autopsy confirmation of specific injuries	815999.9	815999.9	
811000.3	**Amputation [traumatic], partial or complete** between hip and foot, but NFS as to specific anatomical site[s]	811000.3	811000.3	2
	The above descriptor does not apply to feet or toes.			
811001.4	at hip or at buttock	811004.4	811004.4	1
811010.5	bilateral[c]	811004.4[b]	None	1
811002.4	at or above knee, below hip	811004.4	811004.4	2
811012.5	bilateral[c]	811004.4[b]	None	1
811003.3	below knee, at or above ankle	811002.3	811002.3	2
811004.2	foot, partial or complete	811002.3[b]	811002.3[b]	2
811005.2	great toe	853604.2	853604.2	4
811006.2	other toes, single or multiple	853604.2	853604.2	4

[b] Change in severity code in AIS 2005.

[c] In previous editions of AIS, with few exceptions, each injury was coded separately. AIS 2005 introduces "bilateral". Some bilateral injuries may affect severity levels and, therefore, the ISS for patients with those injuries.

[s] Differentiation of specific anatomical sites for this injury category was less detailed in AIS98 than in AIS 2005; hence, the duplication of AIS98 matching codes.

下肢・骨盤・殿部

AIS 2005	損傷内容	⇒ AIS98	⇐ AIS98	FCI

全 域

不確定な情報しか得られない場合には，以下の2つのコードのうちいずれかを選択する。これらのコードは下肢に外傷が存在することを示すが，重症度をもたない。

AIS 2005	損傷内容	⇒ AIS98	⇐ AIS98	FCI
800099.9	**下肢損傷** 詳細不明	815099.9	815099.9	
800999.9	下肢損傷で死亡 詳細な評価や損傷を特定しうる剖検なし	815999.9	815999.9	
811000.3	股関節と足の間の**不完全または完全 [外傷性]，切断** ただし，具体的な場所は詳細不明[s]	811000.3	811000.3	2

上記のコードは足部, 足趾には適用しない。

AIS 2005	損傷内容	⇒ AIS98	⇐ AIS98	FCI
811001.4	股関節または殿部で切断	811004.4	811004.4	1
811010.5	両側[c]	811004.4[b]	なし	1
811002.4	膝関節と股関節の間（膝関節を含む）	811004.4	811004.4	2
811012.5	両側[c]	811004.4[b]	なし	1
811003.3	足関節と膝関節の間（足関節を含む）	811002.3	811002.3	2
811004.2	足部，不完全または完全	811002.3[b]	811002.3[b]	2
811005.2	母趾	853604.2	853604.2	4
811006.2	他の趾，1本または複数本	853604.2	853604.2	4

[b] AIS2005で重症度に変更あり。
[c] 旧版のAISでは一部の例外を除き両側損傷はそれぞれ別にコード選択をしていた。AIS2005では，"両側"を導入した。いくつかの両側損傷は重症度が変化し，その結果ISSが変わることがある。
[s] AIS98のこの損傷に関する部位の記述はAIS2005に比べて少ない。したがってAIS98コードは同じコードを使用している。

LOWER EXTREMITY, PELVIS and BUTTOCKS

AIS 2005	Injury Description	⇒ AIS98	⇐ AIS98	FCI
	Use this category only if no specific injuries to the lower extremity are documented.			
812000.2	**Compartment syndrome** resulting from trauma to soft tissue only, not involving fracture or massive destruction of bone and other anatomical structures, NFS as to specific anatomical site[s]	815000.2	815000.2	5
812001.2	thigh	815000.2	None	5
812002.2	no muscle loss	815000.2	None	5
812003.3	with muscle loss	815000.2[b]	None	5
812004.2	leg	815000.2	None	5
812005.2	no muscle loss	815000.2	None	5
812006.3	with muscle loss	815000.2[b]	None	5
812007.2	foot	815000.2	None	5
812008.2	no muscle loss	815000.2	None	5
812009.3	with muscle loss	815000.2[b]	None	5
813000.3	**Crush Injury** to limb between hip and foot, but NFS as to specific anatomical site[s]	813000.2[b]	813000.2[b]	2
	Must involve massive destruction of skeletal, vascular, nervous and tissue systems. Do not use the above description for feet or toes.			
813001.4	at hip or at buttock	813004.3[b]	813004.3[b]	1
813002.4	at or above knee, below hip	813004.3[b]	813004.3[b]	2
813003.3	below knee, at or above ankle	813002.2[b]	813002.2[b]	2
813004.2	foot, partial or complete	813002.2	813002.2	2
813005.2	great toe	853606.2	853606.2	4
813006.2	other toes, single or multiple	853606.2	853606.2	4
	Assign degloving injuries to External body region for calculating an ISS.			
814000.2	**Degloving injury** NFS	None	None	5
814002.3	entire extremity	814006.3	814006.3	5
814004.2	thigh or calf	814004.2	814004.2	5
814006.2	knee, ankle or foot	814006.3[b]	814006.3[b]	5
814008.2	toe, single or multiple	814002.2	814002.2	5

---

[b] Change in severity code in AIS 2005
[s] Differentiation of specific anatomical sites for this injury category was less detailed in AIS98 than in AIS 2005; hence, the duplication of AIS98 matching codes

下肢・骨盤・殿部

AIS 2005	損傷内容	⇒ AIS98	⇐ AIS98	FCI
	下記のコードは，下肢の外傷について具体的な記述がない場合に選択する。			
812000.2	**コンパートメント症候群** 外傷による軟部組織損傷の結果生じたもの，骨折，または骨その他の解剖学的構造に広範囲な挫滅を伴わないもの。解剖学的部位については詳細不明[s]	815000.2	815000.2	5
812001.2	大腿部	815000.2	なし	5
812002.2	筋肉の欠損を伴わない	815000.2	なし	5
812003.3	筋肉の欠損を伴う	815000.2[b]	なし	5
812004.2	下腿	815000.2	なし	5
812005.2	筋肉の欠損を伴わない	815000.2	なし	5
812006.3	筋肉の欠損を伴う	815000.2[b]	なし	5
812007.2	足部	815000.2	なし	5
812008.2	筋肉の欠損を伴わない	815000.2	なし	5
812009.3	筋肉の欠損を伴う	815000.2[b]	なし	5
813000.3	**挫滅損傷** 股関節と足部の間の下肢，具体的な部位については詳細不明[s]	813000.2[b]	813000.2[b]	2
	骨，血管，神経，組織に広範囲の損傷を伴わなければならない。足部や足趾の場合は上記コードを使用しない。			
813001.4	股関節または殿部	813004.3[b]	813004.3[b]	1
813002.4	膝関節と股関節の間（膝関節を含む）	813004.3[b]	813004.3[b]	
813003.3	足関節と膝関節の間（足関節を含む）	813002.2[b]	813002.2[b]	2
813004.2	足部，部分的または全体	813002.2	813002.2	2
813005.2	母趾	853606.2	853606.2	4
813006.2	他の趾，1本または複数本	853606.2	853606.2	4
	デグロービング損傷は ISS を計算するときは体表で計算する。			
814000.2	**デグロービング損傷** 詳細不明	なし	なし	5
814002.3	下肢全体	814006.3	814006.3	5
814004.2	大腿または下腿	814004.2	814004.2	5
814006.2	膝，足関節または足部	814006.3[b]	814006.3[b]	5
814008.2	足趾，1本または複数本	814002.2	814002.2	5

[b] AIS2005で重症度に変更あり。
[s] AIS98のこの損傷に関する部位の記述はAIS2005に比べて少ない。したがってAIS98コードは同じコードを使用している。

LOWER EXTREMITY, PELVIS and BUTTOCKS

AIS 2005	Injury Description	⇒ AIS98	⇐ AIS98	FCI
	Use this category if penetrating injury does not involve bone or internal structures. Assign to External body region for calculating an ISS. If underlying anatomical structures are involved, code documented diagnoses only and do not use these generic descriptors. Penetrating injury involving a bone is coded as open fracture to the specific bone.			
816000.1	**Penetrating injury** NFS as to specific anatomical site or severity[s]	816000.1	816000.1	5
816002.1	superficial ; minor	816002.1	816002.1	5
816004.2	with tissue loss >25cm^2	816004.2	816004.2	4
816006.3	with blood loss >20% by volume	816006.3	816006.3	4
816010.1	**Penetrating injury** at hip or buttock, NFS as to severity	816000.1	None	5
816011.1	superficial ; minor	816002.1	None	5
816012.2	with tissue loss >25cm^2	816004.2	None	5
816013.3	with blood loss >20% by volume	816006.3	None	5
816014.1	**Penetrating injury** at or above knee, below hip NFS as to severity	816000.1	None	5
816015.1	superficial ; minor	816002.1	None	5
816016.2	with tissue loss >25cm^2	816004.2	None	5
816017.3	blood loss >20% by volume	816006.3	None	5
816018.1	**Penetrating injury** below knee, at or above ankle NFS as to severity	816000.1	None	5
816019.1	superficial ; minor	816002.1	None	5
816020.2	with tissue loss >25cm^2	816004.2	None	5
816022.1	**Penetrating injury** foot, partial or complete NFS as to severity	816000.1	None	5
816023.1	superficial ; minor	816002.1	None	5
816024.2	with tissue loss >25cm^2	816004.2	None	5
816026.1	**Penetrating injury** great toe, NFS as to severity	816000.1	None	5
816027.1	superficial ; minor	816002.1	None	5
816028.2	with tissue loss >25cm^2	816004.2	None	5
816030.1	**Penetrating injury** toe, single or multiple	816000.1	None	5
816031.1	superficial ; minor	816002.1	None	5
816032.2	with tissue loss >25cm^2	816004.2	None	5

---

[s] Differentiation of specific anatomical sites for the injury category was less detailed in AIS98 than in AIS 2005 ; hence, the duplication of AIS98 matching codes.

下肢・骨盤・殿部

AIS 2005	損傷内容	⇒ AIS98	⇐ AIS98	FCI
	下記のコードは穿通性損傷が骨や臓器に及んでいない場合に選択する。ISSを計算するときは体表で計算する。もし創が骨や臓器に達する場合は，損傷した骨や臓器をコード選択し，下記のコードは選択しない。穿通性損傷が骨に及んでいる場合は，該当する骨の開放骨折をコード選択する。			
816000.1	**穿通性損傷** 具体的な部位や重症度[s]については詳細不明	816000.1	816000.1	5
816002.1	表在性；小	816002.1	816002.1	5
816004.2	$25cm^2$を超える組織欠損	816004.2	816004.2	4
816006.3	出血量が全血液量の20％を超える	816006.3	816006.3	4
816010.1	**穿通性損傷** 股関節または殿部，重症度については詳細不明	816000.1	なし	5
816011.1	表在性；小	816002.1	なし	5
816012.2	$25cm^2$を超える組織欠損	816004.2	なし	5
816013.3	出血量が全血液量の20％を超える	816006.3	なし	5
816014.1	**穿通性損傷** 膝関節と股関節の間（膝関節を含む），重症度については詳細不明	816000.1	なし	5
816015.1	表在性；小	816002.1	なし	5
816016.2	$25cm^2$を超える組織欠損	816004.2	なし	5
816017.3	出血量が全血液量の20％を超える	816006.3	なし	5
816018.1	**穿通性損傷** 足関節と膝関節の間（足関節を含む），重症度については詳細不明	816000.1	なし	5
816019.1	表在性；小	816002.1	なし	5
816020.2	$25cm^2$を超える組織欠損	816004.2	なし	5
816022.1	**穿通性損傷** 足部，部分的または全体，重症度については詳細不明	816000.1	なし	5
816023.1	表在性；小	816002.1	なし	5
816024.2	$25cm^2$を超える組織欠損	816004.2	なし	5
816026.1	**穿通性損傷** 第1趾，重症度については詳細不明	816000.1	なし	5
816027.1	表在性；小	816002.1	なし	5
816028.2	$25cm^2$を超える組織欠損	816004.2	なし	5
816030.1	**穿通性損傷** 足趾，単趾または複数趾	816000.1	なし	5
816031.1	表在性；小	816002.1	なし	5
816032.2	$25cm^2$を超える組織欠損	816004.2	なし	5

[s] AIS98のこの損傷に関する部位の記述はAIS2005に比べて少ない。したがってAIS98コードは同じコードを使用している。

LOWER EXTREMITY, PELVIS and BUTTOCKS

AIS 2005	Injury Description	⇒ AIS98	⇐ AIS98	FCI
	Use the following section for blunt soft tissue injury to the lower extremity. Assign to External Body Region for calculating an ISS.			
810099.1	**Skin/subcutaneous/muscle** NFS	810099.1	810099.1	5
810202.1	abrasion	810202.1	810202.1	5
810402.1	contusion ; hematoma	810402.1	810402.1	5
810600.1	laceration NFS	810600.1	810600.1	5
810602.1	minor ; superficial	810602.1	810602.1	5
810604.2	major ; >20cm long <u>and</u> into subcutaneous tissue	810604.2	810604.2	5
810606.3	blood loss >20% by volume	810606.3	810606.3	5
810800.1	avulsion NFS	810800.1	810800.1	5
810802.1	superficial ; minor ; ≤100cm^2	810802.1	810802.1	5
810804.2	major ; >100cm^2	810804.2	810804.2	5
810806.3	blood loss >20% by volume	810806.3	810806.3	5

AIS 2005	損傷内容	⇒ AIS98	⇐ AIS98	FCI
	下記のコードは下肢の鈍的損傷で選択する。ISSを計算するときは体表で計算する。			
810099.1	**皮膚／皮下／筋肉**　詳細不明	810099.1	810099.1	5
810202.1	擦過傷	810202.1	810202.1	5
810402.1	挫傷；血腫	810402.1	810402.1	5
810600.1	裂傷・裂創　詳細不明	810600.1	810600.1	5
810602.1	小；表在性	810602.1	810602.1	5
810604.2	大；長さが20cmを超え，かつ皮下組織に達する	810604.2	810604.2	5
810606.3	出血量が全血液量の20％を超える	810606.3	810606.3	5
810800.1	剥離　詳細不明	810800.1	810800.1	5
810802.1	表在性；小；100cm^{2}以下	810802.1	810802.1	5
810804.2	大；100cm^{2}を超える	810804.2	810804.2	5
810806.3	出血量が全血液量の20％を超える	810806.3	810806.3	5

LOWER EXTREMITY, PELVIS and BUTTOCKS

AIS 2005	Injury Description	⇒ AIS98	⇐ AIS98	FCI
	VESSELS			
	Do not code lower extremity vessel injuries separately when they are directly involved in crush injuries or amputation of a lower extremity unless a vascular injury is higher in severity than the crush injury or amputation. Branches of vessels are not coded unless they are named vessels and/or are listed within a specific vessel descriptor.			
820099.9	**Vascular Injury in Lower Extremity** NFS[f]	None	None	
820299.3	**Femoral artery** and its named branches NFS	820299.3	820299.3	5
820202.3	intimal tear, no disruption	820202.3	820202.3	5
820204.3	laceration ; perforation ; puncture NFS	820204.3	820204.3	5
820206.3	minor ; superficial ; incomplete circumferential involvement ; blood loss≤20% by volume	820206.3	820206.3	5
820208.4	major ; rupture ; transection ; segmental loss ; blood loss >20% by volume	820208.4	820208.4	5
820499.2	**Femoral vein** NFS	820499.2	820499.2	5
820402.2	laceration ; perforation ; puncture NFS	820402.2	820402.2	5
820404.2	minor ; superficial ; incomplete circumferential involvement ; blood loss≤20% by volume	820404.2	820404.2	5
820406.3	major ; rupture ; transection ; segmental loss ; blood loss >20% by volume	820406.3	820406.3	4
820699.2	**Popliteal artery** NFS	820699.2	820699.2	5
820602.2	intimal tear, no disruption	820602.2	820602.2	5
820604.2	laceration ; perforation ; puncture NFS	820604.2	820604.2	5
820606.2	minor ; superficial ; incomplete circumferential involvement ; blood loss≤20% by volume	820606.2	820606.2	5
820608.3	major ; rupture ; transection ; segmental loss ; blood loss >20% by volume	820608.3	820608.3	5
820899.2	**Popliteal vein** NFS	820899.2	820899.2	5
820802.2	laceration ; perforation ; puncture NFS	820802.2	820802.2	5
820804.2	minor ; superficial ; incomplete circumferential involvement ; blood loss≤20% by volume	820804.2	820804.2	5
820806.3	major ; rupture ; transection ; segmental loss ; blood loss >20% by volume	820806.3	820806.3	4

[f] New descriptor in AIS 2005 that allows classification of trauma by body region but does not allow assigning a severity code.

AIS 2005	損傷内容	⇒ AIS98	⇐ AIS98	FCI

血 管

> 下肢の挫滅損傷や切断の場合は血管損傷を別にコード選択しない。ただし，血管損傷の重症度のほうが挫滅損傷や切断の重症度より高い場合はコード選択する。主要な血管の枝はそれが名前をもち，かつ／またはその血管名が列挙されている場合に限り，コード選択をする。

AIS 2005	損傷内容	⇒ AIS98	⇐ AIS98	FCI
820099.9	下腿の血管損傷　詳細不明[f]	なし	なし	
820299.3	大腿動脈　または名前のある分枝　詳細不明	820299.3	820299.3	5
820202.3	内膜剥離，断裂なし	820202.3	820202.3	5
820204.3	裂傷・裂創；穿孔；穿刺　詳細不明	820204.3	820204.3	5
820206.3	小；表在性；非全周性；出血量が全血液量の20％以下	820206.3	820206.3	5
820208.4	大；破裂；断裂；部分欠損；出血量が全血液量の20％を超える	820208.4	820208.4	5
820499.2	大腿静脈　詳細不明	820499.2	820499.2	5
820402.2	裂傷・裂創；穿孔；穿刺　詳細不明	820402.2	820402.2	5
820404.2	小；表在性；非全周性；出血量が全血液量の20％以下	820404.2	820404.2	5
820406.3	大；破裂；断裂；部分欠損；出血量が全血液量の20％を超える	820406.3	820406.3	4
820699.2	膝窩動脈　詳細不明	820699.2	820699.2	5
820602.2	内膜剥離，断裂なし	820602.2	820602.2	5
820604.2	裂傷・裂創；穿孔；穿刺　詳細不明	820604.2	820604.2	5
820606.2	小；表在性；非全周性；出血量が全血液量の20％以下	820606.2	820606.2	5
820608.3	大；破裂；断裂；部分欠損；出血量が全血液量の20％を超える	820608.3	820608.3	5
820899.2	膝窩静脈　詳細不明	820899.2	820899.2	5
820802.2	裂傷・裂創；穿孔；穿刺　詳細不明	820802.2	820802.2	5
820804.2	小；表在性；非全周性；出血量が全血液量の20％以下	820804.2	820804.2	5
820806.3	大；破裂；断裂；部分欠損；出血量が全血液量の20％を超える	820806.3	820806.3	4

[f] AIS2005に加えられた新しいコード。外傷の存在部位を示すことができる。ただし重症度はない。

LOWER EXTREMITY, PELVIS and BUTTOCKS

AIS 2005	Injury Description	⇒ AIS98	⇐ AIS98	FCI
821099.1	**Other named arteries** NFS [e.g., **tibial, peroneal**]	821099.1	821099.1	5
821002.1	intimal tear, no disruption	821002.1	821002.1	5
821004.1	laceration ; perforation ; puncture NFS	821004.1	821004.1	5
821006.1	minor ; superficial ; incomplete circumferential involvement ; blood loss ≤ 20% by volume	821006.1	821006.1	5
821008.3	major ; rupture ; transection ; segmental loss ; blood loss > 20% by volume	821008.3	821008.3	5
821299.1	**Other named veins** NFS [e.g., **saphenous**]	821299.1	821299.1	5
821202.1	laceration ; perforation ; puncture NFS	821202.1	821202.1	5
821204.1	minor ; superficial ; incomplete circumferential involvement ; blood loss ≤ 20% by volume	821204.1	821204.1	5
821206.3	major ; rupture ; transection ; segmental loss ; blood loss > 20% by volume	821206.3	821206.3	4

AIS 2005	損傷内容	⇒ AIS98	⇐ AIS98	FCI
821099.1	その他の名前のある動脈　詳細不明［例：脛骨動脈, 腓骨動脈］	821099.1	821099.1	5
821002.1	内膜剥離, 断裂なし	821002.1	821002.1	5
821004.1	裂傷・裂創；穿孔；穿刺　詳細不明	821004.1	821004.1	5
821006.1	小；表在性；非全周性；出血量が全血液量の20％以下	821006.1	821006.1	5
821008.3	大；破裂；断裂；部分欠損；出血量が全血液量の20％を超える	821008.3	821008.3	5
821299.1	その他の名前のある静脈　詳細不明［例：伏在静脈］	821299.1	821299.1	5
821202.1	裂傷・裂創；穿孔；穿刺　詳細不明	821202.1	821202.1	5
821204.1	小；表在性；非全周性；出血量が全血液量の20％以下	821204.1	821204.1	5
821206.3	大；破裂；断裂；部分欠損；出血量が全血液量の20％を超える	821206.3	821206.3	4

LOWER EXTREMITY, PELVIS and BUTTOCKS

AIS 2005	Injury Description	⇒ AIS98	⇐ AIS98	FCI
	NERVES			
	A diagnosis of nerve palsy or neuropraxia should be coded as a contusion to the specific nerve.			
830099.9	**Nerve injury in lower extremity** NFS[f]	None	None	
830299.1	**Digital nerve** NFS	830299.1	830299.1	5
830202.1	contusion	830202.1	830202.1	5
830204.1	laceration	830204.1	830204.1	5
830399.2	**Femoral nerve** NFS[w]	830699.2	830699.2	5
830302.2	contusion	830602.2	830602.2	5
830304.2	laceration ; avulsion NFS	830604.2	830604.2	3
830306.2	with motor loss	830610.2	830610.2	2
830599.2	**Peroneal nerve** NFS[w]	830699.2	830699.2	5
830502.2	contusion	830602.2	830602.2	5
830504.2	laceration ; avulsion NFS	830604.2	830604.2	3
830506.2	with motor loss	830610.2	830610.2	2
830499.2	**Sciatic nerve** NFS	830499.2	830499.2	1
830402.2	contusion	830402.2	830402.2	3
830404.3	laceration NFS	830404.3	830404.3	5
830406.3	incomplete	830406.3	830406.3	2
830408.3	complete	830408.3	830408.3	1
830699.2	**Tibial nerve** NFS[w]	830699.2	830699.2	5
830602.2	contusion	830602.2	830602.2	5
830604.2	laceration ; avulsion NFS	830604.2	830604.2	3
830606.2	with motor loss	830610.2	830610.2	2

[f] New descriptor in AIS 2005 that allows classification of trauma by body region but does not allow assigning a severity code.
[w] Femoral, peroneal and tibial nerves were combined as one descriptor in AIS98. In AIS 2005, each is a separate injury category ; hence, the duplication of AIS98 matching codes.

下肢・骨盤・殿部

AIS 2005	損傷内容	⇒ AIS98	⇐ AIS98	FCI

神 経

麻痺，神経遮断の診断があれば該当する神経の挫傷としてコード選択する。

(訳者注釈：neuropraxia は，neurapraxia かもしれない。『ステッドマン医学大辞典』の第5版に"よくあるつづりの誤り"とある。ニュラプラキシアとは，神経に沿った伝導の局所的喪失で，軸索変性を伴わない。)

AIS 2005	損傷内容	⇒ AIS98	⇐ AIS98	FCI
830099.9	下腿の神経損傷　詳細不明[f]	なし	なし	
830299.1	趾神経　詳細不明	830299.1	830299.1	5
830202.1	挫傷	830202.1	830202.1	5
830204.1	裂傷・裂創	830204.1	830204.1	5
830399.2	大腿神経　詳細不明[w]	830699.2	830699.2	5
830302.2	挫傷	830602.2	830602.2	5
830304.2	裂傷・裂創；剥離　詳細不明	830604.2	830604.2	3
830306.2	運動麻痺を伴う	830610.2	830610.2	2
830599.2	腓骨神経　詳細不明[w]	830699.2	830699.2	5
830502.2	挫傷	830602.2	830602.2	5
830504.2	裂傷・裂創；剥離　詳細不明	830604.2	830604.2	3
830506.2	運動麻痺を伴う	830610.2	830610.2	2
830499.2	坐骨神経　詳細不明	830499.2	830499.2	1
830402.2	挫傷	830402.2	830402.2	3
830404.3	裂傷・裂創　詳細不明	830404.3	830404.3	5
830406.3	不完全	830406.3	830406.3	2
830408.3	完全	830408.3	830408.3	1
830699.2	脛骨神経　詳細不明[w]	830699.2	830699.2	5
830602.2	挫傷	830602.2	830602.2	5
830604.2	裂傷・裂創；剥離　詳細不明	830604.2	830604.2	3
830606.2	運動麻痺を伴う	830610.2	830610.2	2

---

[f] AIS2005に加えられた新しいコード。外傷の存在部位を示すことができる。ただし重症度はない。
[w] 大腿神経，腓骨神経，脛骨神経の損傷は，AIS98では1つのコードにまとめられていた。AIS2005では，各々が別の神経損傷として分類されている。したがって，(これらのコードを) AIS98に変換すると同じコードになる。

LOWER EXTREMITY, PELVIS and BUTTOCKS

AIS 2005	Injury Description	⇒ AIS98	⇐ AIS98	FCI
	MUSCLES, TENDONS, LIGAMENTS			
840099.9	**Muscle, tendon, ligament injury** NFS[f]	None	None	
840200.2	**Achilles tendon** tear ; avulsion NFS	840200.2	840200.2	4
840202.2	partial disruption	840202.2	840202.2	5
840204.2	complete disruption	840204.2	840204.2	4
840400.2	**Collateral ligament** tear ; avulsion NFS[x]	None	None	5
840402.2	ankle	840402.2	840402.2	5
840403.2	partial disruption	840402.2	None	4
840404.2	complete disruption	840402.2	None	4
840405.2	knee	840404.2	840404.2	5
840406.2	partial disruption	840404.2	None	5
840407.2	complete disruption	840404.2	None	5
840500.2	**Cruciate ligament** [anterior or posterior] tear ; avulsion NFS[x]	840404.2	None	5
840501.2	partial disruption	840404.2	None	5
840502.2	complete disruption	840404.2	None	5
840300.2	**Meniscus** tear ; avulsion NFS	850822.2	850822.2	5
840600.1	**Muscle** tear ; avulsion NFS	840600.2[b]	840600.2[b]	5
840601.1	partial disruption	840600.2[b]	None	5
840603.2	complete disruption	840600.2	840600.2	4
840602.1	contusion ; strain	840602.1	840602.1	
840800.2	**Tendon** [other than Achilles or patellar] tear ; avulsion	840802.2	840802.2	4
840801.2	partial disruption	840802.2	None	4
840802.2	complete disruption	840802.2	None	3
841000.2	**Patellar tendon** tear ; avulsion	841002.2	841002.2	4
841001.2	partial disruption	841002.2	None	4
841002.2	complete disruption	841004.2	841004.2	4

---

[b] Change in severity code in AIS 2005

[f] New descriptor in AIS 2005 that allows classification of trauma by body region, but does not allow assigning a severity code.

[x] Collateral and cruciate ligaments were combined as one descriptor in AIS98. In AIS 2005, each is a separate injury category ; hence, the duplication of AIS98 matching codes.

下肢・骨盤・殿部

AIS 2005	損傷内容	⇒ AIS98	⇐ AIS98	FCI
	筋肉，腱，靱帯			
840099.9	筋肉，腱，靱帯の損傷　詳細不明[f]	なし	なし	
840200.2	アキレス腱　断裂；剥離　詳細不明	840200.2	840200.2	4
840202.2	部分断裂	840202.2	840202.2	5
840204.2	完全断裂	840204.2	840204.2	4
840400.2	側副靱帯　断裂；剥離　詳細不明[x]	なし	なし	5
840402.2	足関節部	840402.2	840402.2	5
840403.2	部分断裂	840402.2	なし	4
840404.2	完全断裂	840402.2	なし	4
840405.2	膝部	840404.2	840404.2	5
840406.2	部分断裂	840404.2	なし	5
840407.2	完全断裂	840404.2	なし	5
840500.2	十字靱帯［前十字靱帯または後十字靱帯］断裂；剥離　詳細不明[x]	840404.2	なし	5
840501.2	部分断裂	840404.2	なし	5
840502.2	完全断裂	840404.2	なし	5
840300.2	半月板断裂；剥離　詳細不明	850822.2	850822.2	5
840600.1	筋肉断裂；剥離　詳細不明	840600.2[b]	840600.2[b]	5
840601.1	部分断裂	840600.2[b]	なし	5
840603.2	完全断裂	840600.2	840600.2	4
840602.1	挫傷；ストレイン（部分的過伸展損傷）	840602.1	840602.1	
840800.2	腱［アキレス腱または膝蓋腱以外］断裂；剥離	840802.2	840802.2	4
840801.2	部分断裂	840802.2	なし	4
840802.2	完全断裂	840802.2	なし	3
841000.2	膝蓋腱断裂；剥離	841002.2	841002.2	4
841001.2	部分断裂	841002.2	なし	4
841002.2	完全断裂	841004.2	841004.2	4

[b] AIS2005で重症度に変更あり。
[f] AIS2005に加えられた新しいコード。外傷の存在部位を示すことができる。ただし重症度はない。
[x] 側副靱帯，十字靱帯は，AIS98では1つのコードで表記されていた。AIS2005では，それぞれの損傷とした。したがって，（これらのコードを）AIS98に変換すると同じコードになる。

LOWER EXTREMITY, PELVIS and BUTTOCKS

AIS 2005	Injury Description	⇒ AIS98	⇐ AIS98	FCI
	JOINTS			
870099.9	Lower extremity joint injury NFS[f]	None	None	
873099.1	**Hip joint** NFS	850699.1	850699.1	5
873089.1	open[a]	850699.1	None	2
873010.1	sprain	850606.1	850606.1	5
873020.1	subluxation	850610.2[b]	None	5
873030.2	dislocation	850610.2	850610.2	4
873031.2	open[a]	850610.2	None	2
873032.2	no articular cartilage involvement	850614.2	850614.2	4
873033.2	open[a]	850614.2	None	2
873034.2	with articular cartilage involvement	850618.2	850618.2	4
873035.2	open[a]	850618.2	None	2
874099.1	**Knee joint** NFS	850899.1	850899.1	5
874089.1	open[a]	850899.1	None	5
874010.1	sprain	850826.2[b]	850826.2[b]	5
874020.1	subluxation	850806.2[b]	None	5
874030.2	dislocation NFS	850806.2	850806.2	2
874031.2	open[a]	850806.2	None	2
874032.2	no articular cartilage involvement	850810.2	850810.2	2
874033.2	open[a]	850810.2	None	2
874034.2	with articular cartilage involvement	850814.2	850814.2	2
874035.2	open[a]	850814.2	None	2
877199.1	**Ankle joint** NFS	850299.1	850299.1	5
877189.1	open NFS[a]	850299.1	None	4
877110.1	sprain	850206.1	850206.1	5
877120.1	subluxation	850210.2[b]	None	5
877130.2	dislocation NFS	850210.2	850210.2	4
877131.2	open[a]	850210.2	None	4
877132.2	no articular cartilage involvement	850214.2	850214.2	4
877133.2	open[a]	850214.2	None	4
877134.2	with articular cartilage involvement	850218.2	850218.2	4
877135.2	open[a]	850218.2	None	3

[a] New descriptor in AIS 2005
[b] Change in severity code in AIS 2005
[f] New descriptor in AIS 2005 that allows classification of trauma by body region, but does not allow assigning a severity code.

下肢・骨盤・殿部

AIS 2005	損傷内容	⇒ AIS98	⇐ AIS98	FCI
	関　節			
870099.9	下肢　関節損傷　詳細不明[f]	なし	なし	
873099.1	**股関節**　詳細不明	850699.1	850699.1	5
873089.1	開放[a]	850699.1	なし	2
873010.1	捻挫	850606.1	850606.1	5
873020.1	亜脱臼	850610.2[b]	なし	5
873030.2	脱臼	850610.2	850610.2	4
873031.2	開放[a]	850610.2	なし	2
873032.2	関節軟骨の損傷を伴わない	850614.2	850614.2	4
873033.2	開放[a]	850614.2	なし	2
873034.2	関節軟骨の損傷を伴う	850618.2	850618.2	4
873035.2	開放[a]	850618.2	なし	2
874099.1	**膝関節**　詳細不明	850899.1	850899.1	5
874089.1	開放[a]	850899.1	なし	5
874010.1	捻挫	850826.2[b]	850826.2[b]	5
874020.1	亜脱臼	850806.2[b]	なし	5
874030.2	脱臼　詳細不明	850806.2	850806.2	2
874031.2	開放[a]	850806.2	なし	2
874032.2	関節軟骨の損傷を伴わない	850810.2	850810.2	2
874033.2	開放[a]	850810.2	なし	2
874034.2	関節軟骨の損傷を伴う	850814.2	850814.2	2
874035.2	開放[a]	850814.2	なし	2
877199.1	**足関節**　詳細不明	850299.1	850299.1	5
877189.1	開放　詳細不明[a]	850299.1	なし	4
877110.1	捻挫	850206.1	850206.1	5
877120.1	亜脱臼	850210.2[b]	なし	5
877130.2	脱臼　詳細不明	850210.2	850210.2	4
877131.2	開放[a]	850210.2	なし	4
877132.2	関節軟骨の損傷を伴わない	850214.2	850214.2	4
877133.2	開放[a]	850214.2	なし	4
877134.2	関節軟骨の損傷を伴う	850218.2	850218.2	4
877135.2	開放[a]	850218.2	なし	3

[a] AIS2005に加えられた新しいコード。
[b] AIS2005で重症度に変更あり。
[f] AIS2005に加えられた新しいコード。外傷の存在部位を示すことができる。ただし重症度はない。

LOWER EXTREMITY, PELVIS and BUTTOCKS

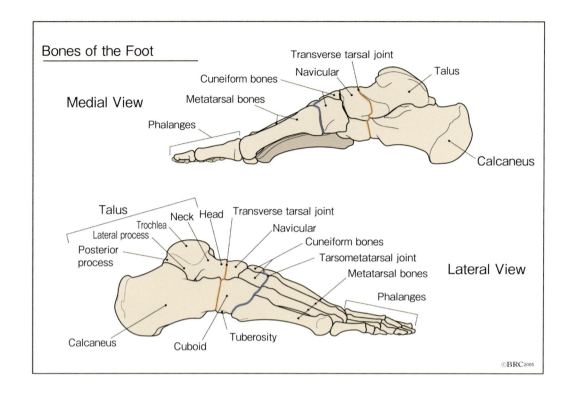

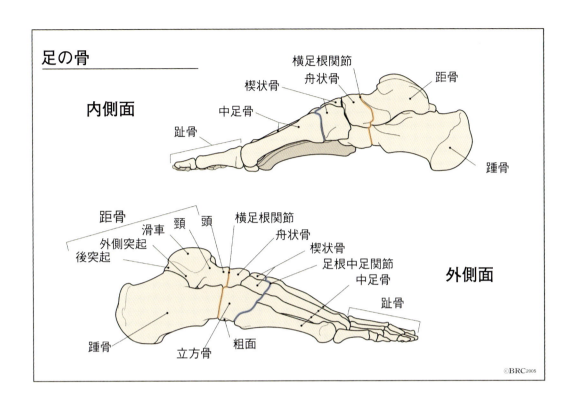

LOWER EXTREMITY, PELVIS and BUTTOCKS

AIS 2005	Injury Description	⇒ AIS98	⇐ AIS98	FCI
	Use the following category if no specific joint of the foot is described.			
870499.1	**Forefoot** joint NFS	850400.1	850400.1	3
870489.1	open[a]	850400.1	None	3
870410.1	sprain	850404.1	850404.1	5
870420.1	subluxation	850402.1	None	5
870430.1	dislocation NFS	850402.1	850402.1	3
870431.1	open[a]	850402.1	None	3
877799.1	**Midtarsal joint** NFS[z]	851299.1	851299.1	4
877789.1	open[a]	851299.1	None	4
877710.1	sprain	851202.1	851202.1	5
877720.1	subluxation	851203.1	None	5
877730.1	dislocation NFS [*Chopart's*]	851203.1	851203.1	4
877731.1	open[a]	851203.1	None	4
877732.1	no articular cartilage involvement	851204.1	851204.1	4
877733.1	open[a]	851204.1	None	4
877734.1	with articular cartilage involvement	851206.1	851206.1	4
877735.1	open[a]	851206.1	None	4
877299.1	**Subtalar joint** NFS[z]	851299.1	851299.1	4
877289.1	open[a]	851299.1	None	4
877210.1	sprain	851202.1	851202.1	4
877220.1	subluxation	851203.1	None	5
877230.1	dislocation NFS	851203.1	851203.1	4
877231.1	open[a]	851203.1	None	4
877232.1	no articular cartilage involvement	851204.1	851204.1	4
877233.1	open[a]	851204.1	None	4
877234.1	with articular cartilage involvement	851206.1	851206.1	4
877235.1	open[a]	851206.1	None	4

---

[a] New descriptor in AIS 2005

[z] Midtarsal (transtarsal or transverse tarsal), subtalar and tarsometatarsal (transmetatarsal) joints were combined as one descriptor in AIS98. In AIS 2005, each is a separate injury category ; hence, the duplication of AIS98 matching codes.

下肢・骨盤・殿部

AIS 2005	損傷内容	⇒ AIS98	⇐ AIS98	FCI
	足部のどの関節か記載されていない場合に選択する。			
870499.1	**前足部関節**　詳細不明	850400.1	850400.1	3
870489.1	開放[a]	850400.1	なし	3
870410.1	捻挫	850404.1	850404.1	5
870420.1	亜脱臼	850402.1	なし	5
870430.1	脱臼　詳細不明	850402.1	850402.1	3
870431.1	開放[a]	850402.1	なし	3
877799.1	**中足根部関節**　詳細不明[z]	851299.1	851299.1	4
877789.1	開放[a]	851299.1	なし	4
877710.1	捻挫	851202.1	851202.1	5
877720.1	亜脱臼	851203.1	なし	5
877730.1	脱臼　詳細不明［Chopart's（ショパール）関節］	851203.1	851203.1	4
877731.1	開放[a]	851203.1	なし	4
877732.1	関節軟骨の損傷を伴わない	851204.1	851204.1	4
877733.1	開放[a]	851204.1	なし	4
877734.1	関節軟骨の損傷を伴う	851206.1	851206.1	4
877735.1	開放[a]	851206.1	なし	4
877299.1	**距骨下関節**　詳細不明[z]	851299.1	851299.1	4
877289.1	開放[a]	851299.1	なし	4
877210.1	捻挫	851202.1	851202.1	4
877220.1	亜脱臼	851203.1	なし	5
877230.1	脱臼　詳細不明	851203.1	851203.1	4
877231.1	開放[a]	851203.1	なし	4
877232.1	関節軟骨の損傷を伴わない	851204.1	851204.1	4
877233.1	開放[a]	851204.1	なし	4
877234.1	関節軟骨の損傷を伴う	851206.1	851206.1	4
877235.1	開放[a]	851206.1	なし	4

[a] AIS2005に加えられた新しいコード。
[z] 中足根部（足根間または横足根）関節，距骨下および足根中足関節は，AIS98では同一の損傷内容にまとめられていた。AIS2005ではそれぞれが別のカテゴリーに分けられたため，AIS98にコードを変換すると重複したコードとなる。

LOWER EXTREMITY, PELVIS and BUTTOCKS

AIS 2005	Injury Description	⇒ AIS98	⇐ AIS98	FCI
878099.1	**Tarsometatarsal joint** NFS[z]	851299.1	851299.1	3
878089.1	open[a]	851299.1	None	3
878010.1	sprain	851202.1	851202.1	4
878020.1	subluxation	851203.1	None	5
878030.1	dislocation NFS [*Lisfranc*]	851203.1	851203.1	3
878031.1	open[a]	851203.1	None	3
878032.1	no articular cartilage involvement	851204.1	851204.1	3
878033.1	open[a]	851204.1	None	3
878034.1	with articular cartilage involvement	851206.1	851206.1	3
878035.1	open[a]	851206.1	None	3
878199.1	**Metatarsophalangeal** or **interphalangeal joint** NFS	851099.1	851099.1	5
878189.1	open[a]	851099.1	851099.1	5
878150.1	**Great Toe** NFS[y]	851099.1	851099.1	4
878151.1	sprain	851002.1	851002.1	5
878153.1	subluxation	851006.1	None	5
878154.1	dislocation NFS	851006.1	851006.1	4
878155.1	open[a]	851006.1	None	4
878156.1	no articular cartilage involvement	851010.1	851010.1	4
878157.1	open[a]	851010.1	None	4
878158.1	with articular cartilage involvement	851014.1	851014.1	4
878159.1	open[a]	851014.1	None	4
878160.1	**Other Toe**, single or multiple, NFS[y]	851099.1	851099.1	5
878161.1	sprain	851002.1	851002.1	5
878163.1	subluxation	851006.1	None	5
878164.1	dislocation NFS	851006.1	851006.1	5
878165.1	open[a]	851006.1	None	5
878166.1	no articular cartilage involvement	851010.1	851010.1	5
878167.1	open[a]	851010.1	None	5
878168.1	with articular cartilage involvement	851014.1	851014.1	5
878169.1	open[a]	851014.1	None	5

[a] New descriptor in AIS 2005
[y] Great toe and other toes were combined as one descriptor in AIS98. In AIS 2005, each is a separate injury category; hence, the duplication of AIS98 matching codes.
[z] Midtarsal (transtarsal or transverse tarsal), subtalar and tarsometatarsal (transmetatarsal) joints were combined as one descriptor in AIS98. In AIS 2005, each is a separate injury category; hence, the duplication of AIS98 matching codes.

AIS 2005	損傷内容	⇒ AIS98	⇐ AIS98	FCI
878099.1	**足根中足関節**　詳細不明[z]	851299.1	851299.1	3
878089.1	開放[a]	851299.1	なし	3
878010.1	捻挫	851202.1	851202.1	4
878020.1	亜脱臼	851203.1	なし	5
878030.1	脱臼　詳細不明［Lisfranc（リスフラン）関節］	851203.1	851203.1	3
878031.1	開放[a]	851203.1	なし	3
878032.1	関節軟骨の損傷を伴わない	851204.1	851204.1	3
878033.1	開放[a]	851204.1	なし	3
878034.1	関節軟骨の損傷を伴う	851206.1	851206.1	3
878035.1	開放[a]	851206.1	なし	3
878199.1	**中足趾節関節または趾節間関節**　詳細不明	851099.1	851099.1	5
878189.1	開放[a]	851099.1	851099.1	5
878150.1	**母趾**　詳細不明[y]	851099.1	851099.1	4
878151.1	捻挫	851002.1	851002.1	5
878153.1	亜脱臼	851006.1	なし	5
878154.1	脱臼　詳細不明	851006.1	851006.1	4
878155.1	開放[a]	851006.1	なし	4
878156.1	関節軟骨の損傷を伴わない	851010.1	851010.1	4
878157.1	開放[a]	851010.1	なし	4
878158.1	関節軟骨の損傷を伴う	851014.1	851014.1	4
878159.1	開放[a]	851014.1	なし	4
878160.1	**他の趾**，単一または複数，詳細不明[y]	851099.1	851099.1	5
878161.1	捻挫	851002.1	851002.1	5
878163.1	亜脱臼	851006.1	なし	5
878164.1	脱臼	851006.1	851006.1	5
878165.1	開放[a]	851006.1	なし	5
878166.1	関節軟骨の損傷を伴わない	851010.1	851010.1	5
878167.1	開放[a]	851010.1	なし	5
878168.1	関節軟骨の損傷を伴う	851014.1	851014.1	5
878169.1	開放[a]	851014.1	なし	5

[a] AIS2005に加えられた新しいコード。
[y] 母趾および他の趾は，AIS98では同一の損傷内容にまとめられていた。AIS2005ではそれぞれが別のカテゴリーに分けられたためAIS98にコードを変換すると重複したコードとなる。
[z] 中足根部（足根間または横足根）関節，距骨下および足根中足関節は，AIS98では同一の損傷内容にまとめられていた。AIS2005ではそれぞれが別のカテゴリーに分けられたため，AIS98にコードを変換すると重複したコードとなる。

LOWER EXTREMITY, PELVIS and BUTTOCKS

AIS 2005	Injury Description	⇒ AIS98	⇐ AIS98	FCI

SKELETAL

Classification of Long Bone Fractures

Long bone fractures are classified as to their location on the bone (i.e., proximal, shaft [diaphyseal] or distal). Proximal and distal fractures are further classified by the extent of articular (joint) involvement, and shaft fractures are classified by their degree of complexity. For long bone shaft fractures, "complex" means multifragmentary. Other clinical descriptions are : spiral, segmental, irregular or comminuted. Selected anatomical drawings and a sample of specific long bone fractures are included to aid the AIS user in becoming familiar with these classification changes and with contemporary orthopedic trauma terminology. The Introduction to the AIS dictionary includes further notes describing the changes.

CODING RULES : Lower Extremities

For patients who die before any radiology is done and no autopsy is performed, a clinical diagnosis of a fracture made by detecting obvious instability of an extremity is acceptable for AIS coding. (Example : leg fracture NFS, 852002.2, if neither tibia nor fibula is named. Alternatively, tibia fracture NFS, 854000.2, or fibula fracture NFS, 854441.2, if known.)

An ankle fracture is a poorly-stated diagnosis. The ankle is a joint and, strictly speaking, cannot be fractured. A diagnosis of ankle fracture with no further detail should be coded as a leg fracture NFS, 852002.2.

Use one of the following three descriptors if specific anatomical information is unknown.

850099.9	**Lower Extremity** fracture NFS[f]	None	None	
852002.2	**Leg** fracture NFS	852002.2	852002.2	5
852004.2	**Foot** fracture NFS	852000.2	852000.2	5

---

[f] New descriptor in AIS 2005 that allows classification of trauma by body region, but does not allow assigning a severity code.

AIS 2005	損傷内容	⇒ AIS98	⇐ AIS98	FCI

骨　格

長管骨骨折の分類

長管骨骨折は骨折のある部位により分類されている（例：近位部，骨幹部，遠位部）。近位部および遠位部の骨折はさらに軟骨（関節）の損傷程度により分類されている。また，骨幹部も複雑度に応じてさらに分類されている。長管骨骨幹部骨折において，「粉砕」とは骨片が複数あることをいう。臨床的に用いられるその他の用語には螺旋状，部分的，不整，粉砕がある。AISのユーザーがこれらの分類の変更に慣れ，かつ整形外科学的用語に慣れるよう，解剖学的図譜や具体的な長管骨骨折の例を取り入れてある。本手引書の序説にこれらの変更についてさらに詳しく記述している。

コード選択のルール：下肢

画像検査なしに死亡し，剖検もされない患者について，四肢の明らかな動揺を認めれば，それを臨床的に骨折と診断し，コード選択を行ってもよい。そのような場合は重症度のもっとも低いコードを選択する。（例：脛骨とも腓骨とも記載されていなければ，下腿骨折　詳細不明，852002.2をコードし，脛骨か腓骨かがわかれば，脛骨骨折　詳細不明，854000.2，または腓骨骨折　詳細不明，854441.2をコードする。）

足関節骨折は不十分な診断である。足関節（足首）は関節であり，厳密にいえば骨折することはない。足関節骨折以外に詳細な記載がなければ，下腿骨折　詳細不明，852002.2をコードすべきである。

他に明確な解剖学的情報がない場合に，以下の3つのコードのうちのいずれかを選択する。

850099.9	下肢の骨折　詳細不明[f]	なし	なし	
852002.2	下腿の骨折　詳細不明	852002.2	852002.2	5
852004.2	足部の骨折　詳細不明	852000.2	852000.2	5

---

[f]　AIS2005に加えられた新しいコード。外傷の存在部位を示すことができる。ただし重症度はない。

LOWER EXTREMITY, PELVIS and BUTTOCKS

BONE: Femur

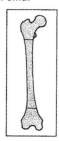

LOCATION: Proximal segment

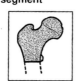

TYPES: Trochanteric area

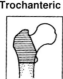

Neck

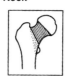

Head

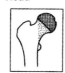

LOCATION: Shaft [diaphyseal] segment

TYPES: Simple

Wedge

Complex

LOCATION: Distal segment

TYPES: Extra-articular

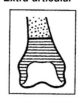

Examples:

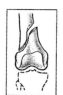

Partial articular

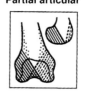

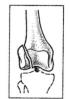

Complete articular

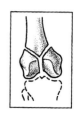

骨：
大腿骨

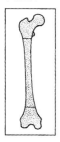

部位：
近位部

型：
転子部

頸部

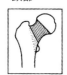

骨頭

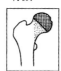

部位：
体（骨幹）部

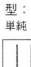

型：
単純

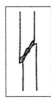

楔状

粉砕

部位：
遠位部

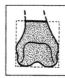

型：
関節外

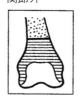

例：

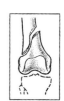

部分関節内

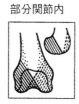

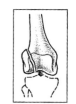

完全関節内

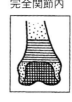

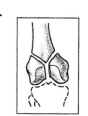

LOWER EXTREMITY, PELVIS and BUTTOCKS

AIS 2005	Injury Description	⇒ AIS98	⇐ AIS98	FCI
853000.3	**Femur** fracture, NFS	851800.3	851800.3	5
853001.3	open NFS	851801.3	851801.3	5
853111.3	**Proximal Femur** fracture NFS	851800.3	851800.3	4
853112.3	open NFS	851801.3	851801.3	4
853151.3	trochanteric ; intertrochanteric	851810.3	851810.3	4
853152.3	open	851810.3[aa]	851810.3[aa]	4
853161.3	femoral neck	851812.3	851812.3	4
853162.3	open	851812.3[aa]	851812.3[aa]	4
853171.3	femoral head ; *Pipkin*	851808.3	851808.3	2
853172.3	open	851808.3[aa]	851808.3[aa]	2
853221.3	**Femur Shaft** fracture NFS	851814.3	851814.3	5
853222.3	open	851814.3[aa]	851814.3[aa]	5
853251.3	simple ; spiral ; oblique ; transverse ; *Winquist I*	851814.3	851814.3	5
853252.3	open	851814.3[aa]	851814.3[aa]	5
853261.3	wedge ; "butterfly" ; *Winquist II or III*	851814.3	851814.3	5
853262.3	open	851814.3[aa]	851814.3[aa]	5
853271.3	complex ; comminuted ; segmental ; *Winquist IV*	851814.3[aa]	851814.3[aa]	4
853272.3	open	851814.3[aa]	851814.3[aa]	4
853331.3	**Distal Femur** fracture NFS	851800.3	851800.3	3
853332.3	open	851801.3	851801.3	3
853351.3	extra-articular ; supracondylar	851822.3	851822.3	3
853352.3	open	851822.3[aa]	851822.3[aa]	3
853361.3	partial articular ; condylar ; *Hoffa*	851804.3	851804.3	3
853362.3	open	851804.3[aa]	851804.3[aa]	3
853371.3	complete articular ; bicondylar ; T-shaped ; Y-shaped	851800.3	851800.3	2
853372.3	open	851801.3[aa]	851801.3[aa]	2

[aa] Also matches with 851801.3

下肢・骨盤・殿部

AIS 2005	損傷内容	⇒ AIS98	⇐ AIS98	FCI
853000.3	**大腿骨**骨折　詳細不明	851800.3	851800.3	5
853001.3	開放　詳細不明	851801.3	851801.3	5
853111.3	**近位部**骨折　詳細不明	851800.3	851800.3	4
853112.3	開放　詳細不明	851801.3	851801.3	4
853151.3	転子部；転子間	851810.3	851810.3	4
853152.3	開放	851810.3[aa]	851810.3[aa]	4
853161.3	大腿骨頸部	851812.3	851812.3	4
853162.3	開放	851812.3[aa]	851812.3[aa]	4
853171.3	大腿骨骨頭；Pipkin（ピプキン）分類	851808.3	851808.3	2
853172.3	開放	851808.3[aa]	851808.3[aa]	2
853221.3	**骨幹部**骨折　詳細不明	851814.3	851814.3	5
853222.3	開放	851814.3[aa]	851814.3[aa]	5
853251.3	単純；螺旋；斜走；横断；Winquist（ウィンクィスト）Ⅰ型	851814.3	851814.3	5
853252.3	開放	851814.3[aa]	851814.3[aa]	5
853261.3	楔状；"蝶形"；Winquist Ⅱ またはⅢ型	851814.3	851814.3	5
853262.3	開放	851814.3[aa]	851814.3[aa]	5
853271.3	複雑；粉砕；分節；Winquist Ⅳ型	851814.3[aa]	851814.3[aa]	4
853272.3	開放	851814.3[aa]	851814.3[aa]	4
853331.3	**遠位部**骨折　詳細不明	851800.3	851800.3	3
853332.3	開放	851801.3	851801.3	3
853351.3	関節外；顆上	851822.3	851822.3	3
853352.3	開放	851822.3[aa]	851822.3[aa]	3
853361.3	部分関節内；顆部；Hoffa（ホッファ）骨折	851804.3	851804.3	3
853362.3	開放	851804.3[aa]	851804.3[aa]	3
853371.3	完全関節内；両顆；T字形；Y字形	851800.3	851800.3	2
853372.3	開放	851801.3[aa]	851801.3[aa]	2

[aa] 851801.3でもよい。

LOWER EXTREMITY, PELVIS and BUTTOCKS

BONE:
Tibia/
Fibula

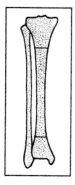

LOCATION: Tibia
Proximal segment

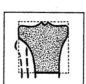

TYPES:
Extra-articular

Parital articular

Complete articular

LOCATION: Tibia
Shaft [diaphyseal]
segment

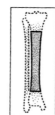

TYPES:
Simple

Wedge

Complex

LOCATION: Tibia
Distal segment

TYPES:
Extra-articular →

Partial articular →

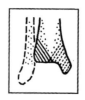

Complete articular →

Examples:

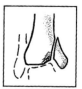

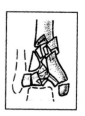

下肢・骨盤・殿部

骨：
脛骨/
腓骨

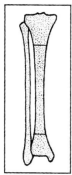

部位：
脛骨近位部

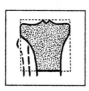

型：
関節外

部分関節内

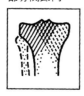

完全関節内

部位：
脛骨骨幹部

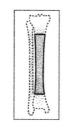

型：
単純

楔状

粉砕

部位：
脛骨遠位部

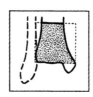

型：
関節外

部分関節内

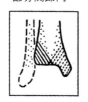

完全関節内

例：

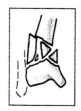

→

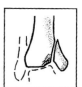

→

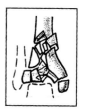

LOWER EXTREMITY, PELVIS and BUTTOCKS

AIS 2005	Injury Description	⇒ AIS98	⇐ AIS98	FCI
854000.2	**Tibia fracture** NFS	853404.2	853404.2	4
854001.3	open	853405.3	853405.3	4
854111.2	**Proximal Tibia** fracture NFS	853404.2	853404.2	4
854112.3	open	853405.3	853405.3	4
854151.2	extra-articular	853404.2	853404.2	4
854152.3	open	853405.3	853405.3	4
854161.2	partial articular ; *Schatzker 1, 2, 3*	853404.2	853404.2	4
854162.3	open	853405.3	853405.3	4
854171.2	complete articular ; plateau ; bicondylar ; *Schatzker 4, 5, 6*	853406.2	853406.2	2
854172.3	open	853408.3	853408.3	2
854221.2	**Tibia Shaft** fracture NFS	853420.2	853420.2	4
854222.3	open	853422.3	853422.3	4
854251.2	simple ; spiral ; oblique ; transverse ; *Winquist I*	853420.2	853420.2	4
854252.3	open	853422.3	853422.3	4
854261.2	wedge ; "butterfly" ; *Winquist II or III*	853420.2	853420.2	4
854262.3	open	853422.3	853422.3	4
854271.2	complex ; comminuted ; segmental ; *Winquist IV*	853422.3[b]	853422.3[b]	4
854272.3	open	853422.3	853422.3	4
854331.2	**Distal Tibia** fracture NFS [includes medial malleolus ; also pilon fracture*]	853404.2	853404.2	2
854332.3	open	853405.3	853405.3	2
854351.2	extra-articular ; isolated medial malleolus	853404.2	853404.2	4
854352.3	open	853405.3	853405.3	4
854361.2	partial articular	853404.2	853404.2	2
854362.3	open	853405.3	853405.3	2
854371.2	complete articular	853404.2	853404.2	2
854372.3	open	853405.3	853405.3	2

[b] Change in severity code in AIS 2005
* Pilon fracture is an intra-articular fracture of the distal end of the tibia that occurs as a result of the talus being pushed upward into the tibial plafond.

下肢・骨盤・殿部

AIS 2005	損傷内容	⇒ AIS98	⇐ AIS98	FCI
854000.2	**脛骨骨折** 詳細不明	853404.2	853404.2	4
854001.3	開放	853405.3	853405.3	4
854111.2	**近位部**骨折 詳細不明	853404.2	853404.2	4
854112.3	開放	853405.3	853405.3	4
854151.2	関節外	853404.2	853404.2	4
854152.3	開放	853405.3	853405.3	4
854161.2	部分関節内；Schatzker（シャツカー）1, 2, 3型	853404.2	853404.2	4
854162.3	開放	853405.3	853405.3	4
854171.2	完全関節内；プラトー；両顆；Schatzker 4, 5, 6型	853406.2	853406.2	2
854172.3	開放	853408.3	853408.3	2
854221.2	**骨幹部**骨折 詳細不明	853420.2	853420.2	4
854222.3	開放	853422.3	853422.3	4
854251.2	単純；螺旋；斜走；横断；Winquist Ⅰ型	853420.2	853420.2	4
854252.3	開放	853422.3	853422.3	4
854261.2	楔状；"蝶形"；Winquist ⅡまたはⅢ型	853420.2	853420.2	4
854262.3	開放	853422.3	853422.3	4
854271.2	複雑；粉砕；分節；Winquist Ⅳ型	853422.3[b]	853422.3[b]	4
854272.3	開放	853422.3	853422.3	4
854331.2	**遠位部**骨折 詳細不明［内果骨折；pilon（ピロン）骨折* を含む］	853404.2	853404.2	2
854332.3	開放	853405.3	853405.3	2
854351.2	関節外；内果単独	853404.2	853404.2	4
854352.3	開放	853405.3	853405.3	4
854361.2	部分関節内	853404.2	853404.2	2
854362.3	開放	853405.3	853405.3	2
854371.2	完全関節内	853404.2	853404.2	2
854372.3	開放	853405.3	853405.3	2

[b] AIS2005で重症度に変更あり。
* Pilon（ピロン）骨折は，距骨が脛骨天蓋に向かって持ち上げられることによって生じる，脛骨遠位端の関節内骨折である。

LOWER EXTREMITY, PELVIS and BUTTOCKS

BONE: Fibula

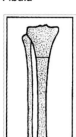

LOCATION: Malleolar segment

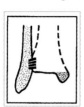

TYPES: Infrasyndesmotic

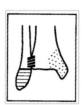

Transsyndesmotic

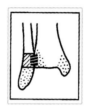

Suprasyndesmotic

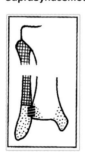

BONE: Patella

TYPES: Extra-articular

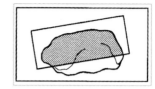

Partial articular

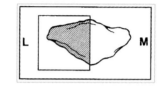 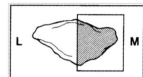

Complete articular

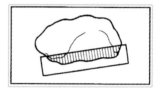

下肢・骨盤・殿部

骨：
腓骨

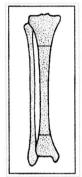

部位：
足関節果部

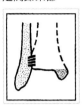

型：
靭帯結合部の下方

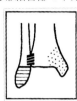

靭帯結合部レベル

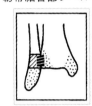

靭帯結合部の上方

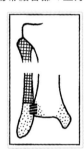

骨：
膝蓋骨

型：
関節外

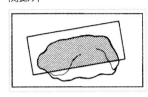

部分関節内

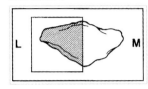 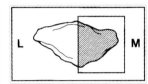

完全関節内

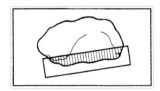

LOWER EXTREMITY, PELVIS and BUTTOCKS

AIS 2005	Injury Description	⇒ AIS98	⇐ AIS98	FCI
854441.2	**Fibula [malleoli]** fracture NFS — Also use this descriptor if specific anatomic location of a bi-malleolar fracture is not known.	851605.2	851605.2	5
854442.2	open	851605.2	851605.2	5
854453.2	below ankle joint (infrasyndesmotic) ; isolated lateral malleolus ; *Weber A*	851608.2	851608.2	5
854454.2	open	851610.2	851610.2	4
854455.2	lateral <u>and</u> medial malleoli (bimalleolar)	851612.2	851612.2	4
854456.3	open	851614.3	851614.3	4
854461.2	through joint (transsyndesmotic) ; *Weber B*	851608.2	None	4
854462.2	open	851610.2	None	4
854463.2	lateral <u>and</u> medial malleoli (bimalleolar)	851612.2	851612.2	4
854464.3	open	851614.3	851614.3	4
854465.2	trimalleolar	851612.2	851612.2	4
854466.3	open	851614.3	851614.3	4
854471.2	above joint (suprasyndesmotic) ; isolated shaft, head or neck ; *Weber C*	851606.2	851606.2	4
854472.2	open	851606.2	None	4
854500.2	**Patella** fracture NFS	852400.2	852400.2	4
854501.2	open	852400.2	852400.2	4
854551.2	extra-articular	852400.2	852400.2	5
854552.2	open	852400.2	852400.2	5
854561.2	partial articular or extensor mechanism intact	852400.2	852400.2	4
854562.2	open	852400.2	852400.2	4
854571.2	complete articular or extensor mechanism disrupted	852400.2	852400.2	3
854572.2	open	852400.2	852400.2	3

下肢・骨盤・殿部

AIS 2005	損傷内容	⇒ AIS98	⇐ AIS98	FCI
854441.2	**腓骨〔足関節果部〕**骨折　詳細不明　　両果骨折でそれ以上に解剖学的部位が不明な場合にもこのコードを選択する。	851605.2	851605.2	5
854442.2	開放	851605.2	851605.2	5
854453.2	足関節の下方（靱帯結合部の下方）；外果単独；Weber A型	851608.2	851608.2	5
854454.2	開放	851610.2	851610.2	4
854455.2	外果および内果（両果）	851612.2	851612.2	4
854456.3	開放	851614.3	851614.3	4
854461.2	足関節部（靱帯結合部レベル）；Weber B型	851608.2	なし	4
854462.2	開放	851610.2	なし	4
854463.2	外果および内果（両果）	851612.2	851612.2	4
854464.3	開放	851614.3	851614.3	4
854465.2	三果	851612.2	851612.2	4
854466.3	開放	851614.3	851614.3	4
854471.2	足関節の上方（靱帯結合部の上方）；骨幹部単独，骨頭または頸部；Weber C型	851606.2	851606.2	4
854472.2	開放	851606.2	なし	4
854500.2	**膝蓋骨**骨折　詳細不明	852400.2	852400.2	4
854501.2	開放	852400.2	852400.2	4
854551.2	関節外	852400.2	852400.2	5
854552.2	開放	852400.2	852400.2	5
854561.2	部分関節内または膝伸展機構損傷を伴わない	852400.2	852400.2	4
854562.2	開放	852400.2	852400.2	4
854571.2	完全関節内または膝伸展機構損傷を伴う	852400.2	852400.2	3
854572.2	開放	852400.2	852400.2	3

LOWER EXTREMITY, PELVIS and BUTTOCKS

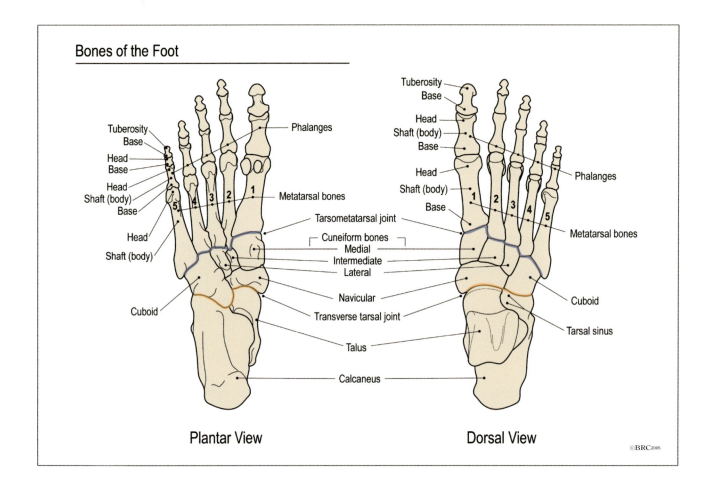

足の骨

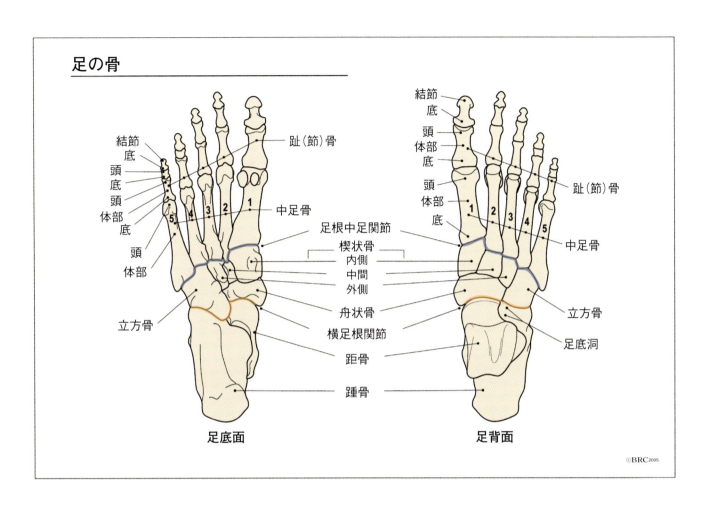

足底面／足背面

LOWER EXTREMITY, PELVIS and BUTTOCKS

AIS 2005	Injury Description	⇒ AIS98	⇐ AIS98	FCI
857200.2	**Talus** fracture NFS[s]	853200.2	853200.2	4
857201.2	open	853200.2	853200.2	3
857251.2	extra articular ; talus neck	853200.2	None	4
857252.2	open	853200.2	None	3
857261.2	fracture line into one joint surface ; talus body	853200.2	None	3
857262.2	open	853200.2	None	3
857271.2	fracture line into ≥ 2 joint surfaces	853200.2	None	3
857272.2	open	853200.2	None	3
857300.2	**Calcaneus** fracture NFS[s]	851400.2	851400.2	3
857301.2	open	851400.2	851400.2	3
857351.2	extra articular	851400.2	None	3
857352.2	open	851400.2	None	3
857361.2	fracture line into one joint surface	851400.2	None	3
857362.2	open	851400.2	None	3
857371.2	fracture line into ≥ 2 joint surfaces	851400.2	None	3
857372.2	open	851400.2	None	3
857400.2	**Navicular** fracture NFS[bb]	852200.2	None	3
857401.2	open	852200.2	None	3
857451.2	extra articular [coronal body split, no joint involvement]	852200.2	None	4
857452.2	open	852200.2	None	4
857461.2	fracture line into one joint surface	852200.2	None	3
857462.2	open	852200.2	None	3
857471.2	fracture line into ≥ 2 joint surfaces	852200.2	None	3
857472.2	open	852200.2	None	3

---

[s] Differentiation of specific anatomical sites for this injury category was less detailed in AIS98 than in AIS 2005 ; hence, the duplication of matching codes.

[bb] Tarsal and metatarsal fractures were combined as one descriptor in AIS98. In AIS 2005, tarsal (navicular, cuboid and cuneiform) and metatarsal fractures are separate categories ; hence, the duplication of AIS98 matching codes.

AIS 2005	損傷内容	⇒ AIS98	⇐ AIS98	FCI
857200.2	**距骨**骨折　詳細不明[s]	853200.2	853200.2	4
857201.2	開放	853200.2	853200.2	3
857251.2	関節外；距骨頸	853200.2	なし	4
857252.2	開放	853200.2	なし	3
857261.2	骨折が1つの関節面に及ぶもの；距骨体部	853200.2	なし	3
857262.2	開放	853200.2	なし	3
857271.2	骨折が2つ以上の関節面に及ぶもの	853200.2	なし	3
857272.2	開放	853200.2	なし	3
857300.2	**踵骨**骨折　詳細不明[s]	851400.2	851400.2	3
857301.2	開放	851400.2	851400.2	3
857351.2	関節外	851400.2	なし	3
857352.2	開放	851400.2	なし	3
857361.2	骨折が1つの関節面に及ぶもの	851400.2	なし	3
857362.2	開放	851400.2	なし	3
857371.2	骨折が2つ以上の関節面に及ぶもの	851400.2	なし	3
857372.2	開放	851400.2	なし	3
857400.2	**舟状骨**骨折　詳細不明[bb]	852200.2	なし	3
857401.2	開放	852200.2	なし	3
857451.2	関節外［冠状の体部の骨折，関節にかからない］	852200.2	なし	4
857452.2	開放	852200.2	なし	4
857461.2	骨折が1つの関節面に及ぶもの	852200.2	なし	3
857462.2	開放	852200.2	なし	3
857471.2	骨折が2つ以上の関節面に及ぶもの	852200.2	なし	3
857472.2	開放	852200.2	なし	3

[s] AIS98のこの損傷に関する部位の記述はAIS2005に比べて少ない。したがってAIS98コードは同じコードを使用している。

[bb] 足根骨および中足骨骨折は，AIS98では1つのコードであった。AIS2005では，足根骨（舟状骨，立方骨，楔状骨）と中足骨骨折はそれぞれを別の損傷として，AIS98の該当コードを反復入力する。

LOWER EXTREMITY, PELVIS and BUTTOCKS

AIS 2005	Injury Description	⇒ AIS98	⇐ AIS98	FCI
857600.2	**Cuboid** fracture NFS[bb]	852200.2	None	5
857601.2	open	852200.2	None	5
857651.2	extra articular [coronal body split, no joint involvement]	852200.2	None	5
857652.2	open	852200.2	None	5
857661.2	fracture line into one joint surface	852200.2	None	5
857662.2	open	852200.2	None	5
857671.2	fracture line into ≥2 joint surfaces	852200.2	None	4
857672.2	open	852200.2	None	4
857500.2	**Cuneiform** fracture NFS[bb]	852200.2	None	3
857501.2	open	852200.2	None	5
857551.2	extra articular [coronal body split, no joint involvement]	852200.2	None	5
857552.2	open	852200.2	None	5
857561.2	fracture line into one joint surface	852200.2	None	5
857562.2	open	852200.2	None	5
857571.2	fracture line into ≥2 joint surfaces	852200.2	None	4
857572.2	open	852200.2	None	4
858100.2	**Metatarsal** fracture NFS[bb]	852200.2	852200.2	4
858101.2	open	852200.2	852200.2	4
858111.2	**First Metatarsal** fracture NFS	852200.2	None	4
858112.2	open	852200.2	None	4
858151.2	extra articular or shaft	852200.2	None	5
858152.2	open	852200.2	None	5
858161.2	partial articular	852200.2	None	4
858162.2	open	852200.2	None	4
858171.2	complete articular	852200.2	None	4
858172.2	open	852200.2	None	4
858121.2	**One of Four Lateral Metatarsals** fracture NFS	852200.2	None	4
858122.2	open	852200.2	None	4
858153.2	extra articular or shaft	852200.2	None	4
858154.2	open	852200.2	None	4
858163.2	partial articular	852200.2	None	4
858164.2	open	852200.2	None	4
858173.2	complete articular	852200.2	None	4
858174.2	open	852200.2	None	4

[bb] Tarsal and metatarsal fractures were combined as one descriptor in AIS98. In AIS 2005, tarsal [navicular, cuboid and cuneiform] and metatarsal fractures are separate categories ; hence, the duplication of AIS98 matching codes.

下肢・骨盤・殿部

AIS 2005	損傷内容	⇒ AIS98	⇐ AIS98	FCI
857600.2	**立方骨**骨折　詳細不明[bb]	852200.2	なし	5
857601.2	開放	852200.2	なし	5
857651.2	関節外［冠状の体部の骨折，関節にかからない］	852200.2	なし	5
857652.2	開放	852200.2	なし	5
857661.2	骨折が1つの関節面に及ぶもの	852200.2	なし	5
857662.2	開放	852200.2	なし	5
857671.2	骨折が2つ以上の関節面に及ぶもの	852200.2	なし	4
857672.2	開放	852200.2	なし	4
857500.2	**楔状骨**骨折　詳細不明[bb]	852200.2	なし	3
857501.2	開放	852200.2	なし	5
857551.2	関節外［冠状の体部の骨折，関節にかからない］	852200.2	なし	5
857552.2	開放	852200.2	なし	5
857561.2	骨折が1つの関節面に及ぶもの	852200.2	なし	5
857562.2	開放	852200.2	なし	5
857571.2	骨折が2つ以上の関節面に及ぶもの	852200.2	なし	4
857572.2	開放	852200.2	なし	4
858100.2	**中足骨**骨折　詳細不明[bb]	852200.2	852200.2	4
858101.2	開放	852200.2	852200.2	4
858111.2	**第1中足骨**　骨折　詳細不明	852200.2	なし	4
858112.2	開放	852200.2	なし	4
858151.2	関節外または体部	852200.2	なし	5
858152.2	開放	852200.2	なし	5
858161.2	部分関節内	852200.2	なし	4
858162.2	開放	852200.2	なし	4
858171.2	完全関節内	852200.2	なし	4
858172.2	開放	852200.2	なし	4
858121.2	**第2〜5中足骨**の1つ　詳細不明	852200.2	なし	4
858122.2	開放	852200.2	なし	4
858153.2	関節外または体部	852200.2	なし	4
858154.2	開放	852200.2	なし	4
858163.2	部分関節内	852200.2	なし	4
858164.2	開放	852200.2	なし	4
858173.2	完全関節内	852200.2	なし	4
858174.2	開放	852200.2	なし	4

[bb] 足根骨および中足骨骨折は，AIS98では1つのコードであった。AIS2005では，足根骨（舟状骨，立方骨，楔状骨）と中足骨骨折はそれぞれを別の損傷として，AIS98の該当コードを反復入力する。

LOWER EXTREMITY, PELVIS and BUTTOCKS

AIS 2005	Injury Description	⇒ AIS98	⇐ AIS98	FCI
858200.1	**Phalange** fracture NFS	853602.1	None	5
858201.1	open	853602.1	None	5
858211.1	**Great Toe** NFS[y]	853602.1	None	4
858212.1	open	853602.1	None	4
858251.1	extra articular or shaft	853602.1	None	5
858252.1	open	853602.1	None	5
858261.1	partial articular	853602.1	None	4
858262.1	open	853602.1	None	4
858271.1	complete articular	853602.1	None	4
858272.1	open	853602.1	None	4
858221.1	**One of Lateral Four Toes** NFS[y]	853602.1	None	5
858222.1	open	853602.1	None	5
858253.1	extra articular or shaft	853602.1	None	5
858254.1	open	853602.1	None	5
858263.1	partial articular	853602.1	None	5
858264.1	open	853602.1	None	5
858273.1	complete articular	853602.1	None	5
858274.1	open	853602.1	None	5

---

[y] Great toe and other toes were combined as one descriptor in AIS98. In AIS 2005, each is a separate injury category; hence, the duplication of AIS98 matching codes.

下肢・骨盤・殿部

AIS 2005	損傷内容	⇒ AIS98	⇐ AIS98	FCI
858200.1	趾(節)骨骨折　詳細不明	853602.1	なし	5
858201.1	開放	853602.1	なし	5
858211.1	母趾(第1趾)　詳細不明[y]	853602.1	なし	4
858212.1	開放	853602.1	なし	4
858251.1	関節外または骨幹部	853602.1	なし	5
858252.1	開放	853602.1	なし	5
858261.1	部分関節内	853602.1	なし	4
858262.1	開放	853602.1	なし	4
858271.1	完全関節内	853602.1	なし	4
858272.1	開放	853602.1	なし	4
858221.1	第1〜第5趾　詳細不明[y]	853602.1	なし	5
858222.1	開放	853602.1	なし	5
858253.1	関節外または骨幹部	853602.1	なし	5
858254.1	開放	853602.1	なし	5
858263.1	部分関節内	853602.1	なし	5
858264.1	開放	853602.1	なし	5
858273.1	完全関節内	853602.1	なし	5
858274.1	開放	853602.1	なし	5

[y] 母趾および他の趾は，AIS98では同一の損傷内容にまとめられていた。AIS2005ではそれぞれが別のカテゴリーに分けられたため，AIS98にコードを変換すると重複したコードとなる。

LOWER EXTREMITY, PELVIS and BUTTOCKS

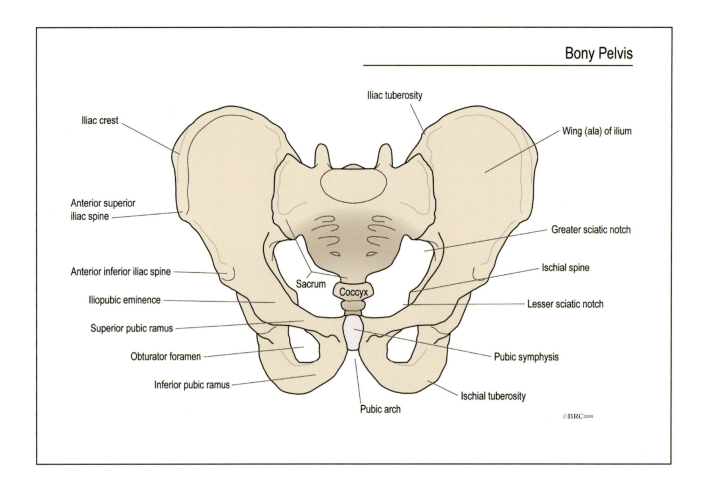

骨盤

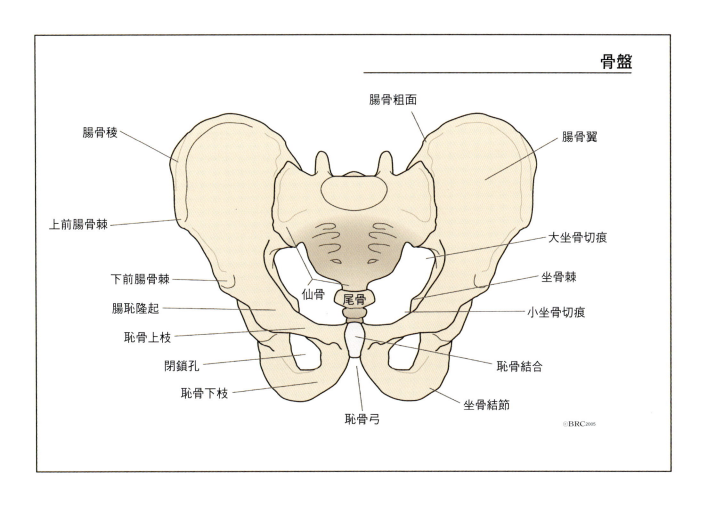

| AIS 2005 | Injury Description | ⇒ AIS98 | ⇐ AIS98 | FCI |

Coding Guidelines : PELVIS

The Pelvis is divided into two anatomic structures for AIS coding : the Pelvic Ring and the Acetabulum. The Pelvic Ring is a single anatomical structure and is assigned only one fracture code depending upon the specific nature of the injury according to each fracture category as described in the dictionary. The Acetabulum may be assigned two fracture codes depending upon whether the injury is unilateral or bilateral.

Pelvic Ring

The Pelvic Ring has two arches : the posterior arch is behind the acetabular surface and includes the sacrum, sacroiliac joints and their ligaments, and posterior ilium ; the anterior arch is in front of the acetabular surface and includes the pubic rami and the symphyseal joint (i.e., the line of union of the bodies of the pubic bones in the median plane).

The severity of a pelvic ring fracture is directly related to the extent of damage to the posterior arch rather than solely to which specific anatomic components are involved. However, because the recording of pelvic ring fractures is not standardized globally, some examples of anatomic descriptors are included in each injury category. These examples are not exhaustive and should be used only as guidelines. To the extent possible, the coder should seek information about the stability or instability of the fracture, described as follows, in assigning an AIS code.

   Stable : fracture not involving the posterior arch ; pelvic floor intact and able to withstand normal physiological stresses without displacement.

   Partially Stable : posterior osteoligamentous integrity partially maintained and pelvic floor intact.

   Unstable : complete loss of posterior osteoligamentous integrity ; pelvic floor disrupted.

CODING RULE : **Pelvis**

For patients who die before any radiology is done and no autopsy is performed, a clinical diagnosis of a pelvic fracture made by detecting obvious instability is acceptable for AIS coding. In such cases, use pelvic ring fracture NFS, 856100.2.

AIS 2005	損傷内容	⇒ AIS98	⇐ AIS98	FCI

コード選択ガイドライン：骨盤

骨盤は AIS コーディングでは2つの解剖学的構造に分類する：骨盤輪と寛骨臼。骨盤輪は単一の解剖学的構造であり，手引書内の骨折のカテゴリーに従って損傷の特徴に合うただ1つのコードを選択すること。寛骨臼については，損傷が両側の場合には2つのコードを選択する。

骨盤輪

骨盤輪は2つの弓がある：後方弓は寛骨臼蓋面の後部から，仙骨・仙腸関節とその靱帯，そして腸骨後部を含む；前方弓は寛骨臼面から恥骨枝と恥骨結合（すなわち，正中の恥骨体部の結合線）を含む。

骨盤輪骨折の重症度は，解剖学的骨折成分だけではなく，後方弓のダメージの広範さに直接相関する。しかし，骨盤輪骨折の分類に世界的標準化がなされておらず，一部の損傷コードでは，お互いの損傷カテゴリーが重なってしまう。こうした例は完全ではないのでガイドラインとしてのみ使用する。可能ならばコーダーは，AIS コードの選択にあたり，以下の分類に従って骨折が不安定型かどうか，さらに情報を求めるべきである。

　安定型：骨折が後方弓を含まない；骨盤底にかからないうえに，通常の生理的ストレスに転位なく耐えられるもの。

　部分不安定型：後方の骨靱帯結合が部分的に保たれ，骨盤底にかからないもの。

　不安定型：完全な骨靱帯結合の破綻；骨盤底の破綻。

コード選択のルール：**骨盤**

画像検査の前に死亡して剖検もされなかった場合，明らかな骨盤動揺の検出による骨折の臨床的診断は許容される。この場合のコードは骨盤骨折 NFS 856100.2を選択する。

PELVIC RING FRACTURES

Types:
Fracture, posterior
Arch intact

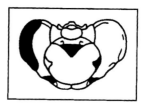

Examples:
Innominate bone
Avulsion fracture

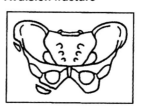

Transverse fracture
Sacrum and coccyx

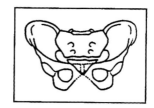

Fracture, incomplete
Disruption of
Posterior arch

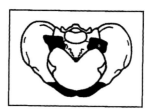

Unilateral, "open
Book" fracture

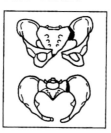

Unilateral, lateral
Compression fracture

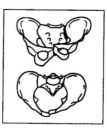

Fracture, complete
Disruption of
Posterior arch

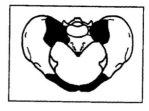

Vertical
Instability

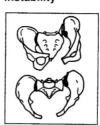

Bilateral, complete
Pelvic floor disruption

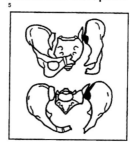

骨盤輪骨折

型：
骨折，後方
骨盤弓に及ばない

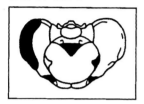

骨折，不完全
後方弓の破綻

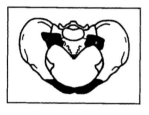

骨折，完全
後方弓の破綻

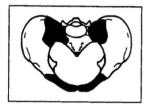

例：
無名の骨
剝離骨折

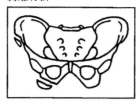

片側
"open book"

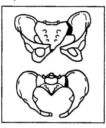

垂直
不安定

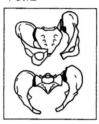

横断骨折
仙骨と尾骨

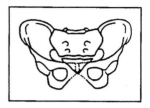

片側
側方圧迫型

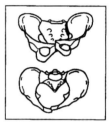

両側
完全型　骨盤底破綻

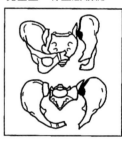

AIS 2005	Injury Description	⇒ AIS98	⇐ AIS98	FCI
856100.2	**Pelvic ring** fracture NFS	852600.2	852600.2	4
856101.3	open but NFS	852604.3	852604.3	2

> Use one of the following two descriptors for any one or combination of the following fracture descriptions *if the fracture is stable* : ischial tuberosity ; pubic ramus with or without symphysis pubis involvement ; undisplaced sacrum ; transverse fracture of sacrum and coccyx with or without sacrococcygeal dislocation.

856151.2	**Pelvic ring** fracture, posterior arch intact ; isolated fracture not destroying the integrity of the pelvic ring	852600.2	None	5
856152.3	open	852604.3	None	5

> Use one of the following four descriptors for any one or combination of the following fracture descriptions *if the fracture is partially or vertically stable* : lateral compression ; "open book" ; symphysis pubis separation ; sacroiliac joint anterior disruption ; anterior compression of sacrum.

856161.3	**Pelvic ring** fracture, incomplete disruption of posterior arch NFS	852604.3	None	4
856162.4	open	852604.3[b]	None	2
856163.4	blood loss ≤20% by volume	852608.4	None	
856164.5	blood loss >20% by volume	852610.5	None	

> Use one of the following four descriptors for any one or combination of the following fracture descriptions *if the fracture is totally unstable* : vertical shear ; pubic rami fractures with sacroiliac fracture/dislocation.

856171.4	**Pelvic ring** fracture, complete disruption of posterior arch and pelvic floor NFS	852606.4	None	2
856172.4	blood loss ≤20% by volume	852608.4	None	
856173.5	blood loss >20% by volume	852610.5	None	
856174.5	open	None	None	2

AIS 2005	損傷内容	⇒ AIS98	⇐ AIS98	FCI
856100.2	**骨盤輪**骨折　詳細不明	852600.2	852600.2	4
856101.3	開放　詳細不明	852604.3	852604.3	2

> 骨折が安定型の場合，以下の骨折の記載について，次の2つのコードのどれか1つのみを用いること：坐骨結節；恥骨枝（恥骨結合の合併の有無にかかわらない）；転位のない仙骨；仙骨と尾骨の横断骨折（仙尾部の転位の有無によらない）。

856151.2	**骨盤輪**骨折，後方弓にかからないもの；骨盤弓連続性が破綻していない単独の骨折	852600.2	なし	5
856152.3	開放	852604.3	なし	5

> 骨折が部分的安定型か垂直安定型の場合，次のような骨折の記載（側方圧迫型；"open book"；恥骨結節離開；仙腸関節の前方破綻；仙骨の前方圧迫）が1つ以上ある場合は，以下の4つのコードのどれか1つのみを用いること。

856161.3	**骨盤輪**骨折，後方弓の不完全破綻　詳細不明	852604.3	なし	4
856162.4	開放	852604.3[b]	なし	2
856163.4	出血量が全血液量の20%以下	852608.4	なし	
856164.5	出血量が全血液量の20%を超える	852610.5	なし	

> 骨折が完全不安定型の場合，次のような骨折の記載（垂直剪断型；仙腸関節離開・骨折のある恥骨枝骨折）が1つ以上ある場合は，以下の4つのコードのどれか1つのみを用いること。

856171.4	**骨盤輪**骨折，後方弓と骨盤底の完全破綻　詳細不明	852606.4	なし	2
856172.4	出血量が全血液量の20%以下	852608.4	なし	
856173.5	出血量が全血液量の20%を超える	852610.5	なし	
856174.5	開放	なし	なし	2

ACETABULUM FRACTURES

Types:

Partial articular, One column
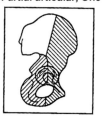

Partial articular, Transverse
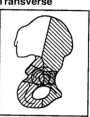

Complete articular, Both columns
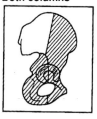

Examples:

Posterior wall
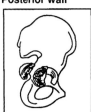

Transverse
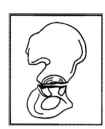

High
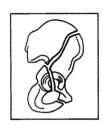

Posterior column
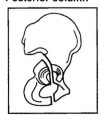

T-shaped
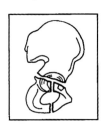

Low
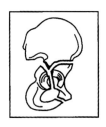

Anterior
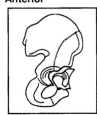

Anterior column, Posterior hemitransverse
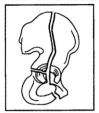

Involving sacroiliac joint
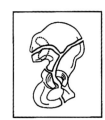

寛骨臼骨折

型:
部分関節内
1つのコラム

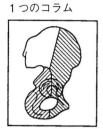

例:
後壁

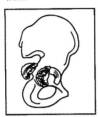

後方コラム

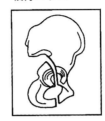

前方

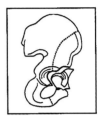

部分関節内
横断型

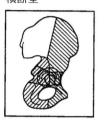

横断型

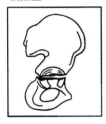

T字型

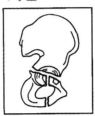

前方コラム
後方半横断型

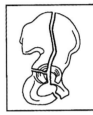

完全関節内
両コラム

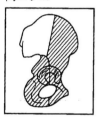

高位

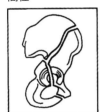

低位

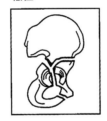

仙腸関節に及ぶ

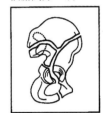

LOWER EXTREMITY, PELVIS and BUTTOCKS

AIS 2005	Injury Description	⇒ AIS98	⇐ AIS98	FCI
856200.2	**Acetabulum** fracture NFS	852600.2	852600.2	5
856202.3	open, but NFS	852604.3	852604.3	5
856251.2	partial articular (involving one column)	852600.2	None	3
856252.3	open	852604.3	None	3
856261.2	partial articular (transverse, "T" shaped)	852600.2	None	3
856262.3	open	852604.3	None	3
856271.2	complete articular (involving both columns, with or without sacroiliac joint involvement)	852600.2	None	2
856272.3	open	852604.3	None	2

Coding Guidelines : ACETABULUM

The acetabulum is classified by anterior or posterior column. The anterior column extends from the anterior half of the iliac crest to the pubis (iliopubic). The posterior column extends from the greater sciatic notch to the ischium (ilioischial).

A partial articular fracture can be one of two types : (a) a fracture involving only one column, either anterior or posterior, with the other column remaining intact ; or (b) a fracture with a transverse component but with a part of the articular surface remaining attached to the ilium.

A complete articular fracture is one in which both columns are disrupted from each other and the attachment between the articular surface and the posterior ilium no longer exists.

下肢・骨盤・殿部

AIS 2005	損傷内容	⇒ AIS98	⇐ AIS98	FCI
856200.2	**寛骨臼**骨折　詳細不明	852600.2	852600.2	5
856202.3	開放　詳細不明	852604.3	852604.3	5
856251.2	部分関節内（1コラムに及ぶ）	852600.2	なし	3
856252.3	開放	852604.3	なし	3
856261.2	部分関節内（横断，T字型）	852600.2	なし	3
856262.3	開放	852604.3	なし	3
856271.2	完全関節内（両コラムに及ぶ，仙腸関節への波及の有無によらない）	852600.2	なし	2
856272.3	開放	852604.3	なし	2

コード選択ガイドライン：寛骨臼

寛骨臼は前方コラムと後方コラムに分類される。前方コラムは腸骨稜の前半分から恥骨までを含む。後方コラムは大坐骨切痕から坐骨までを含む。

　部分的関節面骨折は次の2つのタイプがある。：(a) 前方か後方の，どちらか1つのコラムにのみ及ぶ骨折；(b) 横断型の骨折だが，関節面の一部で腸骨との連続性を維持しているもの。

　完全型関節面骨折は，両コラムに骨折が及び，関節面と腸骨後方との連続性が断たれたもの。

体表（皮膚）および熱傷
その他の外傷

EXTERNAL (Skin) and THERMAL INJURIES

AIS 2005	Injury Description	⇒ AIS98	⇐ AIS98	FCI

Use the following External section if specific lesion or lesion site is unknown, or if assignment of soft tissue (skin) injury to a specific body region is not required. However, the assignment of these injuries to specific body regions, where the information is available, is strongly encouraged. Assign all descriptors in External (Skin) and Thermal Injuries and Other Trauma to External body region for calculating an ISS, unless otherwise stated.

EXTERNAL

AIS 2005	Injury Description	⇒ AIS98	⇐ AIS98	FCI
910000.1	**Soft tissue (skin) injury** NFS[a]	None	None	5

If specific lesion (abrasion, contusion, laceration or avulsion) is unknown or not required, use above for coding any one or more collectively.

AIS 2005	Injury Description	⇒ AIS98	⇐ AIS98	FCI
910200.1	abrasion	910200.1	910200.1	5
910400.1	contusion; hematoma	910400.1	910400.1	5
910600.1	laceration	910600.1	910600.1	5
910800.1	avulsion	910800.2[b]	910800.2[b]	5
914000.1	**Degloving injury**	914000.1	914000.1	5
915000.1	**Frostbite** NFS[a]	None	None	5
915002.1	1st degree; superficial	None	None	5
915004.2	deep; full thickness	None	None	5
915006.3	multiple body sites e.g., fingers, toes, ears	None	None	5
916000.1	**Penetrating injury**	916000.1	916000.1	5

---

[a] New descriptor in AIS 2005
[b] Change in severity code in AIS 2005

体表（皮膚）および熱傷

AIS 2005	損傷内容	⇒ AIS98	⇐ AIS98	FCI

> 特定の損傷や損傷側が不明の場合，または軟部組織（皮膚）損傷を特定の身体部位へ割り当てる必要のない場合，以下の体表の項を使用すること。しかし情報がある場合には，これらの損傷は特定の身体区分に割り当てることが強く推奨される。ISSの計算では，とくに指定のない限り，体表（皮膚）・熱傷・その他の外傷のコードはすべて，体表の身体部位に入れること。

体表

AIS 2005	損傷内容	⇒ AIS98	⇐ AIS98	FCI
910000.1	**軟部組織（皮膚）損傷** 詳細不明[a]	なし	なし	5

> もし損傷の詳細（擦過傷，挫傷，裂創または剝離）が不明，または必要でない場合には，上記のコードをいずれか1つまたはそれ以上の合計で選択する。

AIS 2005	損傷内容	⇒ AIS98	⇐ AIS98	FCI
910200.1	擦過傷	910200.1	910200.1	5
910400.1	挫傷；血腫	910400.1	910400.1	5
910600.1	裂傷・裂創	910600.1	910600.1	5
910800.1	剝離	910800.2[b]	910800.2[b]	5
914000.1	**デグロービング損傷**	914000.1	914000.1	5
915000.1	**凍傷** 詳細不明[a]	なし	なし	5
915002.1	Ⅰ度；表在性	なし	なし	5
915004.2	Ⅱ度；Ⅲ度	なし	なし	5
915006.3	多部位 例：指，つま先，耳	なし	なし	5
916000.1	**穿通性損傷**	916000.1	916000.1	5

---

[a] AIS2005に加えられた新しいコード。
[b] AIS2005で重症度に変更あり。

EXTERNAL (Skin) and THERMAL INJURIES

AIS 2005	Injury Description	⇒ AIS98	⇐ AIS98	FCI

CODING RULES: **Burns**

The following burn descriptions are not a substitute for a comprehensive burn scale, but are only intended as gross estimates of severity. Burns are assigned to the External body region for an ISS. Total body surface area [TBSA] is assessed by using the Diagram of Nines; e.g., one entire upper extremity is 9% of TBSA.

If burns are **only** described as **combined degrees** (e.g., 15% first and second degree) code to the most severe.

When burns occur in **varying degrees** assign an AIS code to the first degree burns separately from second and third degree burns. If second degree burns are less than 10% TBSA and/or third degree burns are ≤ 100cm^2 or > 100cm^2 but < 10%, then both the second and the third degree burns should be coded separately. If the combined second and third degree burns cover ≥ 10% TBSA, assign the AIS code based on their combined TBSA.

Example 1: Adult sustains 40% first degree burns, 5% second degree burns and 2% third degree burns.

Code: 912002.1 for the 1st degree burns
    912006.1 for the 2nd degree burns
    912008.2 for the 3rd degree burns

Example 2: Adult sustains 40% first degree burns, 15% second degree burns and 5% third degree burns.

Code: 912002.1 for the 1st degree burns
    912018.3 for the combined 2nd and 3rd degree burns

If a burn-related amputation occurs at the time of the traumatic event [direct result], code as an amputation in the Extremity body region; do not code the burn separately. If amputation is required after the event, the burn and not the amputation, which is considered treatment, is coded using this section.

Note age breaks at 1 year old for first degree and <5 years old for second and third degree burns.

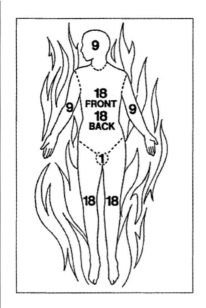

Diagram of Nines

Reprinted with permission of :
American Burn Association
American College of Surgeons

体表（皮膚）および熱傷

AIS 2005	損傷内容	⇒ AIS98	⇐ AIS98	FCI

コード選択のルール：**熱傷**

以下の熱傷の記述は，重症度を大まかに評価したもので，広範囲熱傷の重症度スケールに代わるものではない。熱傷は ISS を計算するときは「体表」として計算する。以下に示すように，熱傷面積（TBSA）は9の法則で評価する。例：一側の上肢全体の TBSA 9 ％である。

もし熱傷の合計面積のみが（カルテに）記載されている場合（例：I 度 II 度あわせて15%），最も重症のコードを選択する。

さまざまな深度の熱傷が混在する場合には，I 度熱傷は II 度・III 度熱傷と別の AIS コードを割り当てる。II 度熱傷が10%TBSA 未満であって，かつ III 度熱傷が100cm^2以下か100cm^2より大きいが10%未満である場合には，II 度と III 度両方を別々にコードする。II 度と III 度熱傷の合計が10% TBSA 以上である場合には，合計面積に基づいてコードする。

例1：40% I 度熱傷，5 % II 度熱傷，および 2 % III 度熱傷を受傷した成人。

コード：I 度熱傷には 912002.1
　　　　II 度熱傷には 912006.1
　　　　III 度熱傷には 912008.2

例2：40% I 度熱傷，15% II 度熱傷，および5% III 度熱傷を受傷した成人。

コード：I 度熱傷には 912002.1
　　　　II 度および III 度熱傷はあわせて 912018.3

受傷時に熱傷に関連した四肢の切断が発生した場合，［直接の結果］は「四肢」の項の切断のコードを使用し，熱傷のコードを使用してはならない。もし，熱傷受傷後に切断を要した場合，「切断」ではなく「熱傷」のコードを選択する。この場合の切断は治療と考える。

注：I 度熱傷では 1 歳未満，II 度・III 度熱傷では 5 歳未満は別コードに分けられる。

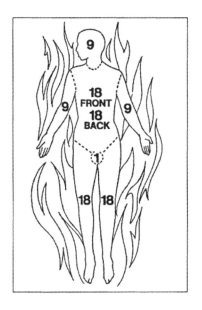

9 の法則

米国熱傷学会，米国外傷学会の許可を得て転載

EXTERNAL (Skin) and THERMAL INJURIES

AIS 2005	Injury Description		⇒ AIS98	⇐ AIS98	FCI
	BURNS				
	Degree	**TBSA**			
912000.1	NFS	NFS	912000.1	912000.1	
912002.1	1st degree; superficial if >1yo	any	912002.1	912002.1	
912003.1	≤1yo	≤50%	912003.1	912003.1	
912004.2	≤1yo	>50%	912004.2	912004.2	
912006.1	2nd degree; partial thickness	<10%	912006.1	912006.1	
912007.1	3rd degree; full thickness	≤100cm^2 [face ≤25cm^2]	912007.1	912007.1	
912008.2	3rd degree; full thickness	>100cm^2; <10% [face >25cm^2]	912008.2	912008.2	
912012.2	2nd or 3rd degree; partial or full thickness	10–19%^{cc}	912012.2	912012.2	
912014.3	<5yo	10–19%^{cc}	912014.3	912014.3	
912018.3	2nd or 3rd degree; partial or full thickness	20–29%^{cc}	912018.3	912018.3	
912020.4	<5yo	20–29%^{cc}	912020.4	912020.4	
912024.4	2nd or 3rd degree; partial or full thickness	30–39%^{cc}	912024.4	912024.4	
912026.5	<5yo	30–39%^{cc}	912026.5	912026.5	
912030.5	2nd or 3rd degree; partial or full thickness	40–89%	912030.5	912030.5	
912032.6	2nd or 3rd degree; partial or full thickness including incineration	≥ 90%	912032.6	912032.6	

^{cc} Any body region

体表（皮膚）および熱傷

AIS 2005	損傷内容		⇒ AIS98	⇐ AIS98	FCI

熱 傷

AIS 2005	熱傷深度	熱傷面積	⇒ AIS98	⇐ AIS98	FCI
912000.1	詳細不明	詳細不明	912000.1	912000.1	
912002.1	Ⅰ度；1歳を超える	熱傷面積を問わない	912002.1	912002.1	
912003.1	1歳以下	50％以下	912003.1	912003.1	
912004.2	1歳以下	50％を超える	912004.2	912004.2	
912006.1	Ⅱ度；非全層性	10％未満	912006.1	912006.1	
912007.1	Ⅲ度；全層性	100cm^{2}以下［顔面の場合は25cm^{2}以下］	912007.1	912007.1	
912008.2	Ⅲ度；全層性	100cm^{2}を超える；10％未満［顔面の場合は25cm^{2}を超える］	912008.2	912008.2	
912012.2	Ⅱ度またはⅢ度；非全層性または全層性	10〜19％^{cc}	912012.2	912012.2	
912014.3	5歳未満	10〜19％^{cc}	912014.3	912014.3	
912018.3	Ⅱ度またはⅢ度；非全層性または全層性	20〜29％^{cc}	912018.3	912018.3	
912020.4	5歳未満	20〜29％^{cc}	912020.4	912020.4	
912024.4	Ⅱ度またはⅢ度；非全層性または全層性	30〜39％^{cc}	912024.4	912024.4	
912026.5	5歳未満	30〜39％^{cc}	912026.5	912026.5	
912030.5	Ⅱ度またはⅢ度；非全層性または全層性	40〜89％	912030.5	912030.5	
912032.6	Ⅱ度またはⅢ度；非全層性または全層性 炭化を含む	90％以上	912032.6	912032.6	

^{cc} 部位を問わない。

OTHER TRAUMA

AIS 2005	Injury Description	⇒ AIS98	⇐ AIS98	FCI
020000.3	**Asphyxia/Suffocation** NFS[a] — Assign this category of injury to Head body region for calculating an ISS.	None	None	
020002.3	without neurological deficit	None	None	
020004.4	with neurological deficit	None	None	
020006.5	with cardiac arrest documented by medical personnel	None	None	
040099.9	**Caustic Agents** NFS[f]	None	None	
	Inhalation injury — Code under Thorax.			
	Ingestion injury — Code to specific organ; e.g., esophagus, stomach.			
060000.3	**Drowning** NFS[a] — Assign this category of injury to Chest body region for calculating an ISS.	None	None	
060002.3	near drowning, no neurological deficit	None	None	
060004.4	near drowning with neurological deficit	None	None	
060006.5	with cardiac arrest documented by medical personnel	None	None	
080000.2	**Electrical injury** NFS	919400.2	919400.2	
080002.3	with muscle necrosis	919402.3	919402.3	
080004.5	with cardiac arrest documented by medical personnel	919404.5	919404.5	
	If electrical burns involve flash, code only the electrical injury and not the associated flash skin burns.			

---

[a] New descriptor in AIS 2005
[f] New descriptor in AIS 2005 that allows classification of trauma, but does not allow assigning a severity code

その他の外傷

AIS 2005	損傷内容	⇒ AIS98	⇐ AIS98	FCI
020000.3	窒息　詳細不明[a]　この損傷区分はISSを計算するときには「頭部」として扱う。	なし	なし	
020002.3	神経脱落症状を伴わない	なし	なし	
020004.4	神経脱落症状を伴う	なし	なし	
020006.5	医療従事者により確認された心停止を伴う	なし	なし	
040099.9	腐食物　詳細不明[f]　吸入損傷　　胸部でコードを選択する。　経口摂取による損傷　　特定の臓器でコードを選択する。例：食道，胃	なし	なし	
060000.3	溺水　詳細不明[a]　この損傷区分はISSを計算するときには「胸部」として扱う。	なし	なし	
060002.3	神経脱落症状を伴わない溺水	なし	なし	
060004.4	神経脱落症状を伴う溺水	なし	なし	
060006.5	医療従事者により確認された心停止を伴う	なし	なし	
080000.2	電撃傷　詳細不明	919400.2	919400.2	
080002.3	筋肉の壊死を伴う	919402.3	919402.3	
080004.5	医療従事者により確認された心停止を伴う	919404.5	919404.5	
	電撃傷が閃光（flash）を伴う場合，電撃傷のみをコード選択し，閃光に合併した熱傷はコード選択しない。			

[a] AIS2005に加えられた新しいコード。
[f] AIS2005に加えられた新しいコード。外傷の存在部位を示すことができる。ただし重症度はない。

OTHER TRAUMA

AIS 2005	Injury Description	⇒ AIS98	⇐ AIS98	FCI
010000.1	**Hypothermia** NFS (primary injury, not treatment-related or sequela)[a]	None	None	
010002.1	>34–35°C	None	None	
010004.2	33–32°C	None	None	
010006.3	31–30°C	None	None	
010008.4	29–28°C	None	None	
010010.5	<27° C	None	None	
012002.2	**Whole Body (explosion-type) Injury** NFS[a]	None	None	
012004.2	minor or superficial to skin, subcutaneous tissue and muscle with or without minor fracture(s)	None	None	
012006.4	major or extensive (>25% TBSA) to skin, subcutaneous tissue and muscle with multiple fractures and/or multiple organ injuries	None	None	
012008.6	massive; multiple organ injury to brain, thorax and/or abdomen with loss of one or more limbs and/or decapitation	None	None	

[a] New descriptor in AIS 2005

その他の外傷

AIS 2005	損傷内容	⇒ AIS98	⇐ AIS98	FCI
010000.1	**低体温症** 詳細不明（主損傷である場合を指し，治療によるものや続発症は除く）[a]	なし	なし	
010002.1	34～35℃	なし	なし	
010004.2	33～32℃	なし	なし	
010006.3	31～30℃	なし	なし	
010008.4	29～28℃	なし	なし	
010010.5	27℃未満	なし	なし	
012002.2	**全身損傷（爆傷）** 詳細不明[a]	なし	なし	
012004.2	軽傷，または皮膚・皮下組織・筋の表在性損傷 軽微な骨折を伴う，または伴わない	なし	なし	
012006.4	広範囲（25% TBSAを超える）の皮膚・皮下組織・筋の損傷，多発性の骨折かつ／または臓器損傷を伴う	なし	なし	
012008.6	重症；脳，胸部かつ／または腹部の多発性の臓器損傷 一肢以上の四肢欠損かつ／または断頭を伴う	なし	なし	

[a] AIS2005で新しく記載。

DICTIONARY INDEX

Page	Anatomical Description	Section
92	Abdomen, whole area [use for Abdominal injury NFS, Penetrating or Skin]	Abdomen
46	Abducens nerve	Head
169	Acetabulum [see Pelvis]	Lower Extremity
148	Achilles tendon	Lower Extremity
46	Acoustic nerve [see Vestibulocochlear nerve]	Head
128	Acromioclavicular joint	Upper Extremity
131	Acromion [see Scapula]	Upper Extremity
97	Adrenal gland	Abdomen
68	Alveolar ridge [see also Teeth]	Face
149	Ankle	Lower Extremity
97	Anus	Abdomen
	Aorta	
93	abdominal	Abdomen
80	thoracic	Thorax
130	Arm NFS	Upper Extremity
46	Auditory nerve [see Vestibulocochlear nerve]	Head
125	Axillary artery	Upper Extremity
125	Axillary vein	Upper Extremity
53	Basal ganglion [see Cerebrum]	Head
41	Basilar artery	Head
97	Bladder (urinary)	Abdomen
125	Brachilal artery	Upper Extremity
110	Brachial plexus	Spine
126	Brachial vein	Upper Extremity
81	Brachiocephalic artery	Thorax
82	Brachiocephalic vein	Thorax
49	Brain stem	Head
79	Breast	Thorax
	Bronchus	
85	distal to main stem	Thorax
85	main stem	Thorax
161	Calcaneus	Lower Extremity
65	Canaliculus (tear duct)	Face
	Carotid artery	
74	common	Neck
63	external	Face
75	〃	Neck
41	intenal	Head
74	〃	Neck
43	Carotid – cavernous fistula	Head
128	Carpal [wrist] joint	Upper Extremity
139	Carpus	Upper Extremity
117	Cauda equina	Spine
43	Cavernous sinus	Head
93	Celiac artery	Abdomen
49	Cerebellum	Head

Page	Anatomical Description	Section
49	Cerebral artery	Head
41	anterior	Head
41	middle	Head
42	posterior	Head
52	Cerebrum	Head
	Chest [see Thorax]	
87	Chordae tendineae [see Intracardiac chordae tendineae]	Thorax
65	Choroid	Face
131	Clavicle	Upper Extremity
167	Coccyx [see Pelvis]	Lower Extremity
148	Collateral ligament	Lower Extremity
98	Colon (large bowel)	Abdomen
65	Conjunctiva	Face
65	Cornea	Face
81	Coronary artery	Thorax
45	Cranial nerve NFS	Head
77	Cricoid cartilage [see Larynx]	Neck
148	Cruciate ligament	Lower Extremity
162	Cuboid	Lower Extremity
162	Cuneiform	Lower Extremity
85	Diaphragm	Thorax
	Digital nerve	
127	hand	Upper Extremity
147	foot	Lower Extremity
	Disc	
112	cervical	Spine
119	lumbar	Spine
115	thoracic	Spine
98	Duodenum	Abdomen
64	Ear canal	Face
64	Ear NFS	Face
128	Elbow	Upper Extremity
	Esophagus	
77	above sternal notch	Neck
86	below sternal notch	Thorax
59	Ethmoid bone [see Skull, base]	Head
65	Eye, whole organ or NFS	Face
62	Face, whole area [use for Penetrating or Skin]	Face
68	Facial bone(s) NFS	Face
46	Facial nerve	Head
103	Fallopian tube [see Ovarian tube]	Abdomen
145	Femoral artery	Lower Extremity
147	Femoral nerve	Lower Extremity
145	Femoral vein	Lower Extremity
155	Femur	Lower Extremity
159	Fibula	Lower Extremity
140	Finger [see Phalange]	Upper Extremity

Page	Anatomical Description	Section
151	Forefoot NFS	Lower Extremity
	Foot	
151	joint NFS	Lower Extremity
153	bone NFS	Lower Extremity
130	Forearm NFS	Upper Extremity
59	Frontal bone [see Skull, vault]	Head
99	Gallbladder	Abdomen
67	Gingiva (gum)	Face
129	Glenohumeral joint [see Shoulder]	Upper Extremity
66	Globe [see Sclera]	Face
47	Glossopharyngeal nerve	Head
130	Hand NFS	Upper Extremity
39	Head, whole area [use for Penetrating, Scalp, Head/Brain injury NFS, Crush]	Head
86	Heart	Thorax
149	Hip	Lower Extremity
133	Humerus	Upper Extremity
78	Hyoid bone	Neck
47	Hypoglossal nerve	Head
49	Hypothalamus [see Brain stem]	Head
99	Ileum (small bowel) [see Jejunum]	Abdomen
93	Iliac artery (common, internal, external)	Abdomen
94	Iliac vein (common, internal, external)	Abdomen
167	Ilium [see Pelvis]	Lower Extremity
64	Inner ear	Face
81	Innominate artery [see Brachiocephalic artery]	Thorax
82	Innominate vein [see Brachiocephalic vein]	Thorax
	Interphalangeal joint	
129	hand [see Metacarpophalangeal joint]	Upper Extremity
152	foot [see Metatarsophalangeal joint]	Lower Extremity
87	Intracardiac valve	Thorax
87	Intracardiac septum	Thorax
40	Intracranial vascular injury	Head
167	Ischium [see Pelvis]	Lower Extremity
99	Jejunum – ileum (small bowel)	Abdomen
137	Joint capsule NFS	Upper Extremity
	Jugular vein	
76	external	Neck
76	internal	Neck
100	Kidney	Abdomen
149	Knee	Lower Extremity
98	Large bowel [see Colon]	Abdomen
77	Larynx	Neck
159	Lateral malleolus [see Fibula]	Lower Extremity
153	Leg NFS	Lower Extremity
66	Lens [see Eye]	Face
102	Liver	Abdomen

Page	Anatomical Description	Section
141	Lower extremity, whole area [use for Penetrating, Skin, Degloving, Amputation, Crush]	Lower Extremity
87	Lung	Thorax
66	Macula	Face
90	Main stem bronchus [see Trachea]	Thorax
159	Malleolus [see Fibula]	Lower Extremity
68	Mandible	Face
70	Maxilla	Face
70	Maxillary sinus [see Maxilla]	Face
127	Median nerve	Upper Extremity
49	Medulla [see Brain stem]	Head
148	Meniscus	Lower Extremity
102	Mesentery	Abdomen
129	Metacarpophalangeal joint	Upper Extremity
139	Metacarpus	Upper Extremity
152	Metatarsophalangeal joint	Lower Extremity
	Metatarsus	
152	joint	Lower Extremity
162	bone	Lower Extremity
49	Midbrain [see Brain stem]	Head
64	Middle ear [see Inner ear]	Face
151	Midtarsal joint	Lower Extremity
67	Mouth NFS	Face
	Muscle NFS	
127	arm	Upper Extremity
148	leg	Lower Extremity
86	Myocardium [see Heart]	Thorax
161	Navicular	Lower Extremity
73	Neck, whole area [use for Penetrating or Skin]	Neck
	Nerve root	
113	cervical	Spine
120	lumbar	Spine
116	thoracic	Spine
71	Nose	Face
59	Occipital bone [see Skull, base or vault]	Head
46	Oculomotor nerve	Head
45	Olfactory nerve	Head
103	Omentum	Abdomen
	Optic nerve	
45	intracranial segment	Head
45	intracananicular segment	Head
64	intraorbital segment	Face
71	Orbit	Face
59	Orbital roof [see Skull, base]	Head
64	Ossicular chain (ear bone)	Face
103	Ovarian tube	Abdomen
103	Ovary	Abdomen

Page	Anatomical Description	Section
67	Palate	Face
103	Pancreas	Abdomen
72	Panfacial	Face
59	Parietal bone [see Skull, vault]	Head
159	Patella	Lower Extremity
148	Patellar tendon	Lower Extremity
167	Pelvis	Lower Extremity
104	Penis	Abdomen
89	Pericardium	Thorax
104	Perineum	Abdomen
147	Peroneal nerve	Lower Extremity
	Phalange	
140	hand	Upper Extremity
163	foot	Lower Extremity
	Phalangeal joint	
129	hand [see Metacarpophalangeal joint]	Upper Extremity
152	foot [see Metatarsophalangeal joint]	Lower Extremity
77	Pharynx	Neck
76	Phrenic nerve	Neck
58	Pituitary gland	Head
107	Placenta [see Uterus]	Abdomen
89	Pleura	Thorax
49	Pons [see Brain stem]	Head
145	Popliteal artery	Lower Extremity
145	Popliteal vein	Lower Extremity
104	Prostate	Abdomen
167	Public ramus [see Pelvis]	Lower Extremity
81	Pulmonary artery	Thorax
87	Pulmonary region [see Lung]	Thorax
82	Pulmonary vein	Thorax
127	Radial nerve	Upper Extremity
136	Radius	Upper Extremity
104	Rectum	Abdomen
92	Rectus abdominus muscle	Abdomen
66	Retina	Face
105	Retroperitoneum	Abdomen
77	Retropharyngeal area [see Pharynx]	Neck
91	Rib cage	Thorax
120	Sacral plexus [see Nerve root]	Spine
167	Sacroilium [see Pelvis]	Lower Extremity
167	Sacrum [see Pelvis]	Lower Extremity
44	Saggital sinus [see Superior longitudinal sinus]	Head
78	Salivary gland	Neck
40	Scalp	Head
131	Scapula	Upper Extremity
147	Sciatic nerve	Lower Extremity
66	Sclera	Face

Page	Anatomical Description	Section
105	Scrotum	Abdomen
87	Septum [see Intracardiac septum]	Thorax
129	Shoulder	Upper Extremity
43	Sigmoid sinus	Head
43	Sinus NFS	Head
72	Skin NFS as to body region	External
	Skull	
59	base	Head
59	vault	Head
59	Sphenoid bone [see Skull, base or vault]	Head
47	Spinal accessory nerve	Head
	Spinal cord	
111	cervical	Spine
118	lumbar	Spine
114	thoracic	Spine
105	Spleen	Abdomen
129	Sternoclavicular joint	Upper Extremity
91	Sternum	Thorax
106	Stomach	Abdomen
43	Straight sinus	Head
81	Subclavian artery	Thorax
82	Subclavian vein	Thorax
151	Subtalar joint	Lower Extremity
44	Superior longitudinal (saggital) sinus	Head
94	Superior mesenteric artery	Abdomen
167	Symphysis pubis [see Pelvis]	Lower Extremity
161	Talus	Lower Extremity
152	Tarsometatarsal joint	Lower Extremity
72	Teeth	Face
59	Temporal bone [see Skull, base or vault]	Head
67	Temporomandibular joint	Face
	Tendon NFS	
127	arm	Upper Extremity
148	leg	Lower Extremity
106	Testes	Abdomen
90	Thoracic duct	Thorax
91	Thoracic wall	Thorax
79	Thorax, whole area [use for chest injury NFS, Penetrating or Skin ; see also Thoracic injury, page 81]	Thorax
140	Thumb	Upper Extremity
77	Thyroid cartilage [see Larynx]	Neck
78	Thyroid gland	Neck
157	Tibia	Lower Extremity
147	Tibial nerve	Lower Extremity
163	Toe [see Phalange]	Lower Extremity
67	Tongue	Face
92	Torso	Abdomen

Page	Anatomical Description	Section
92	Trachea	Abdomen
78	above sternal notch	Neck
90	below sternal notch	Thorax
44	Transverse sinus	Head
46	Trigeminal nerve	Head
46	Trochlear nerve	Head
64	Tympanic membrane (ear drum)	Face
137	Ulna	Upper Extremity
127	Ulnar nerve	Upper Extremity
121	Upper extremity, whole area [use for Penetrating, Skin, Degloving, Amputation, Crush]	Upper Extremity
106	Ureter	Abdomen
106	Urethra	Abdomen
97	Urinary bladder [see Bladder]	Abdomen
107	Uterus	Abdomen
67	Uvea	Face
107	Vagina	Abdomen
	Vagus nerve	
95	abdomen	Abdomen
47	head	Head
76	neck	Neck
84	thorax	Thorax
	Vena Cava	
94	inferior	Abdomen
84	superior [and thoracic portion of inferior]	Thorax
	Vertebra	
112	cervical	Spine
119	lumbar	Spine
115	thoracic	Spine
	Vertebral artery	
42	head	Head
75	neck	Neck
	Vessels	

Each body region, except the Spine and External, has a section titled Vessels. In addition to listing specific arteries and veins, a nonspecific description is included to code vessel injuries when precise information is lacking. The coder is urged to become acquainted with these default codes by body region.

Page	Anatomical Description	Section
64	Vestibular apparatus	Face
46	Vestibular nerve [see Vestibulocochlear nerve]	Head
67	Vitreous	Face
78	Vocal cord	Neck
107	Vulva	Abdomen
174	Whole body injury	Other Trauma
128	Wrist [see Carpal joint]	Upper Extremity

Page	Anatomical Description	Section
72	Zygoma	Face
	The following traumatic events to the whole body or to an entire body region listed as follows:	
90	Air Embolus	Thorax
173	Asphyxia/Suffocation	Other Trauma
172	Burns	Extarnal (Skin) and Thermal Injuries
173	Caustic Agents	Other Trauma
	Compartment Syndrome	
122	arm	Upper Extremity
142	leg	Lower Extremity
61	Concussive Injury	Head
73	Decapitation	Neck
173	Drowning	Other Trauma
173	Electrical Injury	Other Trauma
170	Frostbite	Extarnal (Skin) and Thermal Injuries
90	Hemomediastinum	Thorax
90	Hemopneumothorax	Thorax
90	Hemothorax	Thorax
174	Hypothermia	Other Trauma
89	Inhalation [see Lung]	Thorax
90	Pneumomediastinum	Thorax
90	Pneumothorax	Thorax
173	Suffocation [see Asphyxia]	Other Trauma
174	Whole Body Injury	Other Trauma

●日本外傷学会トラウマレジストリー検討委員会からのお願い
※本書の内容および翻訳に関する疑問等についてのご意見は，下記URLにアクセスしてメールにて送信いただくか，へるす出版まで文書にてお寄せください。
　また，本書発行後に修正すべき点が生じました際には，下記URLにて告知いたしますのでご覧ください。
　　へるす出版ホームページURL：http://www.herusu-shuppan.co.jp

| JCOPY | 〈(社)出版者著作権管理機構 委託出版物〉 |

本書の無断複写は著作権法上での例外を除き禁じられています。
複写される場合は，そのつど事前に，下記の許諾を得てください。
(社)出版者著作権管理機構
TEL. 03-5244-5088　FAX. 03-5244-5089　e-mail：info@jcopy.or.jp

AIS 2005 Update 2008　日本語対訳版

定価（本体価格 18,000 円＋税）

2017 年 3 月 31 日　第 1 版第 1 刷発行
2020 年 2 月 18 日　第 1 版第 2 刷発行

監　訳／一般社団法人日本外傷学会
翻　訳／日本外傷学会トラウマレジストリー検討委員会
発行者／佐藤　枢
発行所／株式会社　へるす出版
　　　　〒164-0001　東京都中野区中野 2-2-3
　　　　電話 03-3384-8035〈販売〉　03-3384-8155〈編集〉
　　　　振替 00180-7-175971
　　　　https://www.herusu-shuppan.co.jp
印刷所／広研印刷株式会社

©2017 Printed in Japan　　　　　　　　　　　　〈検印省略〉
乱丁，落丁の際はお取り替えいたします。
ISBN978-4-89269-903-0